THE OPEN UNIVERSITY

• CENTRE FOR CONTINUING EDUCATION •

A SYSTEMATIC APPROACH TO NURSING CARE

AN INTRODUCTION

Prepared for the Course Team by
Alison Binnie, Senga Bond, Gladys Law,
Karen Lowe, Alan Pearson, Ruth Roberts,
Alison Tierney, Barbara Vaughan

The Open University Press

COURSE TEAM

Open University
Janet Gale BA, MSc, PhD, *Course Team Chairperson*
Monica Howes BSc, *Course Manager*
Kate Robinson BA, SRN, HV, *Course Co-ordinator*
Ian Fordham BA, MA, *Editor*
Ros Porter BA, CertEd, *Designer*
Mark Kesby *Graphic Artist*
Mike Levers AIIP, *Photographer*
Viv Seabright BA, *Project Control*
Paul Smith MA, ALA, *Liaison Librarian*
Antonet Roberts *Secretarial Support*
Vic Finkelstein BA, MA, *Reading Member*
Sue Hurley BSc, PhD, *Reading Member*

Authors
Alison Binnie SRN, SCM, *Nursing Process Co-ordinator, Cambridge Health District*
Senga Bond RGN, BA, MSc, PhD, *Nursing Research Liaison Officer, Northern Regional Health Authority*
Gladys Law SRN, SCM, BTA Cert, RCNT, DN, Dip Adv Nurse Studies, BA, *Adviser and Co-ordinator for the Nursing Process in England and Wales, Department of Health and Social Security*
Karen Lowe SRN, BSc, *Clinical Lecturer in Nursing, Department of Nursing, Manchester University and Ward Sister, Manchester Royal Infirmary*
Alan Pearson SRN, ONC, RNT, Dip N Ed, MSc, *Senior Nurse, Clinical Practice Development, Oxfordshire Health Authority*
Ruth Roberts SRN, SCM, *Nurse Consultant, Services for the Elderly, Cambridge Health District*
Alison Tierney RGN, BSc, PhD, *Nurse author/lecturer*
Barbara Vaughan SRN, RNT, MSc, *Senior Tutor, Nursing Practice Development, Oxfordshire Health Authority*

BBC Open University Production Centre
Ann Pointon BA, Producer
Julia Hardy, Production Assistant

External Assessor
Professor Baroness McFarlane of Llandaff Hon DSc, Hon DEd, MA, Hon MSc, BSc, SRN, SCM, HV Cert, HV Tut Cert, FRCN

Critical Commenters
Charlotte Kratz, Catherine White *Nominees of English National Board for Nursing, Midwifery and Health Visiting*
Sylvia Campbell, Teresa Grant *Nominees of National Board for Nursing, Midwifery and Health Visiting for Northern Ireland*
Christine Chapman, Gillian Stephens *Nominees of Welsh National Board for Nursing, Midwifery and Health Visiting*
Isabel Elliott, Elizabeth Kyle, Mary Theresa McGuiness *Nominees of Department of Health and Social Security, Northern Ireland*
Pat Ashworth *Research Programme Manager, WHO Collaborating Centre, University of Manchester*
Betty Farmer *Research Associate, Nursing Research Unit, University of Edinburgh*
Sheila Mackie Bailey *Clinical Tutor, Addenbrookes Hospital*
Veronica Chapman *Senior Tutor, Professional Development, Maidstone District School of Nursing*
Gill Collinson, Marion Cotton, Louis Gray, Nicola Hunter, Kathy Swift *Post-basic nurses, Royal Marsden Hospital*
Peter Nicklin *Senior Tutor, Continuing Education and Training, North Lincolnshire School of Nursing*
Rod Fletcher *Tutor, Post-basic Education, Wolverhampton*

Developmental Testing of Group Sessions
Group sessions were tested by nurses in groups meeting at:
Bedford General Hospital: leader – Dawn Verrall
Sunderland Royal Infirmary: leader – Kathleen Mawson
St Leonard's Hospital: leader – Trevor Davies
Five groups in S.E. Thames Region: organised by Alan Skeath and Ralph Jordan

The Open University Press
Walton Hall, Milton Keynes MK7 6AA

First published 1984. Reprinted 1984, 1985, 1987

Designed by the Graphic Design Group of the Open University
Printed in Great Britain by Black Bear Press Limited, Cambridge

ISBN 0 335 10515 7

Further information on Open University Continuing Education courses may be obtained from the Learning Materials Service, Centre for Continuing Education, The Open University, Walton Hall, Milton Keynes, MK7 6DH

CONTENTS

INTRODUCTION TO THE COURSE

Welcome to this course. If you are like most people embarking on a new course of study, you are probably feeling some combination of excitement, interest and apprehension. We have produced this course specifically for nurses, midwives and health visitors to give you the opportunity to explore the ideas and practice of the nursing process. This introduction is designed to provide you with information which should help you to have realistic expectations of the course, to use the course materials to their best advantage and to relate them to your own personal experience and situation.

You might like to know something of the history of this course, which the Open University has produced in response to requests from the nursing profession. It is the first course that the Open University has developed specifically for nurses. You can see from the list of Course Team members that these course materials have been produced by people who are highly experienced in using the nursing process, as well as in developing the ideas behind it. As well as the Course Team members, clinical nurses from many specialties throughout the United Kingdom worked through the course during its drafting stages and gave feedback to the Course Team about how it might be improved. Comments were also received from a number of experienced nurse educators and trainers and from representatives of National Boards. Baroness McFarlane of Llandaff was our External Assessor and commented in detail on the academic content of the course. So you can see that many people in many places have helped to develop these learning materials.

AIMS OF THE COURSE

This course has been designed to assist students to:

1 Examine the nature of the relationship between nurse and patient, including the professional attitudes of the nurse and personal attitudes of the patient.

2 Consider systematic approaches to nursing.

3 Consider communications between the nurse and
   - the patient, including the patient's family
   - other health professionals, including others in the nursing profession.

4 Define and describe the steps of the process of nursing in the clinical nursing context.

5 Consider the implementation of systematic approaches to, and conditions for, successful change.

6 Assess the value of a systematic approach to individual care.

STRUCTURE OF THE COURSE

The course consists of:

- this *Workbook*, divided into seven modules

- the *Case Files* containing case material, including notes to use with the audiotape

- an audiotape

- an introductory group meeting

- seven group sessions, each linked to individual modules, five of which include videotape material.

The seven parts of the course, each made up of one module plus a group session, cover the following topics:

Module 1: Nursing practice and the nursing process. This module introduces you to the course and the background against which the steps of the nursing process should be set. Seven themes are established which recur throughout subsequent modules. Three models for nursing practice are described. These, too, are used throughout the rest of the course. Equally importantly, however, this first module asks you to look at your own nursing practice and to think carefully about it.

Module 2: The first step of the nursing process – assessment.

Module 3: The second step of the nursing process – planning. ·

Module 4: The third step of the nursing process – implementation.

Module 5: The fourth step of the nursing process – evaluation.

Modules 2–5 introduce you to the four steps of the nursing process and follow up the themes and models discussed in Module 1.

Module 6: Reviewing the nursing process. This module focuses on a long case study and enables you to see the nursing process in practice as rather more than its four separate steps.

Module 7: Introducing change into nursing practice. This final module helps you to think about developing the nursing process within your own nursing practice.

Your study of these course materials begins with an introductory group meeting which takes place before you read any of the written material. Your individual study of each module in the Workbook will then be followed by a related group session. This will consolidate and extend your study of the Workbook material and will give you an opportunity to sort out any problems which you might have experienced with your individual study. Some of the group sessions require some preparation on your part. Instructions are given for this at appropriate points in the Workbook. Some of the modules also require you to do some preparation before you begin them.

Instructions for this are given at the end of the previous module. So make sure that you read each module in good time and then you will experience no problems.

At the end of some modules, you will find suggestions for optional further reading which you can follow up if you have a particular interest in special aspects or points of the course. References to works cited within each module are collected together at the end of the Workbook.

ORGANISING YOUR STUDY TIME

We have tried to make this course as straightforward as possible for you to use. Nonetheless, you will still have to organise yourself in order to make the most of your study time. To begin with, you need to organise the time itself. Some groups may have a leader who builds your individual study time into a formal timetable for you. But, more often, you will probably be left to study in your own time. On average, each module in this Workbook should take you about four hours to work through. But that's an average: some take longer and some take less time. If a particular module is long, you might wish to spread your study time over more than one occasion. Some modules also ask you to make some initial preparations by gathering information from your work area in advance. So do look ahead in the Workbook and plan your study periods in advance for each module.

As you work through the course, you will often be referred to the *Case Files*. In Modules 2, 3, 4 and 5 you will also be asked to work through sections of the audiotape. Make sure that you have a cassette player to hand when studying these four sections. If you do not possess a cassette player, ask your Group Leader if one is available for borrowing. Or you might be able to come to some co-operative arrangement with a fellow group member who does have one.

Finally, the only items you will need to have with you at every study time or group session, apart from the course materials, are a notebook and pen. Before you begin to study the course, get a notebook to use for this course only, and keep it in your folder with the Workbook at all times. In summary, then:

- look at each module and plan your study time in advance
- give yourself time to make any necessary initial preparations
- arrange to use a cassette player when necessary
- keep a special notebook of your own with the Workbook.

LEARNING ACTIVITIES

Throughout the Workbook and in the *Case Files* you will come across a variety of brief exercises called 'Activities'. These are designed to give you the opportunity to think about, apply and understand more fully the new things you are learning, to use them and relate them to your daily nursing practice and your own work setting. You will see that at the beginning of each activity we suggest the approximate length of time you should spend on it. Each activity is accompanied by a special comment written by the module author which is designed to give you feedback on your answer. You will need to write your responses to most activities in your own notebook, although occasionally space is left for you to write in the Workbook. Sometimes an activity asks for ticks and crosses –these, too, can be written in the Workbook itself, if you like. In most cases, you will find the author's comments immediately after the activity, although a few have been placed at the end of the module text. You might also find it helpful to discuss some of the activities at your group sessions.

The activities are part of the course. They are a crucial and important part of your learning. It is sometimes tempting (especially if time is pressing) not to do the activities properly, but simply to read them, think for a minute or two and then read the author's comment. I would advise you very strongly not to omit the activities in this way, but to spend the allotted time on them. By doing so, your learning will be clearer, your understanding deeper and your ability to relate your studies to your own work situation greatly enhanced.

CONFIDENTIALITY OF PATIENTS' NOTES

For some of the modules, you are asked to gain access to patients' nursing notes for use in an activity or in a group session. This raises a most important issue: patients' notes are confidential documents and must be treated as such.

- To ensure confidentiality, you might want to adopt one of a variety of possible actions. I suggest that you discuss these with your Group Leader so that appropriate action is taken by all group members. But whatever you choose to do always gain permission from the appropriate person in authority to use patients' nursing notes. Depending on your own position, you might decide that this person should be the Ward Sister or the Hospital Administrator, or your group may decide that the relevant Consultant should be asked for his agreement if you are using the medical records of a particular patient.

- Once the appropriate person's approval has been obtained, the patient should be asked for his agreement, stressing that the extracts from his nursing notes are for your personal study only and explaining that they will be kept confidential and destroyed after use.

- Never photocopy notes. Instead, copy them out, omitting all personal information (patient's name, address, telephone number, G.P.) from which the patient could be identified. Also omit the date of birth but keep a record of the patient's age.

- Never show your copy of a patient's notes to anyone outside the group studying this course with you.

- Keep the copied notes in a safe place where no-one will come across them by accident. Do not leave them lying where anyone else might see them.

- Destroy your copied notes as soon as you have finished with them.

Tom Keighley, Nurse Adviser to the Royal College of Nursing Research Society told the 1983 British Computer Society Nursing Specialist Group conference:

> It is essential to remember that the health care records of patients are as precious and private to them as the Pentagon secrets are to the White House.

And we should treat them accordingly.

All the patients and nurses who appear in the course materials are real, and all gave the Open University and the BBC their consent to use the recorded information for educational purposes. Wherever possible, the names of patients have been changed to protect their privacy and ensure that confidentiality is maintained.

Because all the patients and examples are real and the discussions were unscripted, you will find the demonstrations unique. It is not our intention to show perfection, but rather to show and use the reality of trying to implement the nursing process. Much can be learned from others' achievements and errors. We hope that you will approach the course material in this positive way.

THIS COURSE AND YOU

So, what are you expecting to gain from this course? We hope that you will gain a good, practical grounding in the nursing process so that you can go on afterwards to plan how *you* will use it. We do not expect that the course will answer all your questions. It is an introduction to the nursing process, not an end in itself. Indeed, learning about the nursing process, like learning about your own area of nursing, never ends since new knowledge and experience are constantly becoming available. Nonetheless, these seven modules should set you on the right path.

We hope that you will feel that this course is talking to *you* about *your* nursing practice. Clearly, the examples given in the modules cannot cover every area of nursing practice and it is very tempting to say "Well, it might be all right for them. But it's not like that in my specialty". If you find yourself thinking or saying that, stop and try to see beyond the general nursing or specialist examples given and apply the principles to *your* situation and specialty.

To help you to relate the course to your situation, we have asked you to use relevant materials (notes and records) from your own work setting while doing the activities. The group sessions will also ask you to think specifically about your own nursing experiences.

I hope you will feel that this course is personally relevant to you, and that it gives you a good grounding in the nursing process. I hope, too, that you will enjoy the course and come out of it with a new enthusiasm for nursing and a deeper understanding of the nursing process and some of the skills and attitudes on which it rests. It should stimulate a desire to analyse your practice and identify parts which are suitable for development, and a wish to share your thoughts with the other members of your team.

Finally, I do hope that, while you are working through this course, you will feel free to send me any comments you might have:

Dr Janet Gale
Course Team Chairperson
Centre for Continuing Education
Health and Social Welfare Section
Open University
Walton Hall
Milton Keynes
MK7 6AA

ACKNOWLEDGEMENTS

Our special thanks go to Dr Jim Leeming and Dr J. B. Pearce for general comments on the course, to Betty Farmer and Alison Tierney for their assistance with Module 1 and to Pat Ashworth and Margaret Scholey for their assistance with Module 6.

We are very grateful to all the patients, nurses and other health staff who contributed to the production of this course – either by being photographed or by allowing their personal details and experiences to be used for teaching purposes. We especially appreciate that some nurses deliberately worked at less than their best, at our request, in order to illustrate a teaching point. We are also grateful to those hospitals which permitted photographs to be taken and audio and video recordings to be made in their wards, and to those patients and staff who participated.

Throughout the text nurses are referred to as "she", patients as "he" and, sometimes, people as "Man". After much debate, the Course Team agreed to this convention. However, we regret that the English language has not yet evolved a non-sexist terminology which is suitable.

MODULE 1
NURSING PRACTICE AND THE NURSING PROCESS

Prepared for the Course Team by Alan Pearson and Barbara Vaughan

CONTENTS

OBJECTIVES

After studying this module, you should be able to:

1 Explain the meaning of the word 'holism' and describe how it relates to a systematic approach to care.

2 Discuss the role of the nurse by outlining:
 ● the unique and collaborative aspects of the role
 ● the clinical, managerial and teaching aspects of the role.

3 Differentiate between a *directorship* and a *partnership* nurse-patient relationship, and describe how the steps in the nursing process can be approached with the patient as partner.

4 List the three elements included in a model designed to give direction to nursing practice.

5 Briefly describe the three models of nursing developed by:
 ● Roper, Logan and Tierney
 ● Orem
 ● Saxton and Hyland.

6 Define accountability and discuss how this relates to the nursing process.

7 List the four steps in problem solving.

8 Critically discuss introducing a nursing process approach within the context of the multi-disciplinary team.

9 Demonstrate an appreciation of the broad perspective from which the nursing process is viewed in this module when discussing its relevance to your day-to-day practice.

NURSING PRACTICE AND THE NURSING PROCESS

In the introductory group meeting, you have been able to think and talk about nursing and to identify some of the major principles on which we base our practice. The nursing process is a systematic organised way of approaching nursing. The *process* itself does not tell us anything about the content of nursing. In fact, it is something which is shared by many other groups of people such as teachers or engineers. What makes it special in this context is the word 'nursing'.

Future modules will concentrate on the process as it applies to nursing. The purpose of this module is to discuss in greater detail some of the underlying principles of nursing which you have already begun to identify. You will probably be familiar with some of them. If this is so, it will give you the opportunity to reconsider them in the light of your current practice. Other principles may not be so familiar to you and may give you fresh food for thought.

Seven basic themes which recur throughout all the modules of the course are discussed. These themes are:

- problem solving
- people as patients
- the role of the nurse
- the nurse-patient relationship
- models for practice
- accountability
- nursing in an organisation.

In order to complete this module you will require the case notes on Mrs Dickenson in Part I of the *Case Files*.

PROBLEM SOLVING

The basis of this course is the nursing process, which is often described as a systematic problem-solving approach to care. We prefer to use the term 'problem-oriented' when referring to nursing. This is a broader concept than problem solving and is preferred, since not all problems can be solved. In some instances, once problems have been identified it may be more appropriate to offer a patient support in coping with them rather than unrealistically trying to solve them.

A problem-oriented approach, however, is based on the problem-solving technique. This is a technique which is commonly applied both in everyday life and in many different types of occupation. Even within the health care team this approach to practice is found in medicine, physiotherapy, occupational therapy, social work and dietetics, to give examples. Outside health care teachers, probation officers, architects and many others use it. Teachers often refer to the problem-solving approach in their work as 'the teaching process', and similarly its application to nursing has come to be known as 'the nursing process'. Thus problem solving in itself is not new, nor is it unique to nursing. As many other health workers are familiar with this approach to care, the use of the nursing process often helps to improve inter-team communication. Nurses and others begin to 'talk in the same language' and can be seen to be involved in a rational decision-making process.

The problem-solving process has been described by many people as being made up of various steps. The number of these steps varies from four to ten, according to the different interpretations. However, the principle remains the same. The steps used in the problem-solving process may be summarised as:

1 Collecting relevant information or data, and identifying the problem(s). This step is often referred to as **assessment.**

2 Listing possible courses of action which may be taken to resolve the problem in some way, suitable to the specific situation. One particular course of action is then chosen, taking into account such considerations as resources, constraints and priorities. This step also includes the setting of goals towards which the chosen course of action will aim and is usually referred to as **planning.**

3 The plan is then put into action. Again, it is essential to consider the available resources, the constraints and the priorities. This step is known as **implementation.**

4 The final step is to see whether the goal which was set initially has been achieved by implementing the plan of action. This step is known as **evaluation.** It is also sometimes regarded as reviewing the situation to see whether or not the problem still exists and to identify whether any new problems have arisen. Evaluation leads back to a need to re-assess, to re-plan and if necessary, to take new actions.

The nursing process, then, consists of:

- **nursing assessment**
- **planning nursing**
- **implementing nursing**
- **evaluating outcomes of nursing.**

Future modules will deal with each of these stages in more detail.

Although we have separated the stages of the nursing process for the purposes of description, in practice the whole process is integrated. The sequence of steps follows a spiral route rather than a climb up the four steps of a ladder, as shown in Figure 1.1.

Whilst these four steps are the process through which nursing can be provided, they cannot stand alone but need to be considered alongside many other issues. The remainder of this module is devoted to looking at some of them. There may be other issues which you think are particularly relevant to nursing in the place where you work. However, the relevance of the themes which we will discuss are common to all nurses, regardless of the setting in which they practise.

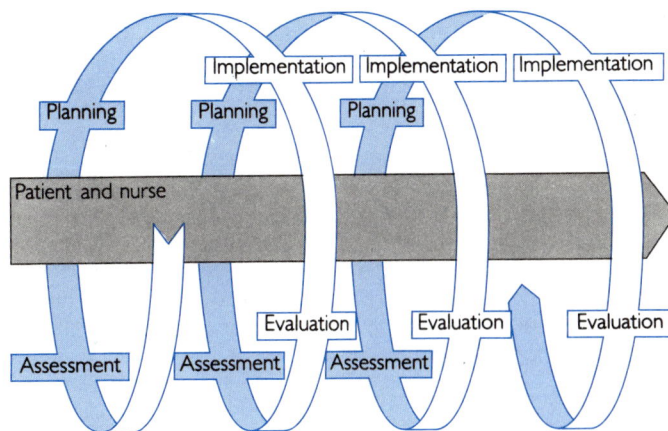

Fig. 1.1 The problem-solving process

PEOPLE AS PATIENTS

One of the special contributions that nursing has to offer health care is that nurses have always considered patients as people with individual needs. Whilst other health care workers would all say that they, too, see patients as individuals, nurses are often regarded as the ones who are closest to the patient. They are the ones who provide the small intimate services which are special to individuals, respecting their personal preferences and providing a link with other health workers as well as with friends and relatives. In many settings nurses provide a twenty-four hour service. They are in a position to co-ordinate the activities in a patient's day, so that all other members of the team can make their contributions without them overlapping. For instance, the contribution of the occupational therapist may not be so effective if her work follows immediately after a patient has spent a tiring session with the physiotherapist.

If this idea is accepted, we must first consider the nature of people in order to be able to recognise their needs. Each person is an individual with a personal view of life which will be reflected in his response to a given set of circumstances. Some responses, such as the physiological response to the loss of blood, will be shared by all. Others, such as reacting to the loss of blood with panic, calmness or acceptance, are unique to an individual. They are dependent on many factors such as past experience, knowledge, social background and the stage of development.

Activity 1.1   **Allow 10 minutes**

Meet Mrs Dickenson

In this activity we would like you to consider the needs of one particular person as a patient.

Read the case notes on Mrs Dickenson, and answer the following questions:

1 What information have you obtained about Mrs Dickenson which would be common to many people with the same condition?

2 What information have you obtained about Mrs Dickenson which is unique to her?

From the information you have discovered in this exercise you will see that Mrs Dickenson has some needs which are common to many people with the same condition. However, there are other things about her responses to her illness and to hospital admission which are specific to her and which therefore create individual needs.

In fact, Mrs Dickenson is unique. She is an individual who is a mother, living in a particular social setting with members of her family. She has a personality of her own and a way of viewing the world which is special to her. She, like all of us, is made up of many different components, all of which contribute to her as a whole being. Some of these components are shown in Figure 1.2.

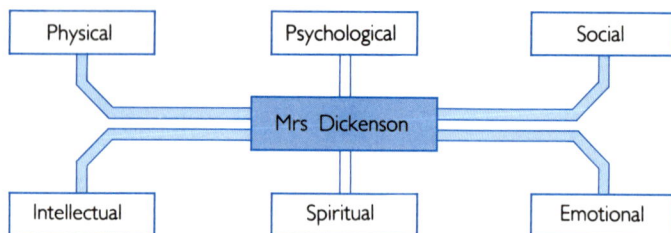

Fig. 1.2 Some of the components of a 'whole' being

What is unique about Mrs Dickenson is the balance and inter-relationship of the various components. It is not sufficient to view each one independently; rather we should see her as a whole, made up of these parts. Let's think of an analogy described by Byrne and Thompson (1978). Water is made up of two parts: oxygen and hydrogen. If we view these parts separately they have a common quality, namely that each will support fire. However, if we combine them in the right quantities to make water, that quality will alter and they will, in combination, extinguish fire. Similarly, Mrs Dickenson is made up of various components, some of which we have identified.

What is unique about Mrs Dickenson is the manner in which they are combined. This concept has been called *holism*. It was first described by a South African statesman called Jan Christiaan Smuts in 1926. Byrne and Thompson have summarised clearly the two major features of holism in relation to Man as:

– Man always responds as a unified whole.
– Man as a whole is different from and more than the sum of his component parts.

This concept moves away from a fragmented and disease-oriented approach to care towards viewing patients as whole people. It means considering how they, as individuals with their own needs, respond to the situations in which they find themselves.

NEEDS

Mrs Dickenson's individuality means that she has individual needs. By needs, we mean those requirements which must be satisfied in order that an individual may survive and find living purposeful, acceptable and fulfilling, or may peacefully approach death. Human needs are complex and have been the subject of study by many experts. Some suggest that all individuals share a number of basic needs necessary for survival and that, once these are met, other needs relating to higher things – such as belonging and the need to feel good about oneself – arise. Maslow (1954), for example, described a hierarchy of needs which are arranged, as shown in Figure 1.3, in a pyramid of less or greater priority or potency.

Needs are discussed further in Module 2, but seeing individuals *holistically* means that a whole variety of needs are recognised. Whilst the hierarchy of needs described by Maslow is a useful guide to the recognition of human needs, not all individuals respond in the precise order given. For instance, a mother may deny her own needs for safety in order to protect her child. Similarly a severely depressed person may deny his need for food and water. Some people prefer to think more in terms of a series of needs placed on

Fig. 1.3 A hierarchy of human needs (after Maslow, 1954)

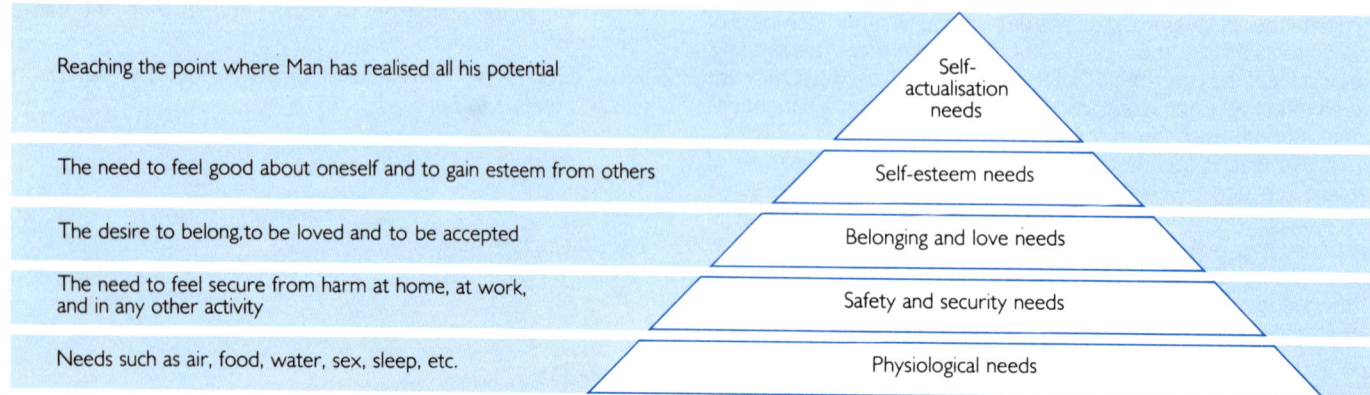

Reaching the point where Man has realised all his potential	Self-actualisation needs
The need to feel good about oneself and to gain esteem from others	Self-esteem needs
The desire to belong, to be loved and to be accepted	Belonging and love needs
The need to feel secure from harm at home, at work, and in any other activity	Safety and security needs
Needs such as air, food, water, sex, sleep, etc.	Physiological needs

an equal footing rather than in a hierarchy, as different ones may take priority at different times.

Surveys which have sought the views of patients on nursing, such as those conducted by the Central Health Services Council (1963) and the Royal Commission on the National Health Service (1978), have found that the way in which nurses sometimes practise actually 'de-personalises' those for whom they care. In other words, the person's individuality and background can be forgotten, and only those needs common to all patients with similar conditions are recognised. However, if we believe that a holistic view of patients is important then their individuality cannot be ignored. Every person has the right to be seen from this holistic viewpoint and the nursing process is a system which can help nurses to put this view into practical use.

THE ROLE OF THE NURSE

DEFINING NURSING

Having sketched an outline of patients as people, taking a holistic point of view, let us now consider the role of the nurse. Nursing is a complex activity which varies considerably according to the place in which you work. Defining what nursing is has always been found to be difficult, since its whole essence is its adaptability to both varying needs and varying settings. Yet as McFarlane (1980) says, "it is important to identify the particular contribution of nursing to health care delivery".

Activity 1.2	Allow 5 minutes

What is nursing?

This activity is designed to help you think about your own definition of nursing.

Imagine that a visitor from Mars has just arrived. He has no understanding of the word 'nursing' (although he does understand English) and asks you what it means. Without being specific about the individual acts of nursing, give an explanation of nursing.

Authors' comment

This is a difficult exercise which many people have attempted over many years. Probably the most widely accepted definition of nursing is that offered by Virginia Henderson (1966): "The unique function of the nurse is to assist the individual, sick or well, in the performance of those activities contributing to health or its recovery (or to peaceful death) that he would perform unaided if he had the necessary strength, will or knowledge. And to do this in such a way as to help him gain independence as rapidly as possible".

From this well-known statement, McFarlane (1980) has extracted some important points about the role of the nurse:

- nursing consists essentially of acts of helping or assistance
- there is a nursing role in respect of well people (preventive) as well as sick people
- the major focus of nursing is on activities which people normally do for themselves; other authors call these 'self-care activities' or 'daily living activities'
- the conditions which validate nursing action are lack of strength, or will or knowledge. The nursing role therefore takes in physical and psychological assistance and it has a teaching function.

NURSING AND THE ACTIVITIES OF LIVING

Having considered a broad definition of nursing, it may be helpful to break it down into some of its component parts. Whilst the elements of care offered to each patient will always be unique if they are to meet the needs of an individual, it is helpful to have some frame of reference to guide practice.

Activity 1.3	Allow 10 minutes

Nursing activities

The purpose of this activity is to help you identify components of nursing which are universally applicable.

List some of the nursing activities which form the 'core' of nursing and are common to all areas of practice.

Henderson (1969) has defined fourteen activities of daily living which she sees as areas of patient need which may usually be met by the nurse. She summarises these areas of need as being able to:

1 Breathe normally
2 Eat and drink adequately
3 Eliminate by all avenues of elimination
4 Move and maintain desirable posture
5 Sleep and rest
6 Select suitable clothing, dress and undress
7 Maintain body temperature . . . by adjusting clothing and modifying the environment
8 Keep the body clean and well groomed and protect the integument [skin]
9 Avoid dangers in the environment and avoid injuring others
10 Communicate with others in expressing emotions, needs, fears, questions and ideas
11 Worship according to his faith
12 Work at something that provides a sense of accomplishment
13 Play, or participate in various forms of recreation
14 Learn, discover or satisfy the curiosity that leads to 'normal' development and health.

Henderson also suggests that when the nurse is considering these basic needs she must take into account various conditions which will affect the patient as an individual. These include:

● age

● temperament, emotional state or passing mood

● social and cultural status

● physical and intellectual capacity.

If each of the components which goes towards making up nursing is considered with these conditions in mind, the individuality of each patient will not be lost.

COMPONENTS OF NURSING

Another way of looking at the role of the nurse is to break it down into the different types of service which are offered. Whilst there is frequently an overlap in the different aspects, they can be identified separately for the purpose of discussion. One way of categorising the activities which contribute to nursing is to group them into those related to:

Clinical care: by clinical care, we mean the nurse's direct role in doing for the patient those things which he is unable to do for himself. Such activities as assisting with mobility, measuring blood sugar levels, or giving the correct medication at the right time may be included in this category.

Management of care: there are two elements within this category. Firstly there is the aspect of managing or organising the care for an individual patient. This may include such things as co-ordinating the care provided by the nurse with that provided by other health care workers, in order that the patient can have sufficient rest. The second aspect is related to managing resources in order that care can be given most effectively: for example, the allocation of work, the provision of resources or communications.

Teaching: the aspects of the nurse's role related to teaching include helping the patient to adapt physically, mentally and socially to his condition. They also include giving information to help the patient to stay healthy or to prevent a recurrence of a recent illness. In other words, there is a health education role. The third aspect of teaching is the nurse's responsibility for passing on knowledge to professional colleagues with less experience.

Activity 1.4   **Allow 10 minutes**

How your time is allocated

In this activity we ask you to consider the balance of these three broad components of nursing in your work.

List some of the activities which you perform in your daily work under the following three headings:

1 Clinical care
2 Management of care
3 Teaching.

THE COLLABORATIVE ROLE

The components of nursing we have discussed so far have been those which are unique to nursing and for which the nurse holds total responsibility. There are, however, other aspects of patient care with which the nurse is involved but which stem from other health care workers. As McFarlane (1980) says "Besides her unique role she [the nurse] also has a collaborative role with doctors and other health professionals".

The degree of collaboration between the doctor and the nurse is obviously dependent on both the individual needs of the patient and the type of setting in which the nurse is working. Much of the work which nurses undertake arises out of medical needs and is based on the diagnosis and medical treatment of disease.

Obviously the nurse is dependent on the doctor for his contribution to this aspect of patient care, since it is not within the nurse's role to diagnose disease. However, her knowledge of the patient as a holistic individual can assist the doctor in making his decision about the medical management most suitable for the patient. In this situation she will collaborate with him. For instance, nurses who are with patients for long periods of the day are in a position to observe the effects of a particular drug on a patient and to share this information with their medical colleagues. Whilst the responsibility for prescribing that drug remains with the doctor, the nurse's contribution will be to ensure that the patient receives the medication and to observe its effects.

In some instances nurses will be asked by other health care workers, and in particular doctors, to take on the responsibility for performing some of the tasks arising out of their management. For instance, in some settings nurses take venous blood, a task which is traditionally medical and related to the medical management of the patient. McFarlane (1980) fears that because of this "the unique caring role of the nurse may be crowded out . . . [or] delegated to the less skilled".

Whilst this point must never be forgotten, it is sometimes in the interests of all concerned that nurses should be prepared to perform some medical tasks, provided that they have the necessary knowledge and skills. However, it would be detrimental to patient care if these sorts of tasks were to take precedence over the unique caring aspects of nursing.

Activity 1.5	Allow 10 minutes

Working with others

This activity enables you to examine the independent and collaborative aspects of your work.

List some of the activities which you carry out in each of the following two categories:

1 Collaborative work with other health care workers
2 Work which is assessed, initiated and controlled by you.

Authors' comment

Since the role of the nurse is so complex it is not only a very difficult subject to define but also a very difficult role to fulfil. The nursing process, that is a systematic problem-oriented approach to nursing, offers a very useful way of structuring such a complex area of work. Whilst it will not tell you what nursing is, it will help you to translate your own thoughts about nursing into the care you offer patients.

THE NURSE-PATIENT RELATIONSHIP

We have referred to people as patients with unique and individual needs. We have also considered nursing and both the unique and collaborative contributions which it has to offer people. In this section we would like to combine the two and consider the nurse-patient relationship.

The nurse can be seen as a *partner* in care – someone who, in the widest sense, supports the patient's own ability to overcome his problems. Your contribution may include filling in any gaps in knowledge so that the patient can be aware of factors which inhibit him from reaching towards his full potential. Similarly, it offers the patient the opportunity to make informed suggestions and decisions for himself.

You may have observed a mother who will smother a child with her love and attention, giving him everything he asks for and doing everything for him because she cares for him so much. In fact, she

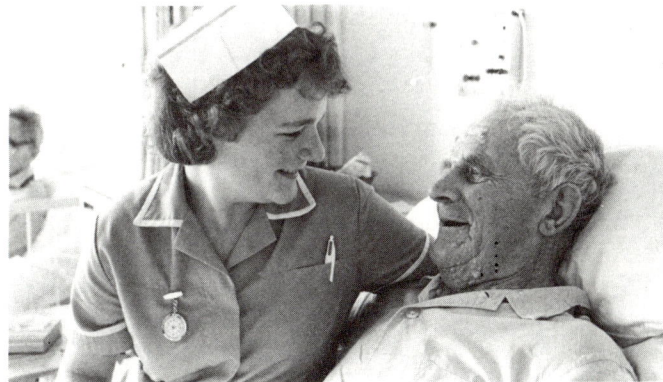

Nurse and patient working together in partnership

may be inhibiting his development, and in adult life he is likely to experience great difficulty in living an independent life. Alternatively, there is the mother who will allow her child to share in, and contribute to, decision making. Although she will use her greater experience and knowledge in order to support and guide the child, she will allow him freedom to make choices and experience doing things for himself. In this way he can develop independence.

Similarly in nursing, care and concern for the patient *can* be interpreted as meeting all a patient's needs for him and directing his activities. However, if nurses perceive their role as assisting an individual to develop, to learn and to grow, the relationship fostered will be that of *partnership*. They may offer their knowledge and experience to the patient as a source of support from which he can, as far as possible, control his own future. The Oxford Dictionary includes in its definition of nursing the word 'nurture', meaning to 'nourish, rear, foster, train and educate'. Thus nurturing may well be an apt word to describe the sort of relationship which ideally exists between nurse and patient.

The development of a relationship based on partnership will vary according to circumstances; for example, the setting in which nursing is taking place has an effect on the relationship. The hospital patient is a stranger in an environment unfamiliar to him. The patient being nursed at home receives the nurse into his home as a visitor. Similarly, the actual physical and mental condition of the patient determines how much he can be involved in his own care. The unconscious patient is highly dependent on the nurse to assist him in meeting his needs, whilst the patient learning to cope with a colostomy under the supervision of a district nurse visiting weekly may be virtually independent of the nurse; many patients fall between these two extremes. Figure 1.4 indicates the range of the relationship possible between a nurse and a patient – from the nurse assuming control and directing care through to the nurse and patient working together in partnership.

Bearing these important variations in mind, the crucial goal of nursing can still be seen as creating a partnership through which patient problems can be overcome and patients' needs met. The nursing process can be an effective way of involving the patient in his care. This can be achieved both by giving an explanation of how nursing can help him and by including the patient's contribution in the plan of care designed for him as an individual.

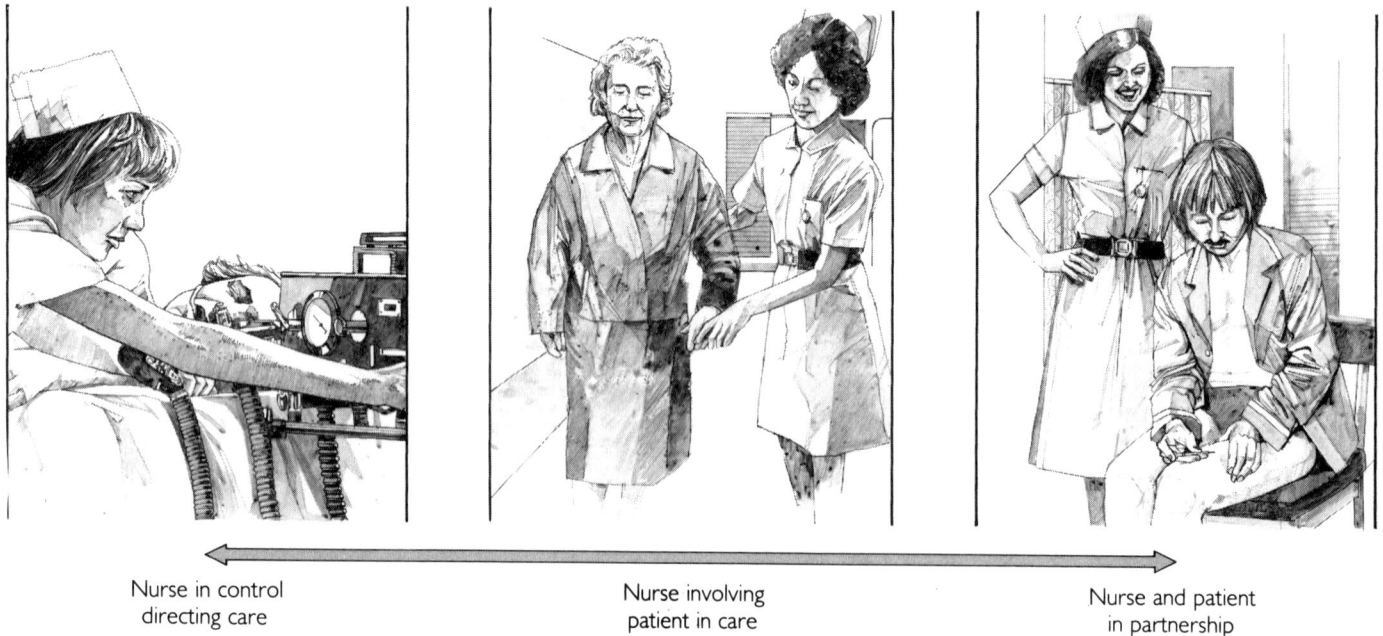

Nurse in control
directing care

Nurse involving
patient in care

Nurse and patient
in partnership

Fig. 1.4 Directorship/partnership continuum

MODELS FOR PRACTICE

We have already spent some time in this module discussing what nursing is and the role of the nurse. You may personally have experienced some of its complexity when attempting Activity 1.2. Roper (1976) and McFarlane (1980) suggest that because attempting to define nursing is so complex it may be helpful to construct a 'picture' of all the ideas that go towards making up nursing. A picture of this sort can be referred to as a *model*.

A model is a framework or pattern that we follow, reflecting and giving direction to the way we act. For instance, what we eat will reflect our views about our weight, our personal likes and dislikes, our ethical and religious views and our beliefs about the value of certain foods. It will also reflect what we hope to achieve through eating – survival, a change in weight or the pleasure derived from the taste and sight of food. It has been said that some people eat to live whilst others also live to eat. The way we select our food to achieve our goals is based on such things as our knowledge of the nutritional content and value of various foods, their availability and our past experience of their flavour and smell. In other words we base our choice of food on our beliefs about certain foods, what we hope to achieve by eating and what we know about the food we choose.

If you live alone or your choice of food is not influenced by those around you there is no reason for you to discuss your ideas with others. However, in a family unit or in a society where eating is a communal activity, the beliefs, goals and knowledge have to be broadly agreed upon by all concerned.

In the same way nursing is frequently an activity which is shared by many people. In order that groups of people working together do not practise in conflicting ways they need to share their ideas and thoughts concerning their beliefs about Man, who is the recipient of nursing; what they hope to achieve, or the goals of their nursing; and the knowledge on which they base their practice.

These three components – beliefs about Man, the goals or expected outcomes of practice and the knowledge needed to achieve the goals – are essential to any model for practice.

The existence of nursing models must be included in any discussion about the nursing process. All of us already operate from the basis of some kind of personal model, but frequently it remains *implicit*. In order to carry out the process of nursing meaningfully and rationally the model must be made *explicit*, so that care is goal-directed. Carrying out the nursing process without having established and explained a model on which to base practice can lead to disjointed activities and lack of team unity.

You may be familiar with a situation where a new nurse has joined the team with which you work. Although there is nothing specific that you can criticise about either her practice or her as a person, she does not 'fit' in your team. One of the reasons for her inability to fit may be that she is practising from a different model of nursing than the one your team uses. Over a period of time she may adopt the team's beliefs and goals. Sometimes, however, this does not happen and, if she does not leave, the differences may lead to conflict and confusion for patients and nurses alike. Agreement on a model would have provided a "unifying framework for an organised way of looking at nursing" (Pearson, 1983). In this way the conflict and confusion could have been avoided.

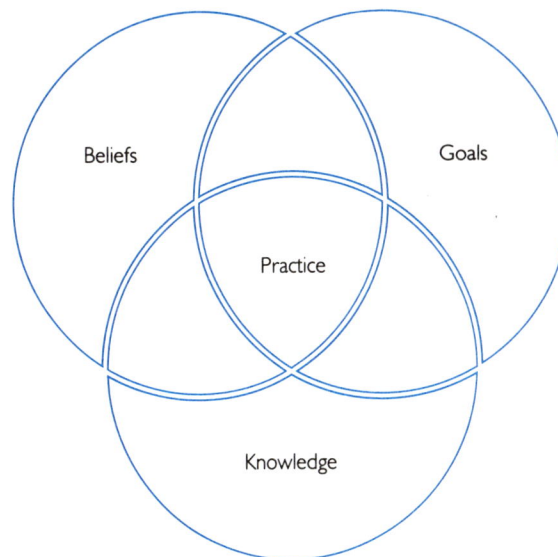

Fig. 1.5 *Components of a model for practice*

Pearson continues to say "until recent years, and in many parts of the world now, nursing has been practised from the basis of disease/medical/hospital oriented models". In the medical model,

- **Man** is seen as a biological being whose integrity is disturbed by disease
- the **goal of care** is to cure that disease through medical treatment
- the **knowledge base** needed to achieve this goal is mainly made up of the biophysical sciences such as physiology, pathology and microbiology.

NURSING MODELS

In recent years, there has been an emergence of models specifically for nursing and, as Orem (1980) says, the nurse's role is now "emerging from the obscurity imposed by an overemphasis on the relationship between the physician and the nurse...Nurses are coming to recognise that an item of information about a patient may have one meaning for a physician but quite a different meaning for a nurse".

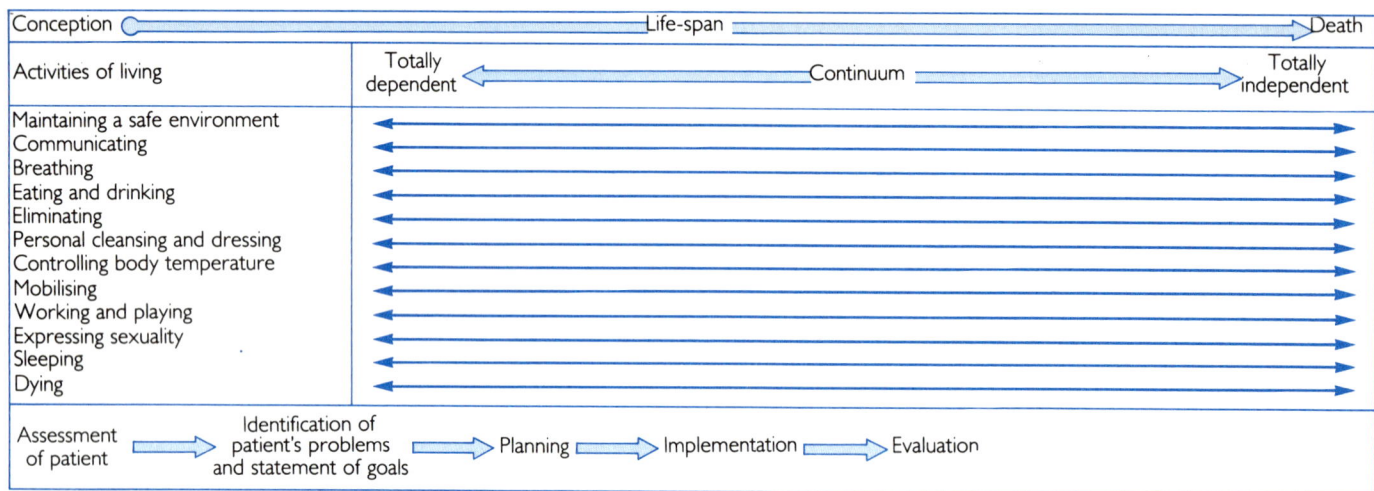

Fig. 1.6 (a) The Activities of Living Model (adapted from Roper, Logan and Tierney, 1983)

Whilst using the nursing process as a way of organising work, a nursing model will help you to decide on the content of nursing. It will give structure to the nursing assessment, and to the planning, implementation and evaluation of care.

Many nursing models have been described over recent years. We intend to outline three, although this does not mean that these are the only ones or the best ones available. We have summarised them under the three headings mentioned previously, namely beliefs about Man, the goals of nursing and the knowledge on which practice is based. In order to indicate the variety of approaches which different people have taken, the third model we describe is intentionally very different from the first two.

The idea of a nursing model is sometimes difficult to grasp because nurses in the past have often not been used to conceptualising their views of what constitutes nursing nor to making their thoughts explicit. You may therefore find it necessary to read the description of each model two or three times and spend some time considering its application in the place where you work before the relevance of the ideas becomes clear. You may find that one or more of the models is totally inappropriate either to your own beliefs or to the place in which you work. Whilst one of the models may suit you and your place of work well, an alternative approach may be to take elements from several different models in order to build your own particular model. A model should reflect your own beliefs and be suitable for the place in which you work.

Model 1 The Activities of Living Model: Roper, Logan and Tierney

The Roper, Logan and Tierney model for nursing is based on a model of living which focuses on twelve *activities of living* (ALs).

You may well be familiar with this model because, unlike most nursing models which have their origins in North America, this one has been developed by British nurses. The model, first presented in a nursing research monograph by Roper (1976), is described in full in *The Elements of Nursing* (Roper, Logan and Tierney, 1980). The model actually incorporates the four steps of the nursing process and in their second book *Learning to Use the Process of Nursing* (1981), the authors illustrate how their model can be used as a framework for the nursing process. Subsequently, they set up a project to test the relevance of the model in the real world of nursing – in practice. A number of nurses, working in nine very different health care settings, were invited to try out the model and contribute their patient studies to the third book in the series *Using a Model for Nursing* (1983). So, although consideration of 'models' may seem to be essentially an academic exercise, this model for nursing has been taken beyond the realms of theory and subjected to the realities of nursing in practice.

A diagrammatic representation of the Roper, Logan and Tierney model (slightly simplified by permission of the authors) is shown, with an example, in Figures 1.6 (a) and 1.6 (b).

The beliefs about Man on which this model is based are that individuals are engaged in a process of living – 'living' being described as an amalgam of twelve activities of living – throughout their lifespan from conception to death. The life-span is shown in the diagram of the model, an arrow indicating the direction of movement along it. In moving through the life-span, the individual is continually changing and every activity of living is influenced by physical, psychological, sociocultural and economic factors.

Related to, but not entirely dependent upon, the life-span is a dependence/independence continuum. This is included in the model to acknowledge that there are periods in life when a person cannot yet, or can no longer, perform certain activities of living independently. Unlike the life-span, movement along this continuum can take

Conception ──────────────── Life-span ──────────────── Death

Activities of living	Totally dependent ←────── Continuum ──────→ Totally independent
Maintaining a safe environment	
Communicating	
Breathing	
Eating and drinking	
Eliminating	
Personal cleansing and dressing	
Controlling body temperature	
Mobilising	
Working and playing	
Expressing sexuality	
Sleeping	
Dying	

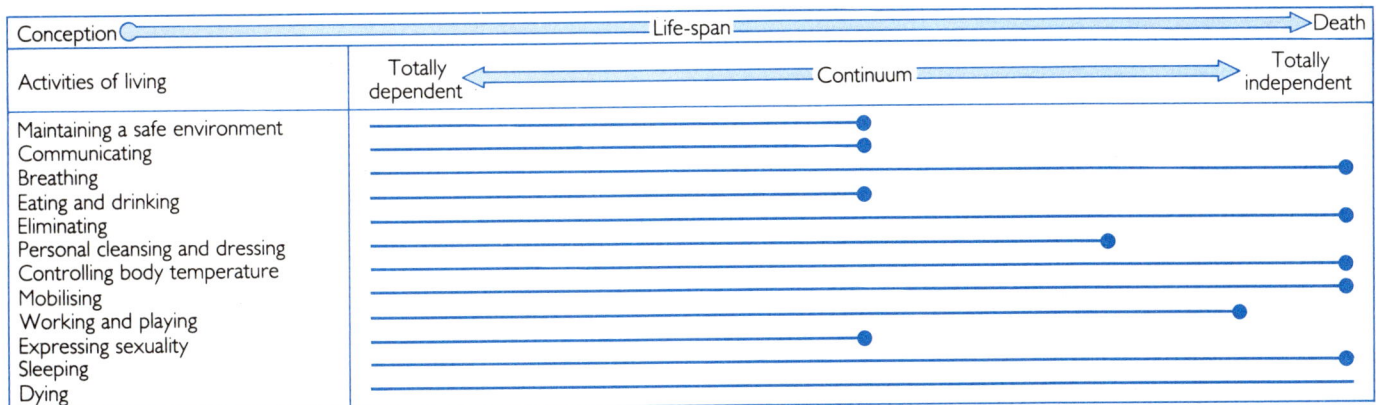

Fig. 1.6(b) An example showing dependence/independence at five years old (adapted from Roper, Logan and Tierney, 1983)

place in either direction, as shown in the diagram of the model. A person's position on the dependence/independence continuum may be relative to position in the life-span, as in the case of the very young or the very old, or may be determined by current circumstances, such as ill-health or accident.

In the model, beliefs about people as individuals are based on the premise that a person's individuality is reflected in the highly individualised performance of activities of living. The twelve activities specified are:

- maintaining a safe environment
- communicating
- breathing
- eating and drinking
- eliminating
- personal cleansing and dressing
- controlling body temperature
- mobilising
- working and playing
- expressing sexuality
- sleeping
- dying.

The goals of nursing derived from this model are developed from the link between *nursing* and *living*. Because most people only require nursing from time to time during their lifetime, the rationale for linking nursing with living is the belief that this would encourage minimal disruption to a person's usual style of living during the period when nursing is required, and that goals of nursing would reflect the individual's goals of living. Nursing thus focuses on the individual's activities of living, enabling the person to retain or regain independence in the ALs or helping that individual to cope with dependence if independence is not possible or desirable. Nursing,

then, is viewed as helping the patient/client to solve, alleviate, cope with, or prevent problems related to activities of living. Concern with a patient's 'problems' does not preclude consideration, using this model, of goals related to prevention of ill-health and promotion of health: the model is as applicable to 'well' people as to patients who are 'ill'.

The knowledge base needed for nursing using this model also centres on the twelve activities of living. The complexity of the activities of living is apparent from the chapter devoted to each in *The Elements of Nursing*. It is essential before using the model for nurses to familiarise themselves with the ALs – their nature and purpose, the body structure and function required for each, and the factors which influence the way a person carries out each AL. The person's point on the life-span influences ability to carry out ALs and the style of doing so. The patient's degree of dependence/independence is an equally important consideration, the model alerting nurses to pay attention to what patients can do independently as well as what they cannot do.

Considerable knowledge and skill is required to:

- assess patients' levels of independence in all the ALs
- judge in which direction, and by what amount, they should be assisted to move along the dependence/independence continuum for each AL
- decide which nursing interventions are required to meet the goals set in relation to problems, actual and potential, associated with the ALs.

Model 2 The Self-Care Model: Orem

The Self-Care Model, described by Orem in *Nursing: Concepts of Practice* (1980), is similar in emphasis to the Activities of Living Model.

The beliefs about Man on which this model is based are that all individuals have self-care needs, and that they have the right to meet these needs themselves if it is at all possible. Self-care is care given by oneself for oneself. Self-care is deliberate action which has as its purpose the meeting of individual requirements for effective living. Self-care is learned behaviour; its development is aided by intellectual curiosity, by instruction and supervision from others, and by experience in performing self-care measures. Orem's concept of self-care is grounded in the belief that self-maintenance and self-regulation are valued as first-line strategies for effective human functioning in society.

The goals of nursing are to meet self-care needs, either through supporting the patient in meeting his own self-care needs, through enabling a relative or friend to be the self-care agent or through the nurse acting as the self-care agent.

The knowledge base for nursing centres on self-care – that is, those actions which people take in order to function as a whole being. Orem identifies eight categories of needs which form a common core of requirements for effective living. These categories, which are interrelated, are:

- **air**
- **water**
- **food**
- **elimination**
- **activity and rest**
- **solitude and social interaction**
- **prevention of hazards**
- **promotion of normality** as this relates to social standards and personal potential.

The individual's capacity for meeting the requirements for effective living is influenced by certain factors which are illustrated in Figure 1.7 above.

Orem categorises certain of the influences on self-care ability and performance which present particular challenges in relation to meeting the common requirements for effective living. The first

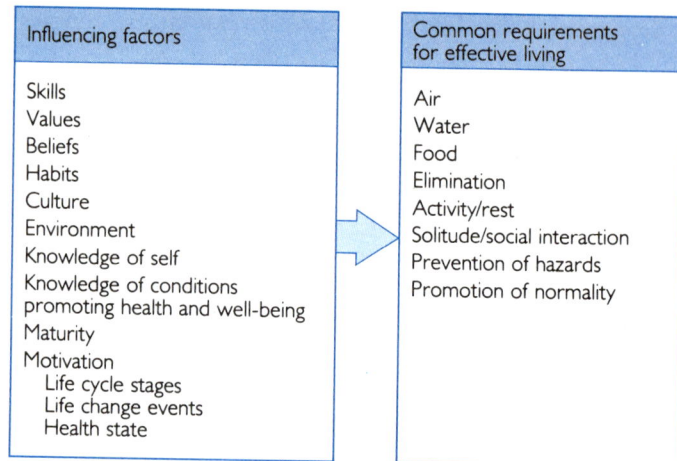

Fig. 1.7 Influences on self-care ability and performance in relation to the requirements for effective living

category is created out of the life-cycle stages and life change events. These comprise the developmental factors which may alter the requirements for effective living (Figure 1.8).

The second categorisation of influence on self-care is concerned with health state, and in particular with deviations from health. Health deviations challenge existing self-care patterns, or demand the establishment of new self-care practices, in order to correct the imbalance between the need and the existing capacity of the individual to meet the need.

Where there is a balance between the demand to attend to oneself and the ability to meet that demand, the person is capable of self-care. Where the demand outweighs the ability to meet it, the person has a self-care deficit (Figure 1.9). The type of action required to meet the need will determine *who* should meet the need. When the self-care deficit is made good by a relative or

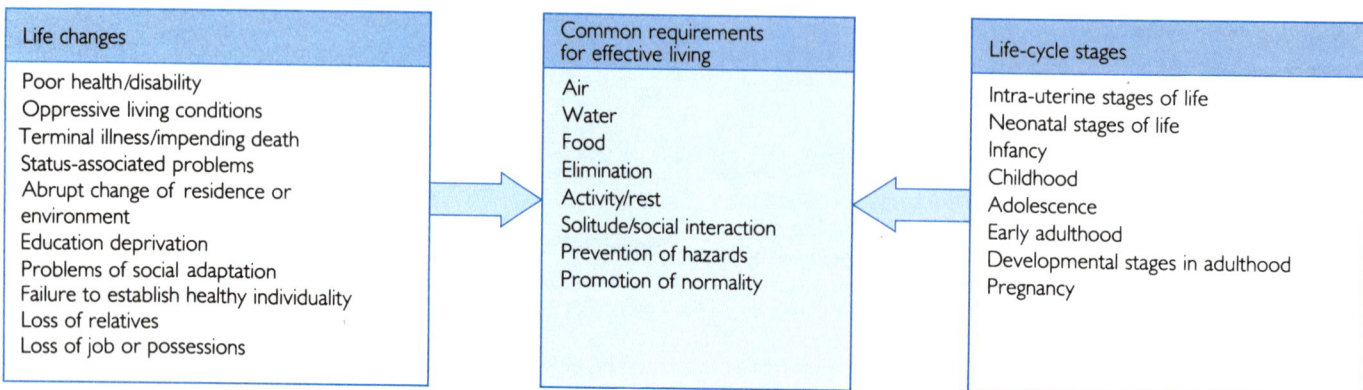

Fig. 1.8 Developmental influences on self-care in relation to the requirements for effective living

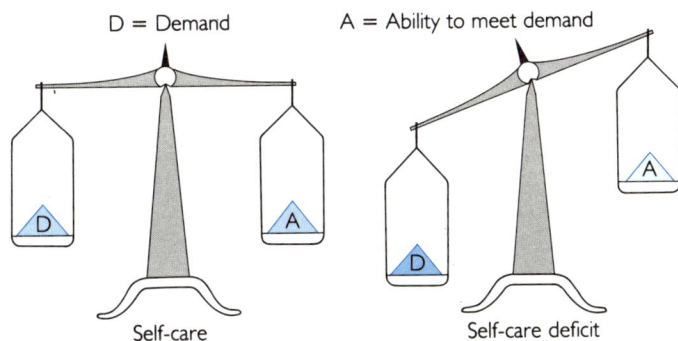

Fig. 1.9 Balance between demand and self-care ability

guardian, then the care given is described as 'dependent care', for example, the care provided by a mother for an infant or the care provided by a family for an ageing relative. Where the deficit exceeds the capacity for self-care *and* dependent care, a nursing service is required.

Nurses establish helping relationships with individuals who have a self-care deficit. The help which is given is directed toward the maintenance of life, recovery from disease or injury, or developing the ability to cope with the effects of disability. Orem identifies five helping methods:

- acting for or doing for another
- guiding another
- supporting another (physically or psychologically)
- providing an environment that promotes personal development
- teaching another.

The development of self-care actions, or the restoration of existing patterns of self-care, is often accomplished in stages. Different helping methods, or different combinations of helping methods, will be necessary at different stages. The selection of appropriate helping methods is assisted by considering whether or not the person in need of help occupies an active or passive role in relation to meeting the need. For example, the unconscious patient is unaware of his needs, cannot make judgments or decisions, and cannot act on his own behalf. In this situation, the nurse will fully compensate for the self-care deficits, and her actions will be 'acting for or doing for'.

In the case of the unconscious patient, on regaining consciousness he may be able to make judgments and decisions and to carry out some actions toward meeting his needs. In this situation the nurse may, for example, adjust the environment to facilitate some aspects of self-care, and continue to carry out the actions which the person cannot yet accomplish on his own behalf; the nurse partially compensates for the patient's deficit.

Finally, the person may have the necessary skills to meet his requirements, but may be in need of psychological support. The nurse then occupies a supportive/educative role.

Model 3 The Stress-Adaptation Model: Saxton and Hyland

This model was originally described by the American authors, Saxton and Hyland, in *Planning and Implementing Nursing Intervention* (1979). It is based on a belief that throughout his life cycle an individual is constantly subjected to stresses to which he must make adaptive responses as a whole person. At times, these responses can be detrimental to the total organism. They suggest that knowledge of the adaptive responses an individual makes to stress – according to his past experience, present state and future needs – enables nurses to assess and plan nursing interventions. They feel that a framework of this kind is sufficiently flexible to incorporate new knowledge and health care concepts as they become available and can be applied regardless of a patient's diagnosis or environment.

This approach varies considerably from the previous two described and offers you insight into an alternative model where the emphasis is on adaptation.

The beliefs about Man on which this model are based are that Man has both physical and psychological aspects which develop interdependently through adaptive responses to normal stresses. There is, however, a limit to an individual's innate capacity to adapt, which is dependent on the personal resources he has to draw upon, and the degree and types of stress – either physiological or psychological – that he experiences at any one time. If this limit is exceeded he may require help in adapting to the circumstances in which he finds himself.

The goals of nursing in this model are to assist Man to respond to stress by making healthy adaptations which will lead to development. They are also concerned with assisting Man in limiting, altering or preventing unhealthy or inappropriate adaptations.

The knowledge base for this model is derived from theories of stress and the adaptive responses that an individual makes to stress. *Stress* is defined as any "factor or factors that require some response or result in some change within an individual". These stresses may be categorised as:

- physical: temperature, sound, pressure, light, motion, gravity and electricity
- chemical: acids, alkalis, drugs, toxic substances, hormones, gases, water and nutrients
- microbiological: viruses, bacteria, moulds and parasites
- physiological: disturbances in structure or function of any tissue, organ, system or body part
- developmental: genetic endowment, prematurity, immaturity, growth and ageing
- emotional: real or imagined threats to values, self-image or self-concept and sociocultural/religious interpersonal pressures.

Stress is a normal and necessary part of everyday life and adaptive response to it normally leads to development. However, should the degree of everyday stress increase, or if an unusual stress such as an infection, a bereavement or an accident is added, an individual's ability to make adaptations may be impaired.

Adaptation

Saxton and Hyland suggest that "adaptation can be simply defined as the anatomical, physiological or psychological responses or changes in an individual that occur as a reaction to stress". The purpose of such adaptations is to allow an individual to continue functioning effectively. They suggest that adaptations are "defences with which the individual attempts to counter a stress by limiting its site, lessening its impact or neutralising its effects so that the body can continue to function".

Adaptations may be inherent, as in the case of the physiological response to exposure to heat. Alternatively, they may be learnt or acquired as in the case of the many different behaviours one sees in an individual as a response to grief. They are dependent upon an individual's learned or acquired responses, the level of development and his genetic makeup. They are also dependent upon the total degree of stress experienced at any one time. Numerous small stresses may be as harmful as one major stress and it may be that one small extra stress is the 'last straw' with which an individual cannot cope.

Whilst many of the adaptations that an individual makes to a stress are appropriate, in some circumstances they may be either inefficient or inappropriate. For instance, an individual may respond to the pressure of a broken marriage by smoking excessively. This 'coping mechanism' can in itself be harmful and lead to further stresses, such as lung or heart disease. Similarly, an individual may respond to the stress of a broken arm by keeping the shoulder still. In the long term, this may result in a stiff shoulder which will act as an additional stress.

Stress-adaptation cycle

The authors of this model suggest that stress may be divided into two categories:

- **primary stresses** are those which result from a person's interaction with the environment and are external in nature. They lead to a direct adaptation.

- **secondary stresses** are those which result from an ineffective adaptation to the primary stress. A circular relationship can be identified, which may remain unbroken without appropriate nursing intervention.

Their relationship is shown in Figure 1.10 (bottom of page).

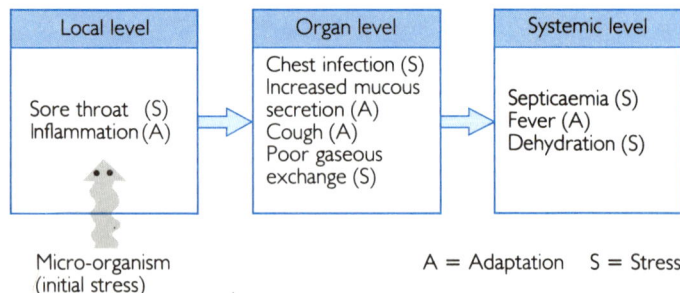

Fig. 1.11 Potential progress of initial stress if not contained

Adaptive processes usually occur at a *local* level initially, but if they are ineffective the effects of the primary stress may spread to invade an *organ*. At this level secondary stresses may occur, leading to further adaptations. If uncontained at this level, stresses may affect the *whole system*. Figure 1.11 gives an example of the progress which may occur if initial adaptations are inadequate in containing a stress.

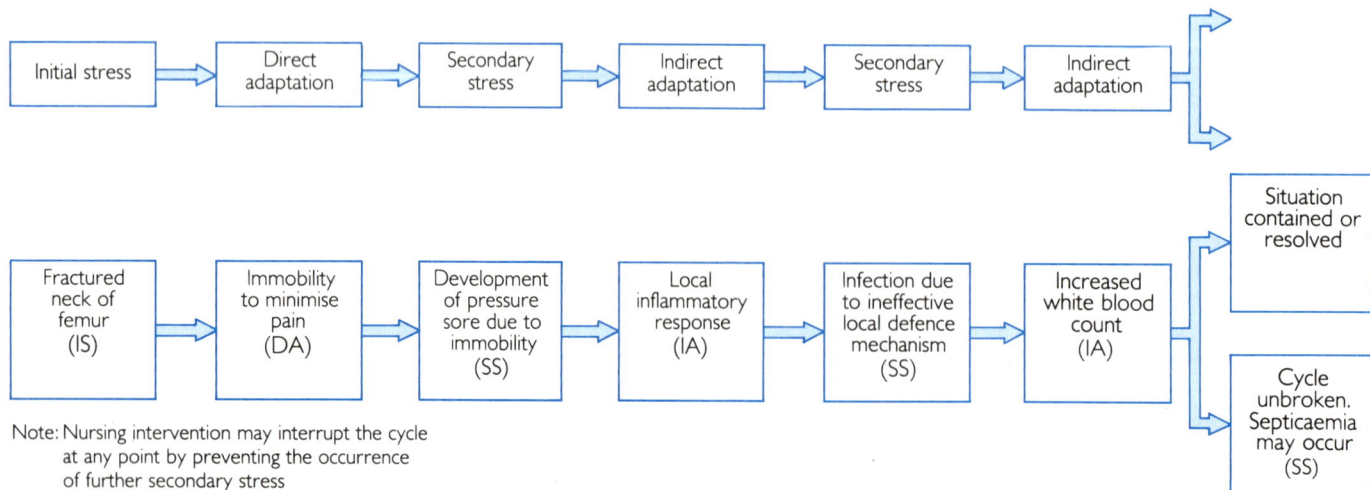

Note: Nursing intervention may interrupt the cycle at any point by preventing the occurrence of further secondary stress

Fig. 1.10 Stress-adaptation cycle (adapted from Saxton and Hyland, 1979)

Levels of adaptation

Saxton and Hyland describe five different levels of adaptation which an individual makes in response to stress although, as they point out, frequently there is overlap or movement between the levels. These five levels are:

First level: these are the responses we all make continuously to the stresses of everyday life and we are rarely aware of them. They include reflex responses, for instance the maintenance of blood pressure following a change in position. They generally aim at protecting, restoring or maintaining the status quo.

Second level: when first level responses have been unable to cope with a stress, we may become aware of the presence of that stress and consciously or unconsciously bring into action another adaptation. When there is excessive fluid loss in very hot weather or after eating a salty meal, we may feel thirsty and drink extra fluid to compensate. Psychologically, we may take such actions as seeking company or avoiding a particular situation. The individual is still able to cope but is more aware of his actions.

Third level: at the third level of adaptation signs and symptoms occur because our normal defence mechanisms have failed to reduce, limit or control a stress. They include such responses as swelling and pain in response to trauma or sleeplessness in response to anxiety. They usually prompt the individual to seek assistance.

Fourth level: at this level the adaptation itself will create additional stresses. An adaptive response of vomiting in response to a gastric irritant can in itself lead to dehydration and electrolyte imbalance. Psychologically, responses may include such activities as withdrawal and lethargy, leading to a failure to eat and new stresses caused by poor nutrition.

Fifth level: at the final level of adaptation the response that an individual has made to a stress becomes life-threatening. For instance, the swelling of brain tissue following trauma may be extensive enough to cause pressure on the respiratory control centre and inhibit an ability to breathe. Psychologically, adaptations at this level may include psychotic or neurotic states. This level of adaptation is life threatening and requires urgent intervention.

In assessing an individual's level of adaptation the nurse must take into account the individual's specific complaints, level of development, past history, as well as laboratory reports and personal observations.

Saxton and Hyland suggest that, when planning nursing care, nurses can use their knowledge of the potential progress of the stress-adaptation cycle and of possible measures which may be taken to contain or reduce stress or make appropriate adaptations. They suggest five objectives for nursing intervention which match the five different levels of adaptation. They add two more objectives which are common to all situations:

1 Support the individual's first-level adaptations to assist in sustaining and maintaining the defensive responses
2 Limit the individual's second-level adaptations to confine or restrict the compensatory responses
3 Alter the individual's third-level adaptations to modify or reduce the symptoms of response
4 Interrupt the individual's fourth-level adaptations to redirect or stop the responses that have become stresses
5 Supplement the individual's fifth-level adaptations to complement or replace the responses that are threatening life functions.

Additional objectives:

1 Reduce or limit the extent and intensity of the present stress affecting the patient
2 Prevent additional stress for the patient whenever possible.

Saxton and Hyland use the nursing assessment graph shown in Figure 1.12 to show the relationship between the levels of adaptation and nursing intervention. Following the nursing assessment, a patient's position can be plotted on the chart to act as guidance in planning the level of nursing intervention required.

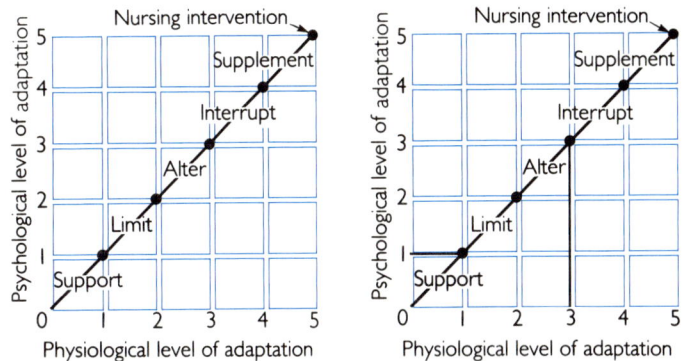

Fig. 1.12 (Left) Nursing assessment graph. (Right) Nursing assessment graph completed for an unconscious patient, aged 33, with fractured skull (Saxton and Hyland, 1979)

A CHOICE OF WORKING MODELS

The three nursing models which have been described reflect the same underlying themes: a recognition of a patient at an individual stage of development, the capability for self-care, common daily living needs, and the reaction to stress and the ability to adapt. The variation in the models comes in the different emphasis given to each component, reflecting the authors' ways of expressing their individual views of nursing. In selecting a model you may prefer to use one which has not been described here as a framework on which to base your practice. You may prefer to take elements from various models and incorporate them in a model of your own, which can guide and direct your practice. All of us already have some ideas about nursing which determine the ways in which we practise. A unit within a hospital, or in the community nursing services, may have its own model. For example, in hospital the nurses working on an acute surgical ward may collectively operate using a stress-adaptation framework, whilst those working on a ward for the mentally handicapped may use an approach based on a self-care framework.

Conflict can arise if the individual members of a nursing team within one unit base their practice on different models, and it is therefore useful if the team can come to some common agreement on an appropriate model. For example, if one nurse's belief is that Man is a biophysical creature and the goals of her care are solely aimed towards curing disease, her approach would vary from the nurse who holds a holistic view of Man and sees her goal as being one of assisting him in becoming independent and fulfilled. If both shared a similar model such a difference would be less likely to occur. Thus, establishing a common model within a unit can help to give a type of care which is consistent and which gives a clear picture of the overall goals of nursing to the whole team.

NURSING MODELS AND THE NURSING PROCESS

Once a model has been identified, it will guide the way in which the process of nursing is put into action. How each step of the nursing process is carried out is influenced by the model on which practice is based. The link between the nursing model and the nursing process is of extreme importance since the model will, for example, reflect the sort of information sought during assessment and hence the way a form for recording such information will be structured. It will also give guidance to the identification of goals, the way in which nursing actions are planned and implemented and the aspects of care to be evaluated. In other words, a nursing model influences the content of each stage of the nursing process, giving it direction and making it purposeful.

Activity 1.6   **Allow 15 minutes**

A model for you?

You might have found the section on models contained a lot of ideas which are new to you and which may need further thought. This activity is intended to assist you in understanding the concept of nursing models.

Consider the three major elements which go towards making a model for practice and, using the following headings, briefly outline your own ideas about a nursing model. They may reflect those described in the text or have arisen from other sources.

1 Beliefs about Man
2 Goals of care
3 Knowledge for practice

Authors' comment

It is difficult to put a time limit on an activity of this kind as ideas often emerge over a long period. However, having considered some of your own thoughts, you may find it helpful to spend some further time discussing and comparing them with those colleagues with whom you work.

ACCOUNTABILITY

Nursing has been described by many as a service-oriented profession. In other words, it offers a specific service to clients or patients which is associated with their health. You may have discovered in working through this module that it is difficult to define exactly for which aspects of health care nurses are specifically responsible. However, once you have clarified in your own mind what a patient's needs are, and in what ways the nurse may help to meet those needs, you can identify areas which clearly belong to nursing care.

If you, as a nurse, offer a service for which you are uniquely responsible, you must be prepared to stand accountable for your actions. Accountability may be described as being personally responsible for the outcome of one's own professional actions. Lewis and Batey (1982) emphasise that accountability implies "a formal obligation to *disclose*" what you have done, why you did it and what the results of your actions were. The disclosure can take place before, during or after a particular action, and *"initiating the disclosure is the responsibility of the one accountable and not of others"*.

In order to be able to achieve accountability, nurses' actions must be *explainable, defendable,* and *based on knowledge* rather than on tradition or myth. They must be able to explain how a particular difficulty was identified and the reason for the action taken. If nurses are willing to be held accountable for nursing actions there are two major criteria to be met. Firstly, a statement must be made of the *expected outcome* of the actions or the goals which are being sought. Secondly, a *system of evaluation* must be established by which the nurse can assess whether these outcomes have been achieved.

RESPONSIBILITY

Although some people use the words 'accountability' and 'responsibility' interchangeably, there is a difference between the two. Whilst accountability suggests that one has made a decision to carry out an action oneself, responsibility implies that one has been requested to carry out an action by another. The request can come from other nurses, for instance a senior nurse giving a junior nurse responsibility to undertake certain activities. In other instances the request might be made by people other than nurses, such as doctors or administrators.

The first person, or initiator, is accountable for deciding upon the action and the ability of the person to whom she has delegated the task. The second person is responsible for its safe completion. She can, however, be held accountable if she performs a task for which she knows she has not acquired the necessary knowledge or skills. Similarly she is expected to act 'reasonably'. For instance, if a senior nurse asks a junior nurse to assist a patient with bathing, it is the senior nurse who is accountable for that decision. If, however, the junior nurse makes the bath water too hot and the patient is scalded she is personally accountable, since it is 'reasonable' to expect an adult to know that the water is too hot.

In the past nurses have often accepted without question responsibilities laid on them by others. For instance, we have accepted the responsibility for carrying out some procedures traditionally undertaken by doctors. Similarly we have accepted some administrative procedures which are not always appropriate to nursing. As we become more certain about the nature of nursing itself and those actions for which we are accountable, we may become more critical about those actions for which we are prepared to take responsibility. Before accepting the responsibility we have to ask whether the action is appropriate to nursing and whether it will benefit the patient if it is accepted by nurses. We also have to ask whether we have the necessary knowledge or skills to take the action requested.

AUTHORITY

In order to be accountable, nurses must also have authority to act. Authority is the rightful power to act and as Batey and Lewis (1982) suggest, it is derived from at least three sources in nursing:

Authority of a situation: this is most striking in an emergency situation where a nurse may respond by fulfilling actions which she would not undertake at a less acute time.

Authority of expert knowledge: a nurse's professional qualification gives her the authority to undertake certain activities. It implies that she has attained the knowledge and skills to act. In the past nurses have sometimes, at the request of others, taken on the responsibility for some actions for which they have not acquired the necessary knowledge. In this situation, they are not in a position to take authority for their actions. In the same vein, there is a need for nurses to extend their knowledge and keep up-to-date with new ideas and research findings. This will ensure that their authority is soundly based and will in some instances, as new knowledge is gained, extend that authority.

Authority of position: this is the authority that is linked to a formal position in an organisation. It is often expressed explicitly in a job description. Whilst authority of position may, in some circumstances, be delegated to others, authority of expert knowledge can only rest with those who hold that expert knowledge.

AUTONOMY

In order to be accountable for their actions it is necessary for nurses to hold a degree of autonomy. Autonomy which is related to work may be described as "freedom for the professional to practise the profession in accordance with his/her professional training" (Engel, 1970).

Autonomy exists in nursing when nurses use their own judgment to decide what actions are necessary to achieve identified patient goals. This is followed by the nurse implementing the action that she has decided is appropriate. An example may be a nurse's autonomous decision about how often and in what way a patient may be given assistance with oral hygiene. Her goal will be that the patient's mouth will be moist and clean, and her actions are planned from her knowledge of the ways in which this goal may be achieved.

This does not imply absolute independence since it is "confined to that for which the professional (the nurse) holds authority derived from expert knowledge and position" (Batey and Lewis, 1982).

If nurses are truly autonomous professionals in their own right, no-one can stop them from taking action following independent decisions they have made about nursing matters. This does not mean that others cannot challenge their decisions nor that nurses should ignore such challenges.

Activity 1.7   Allow 5 minutes
What are you accountable for?
In this activity we ask you to think about your own practice in relation to the preceding discussion.

Think back to the last time you were working in your own area and consider one clinical decision which you made during your span of duty, for example the action you prescribed to prevent the formation of deep venous thrombosis. Consider how you would defend that decision to your own peer group and the reason why you thought that action was necessary.

Authors' comment
We hope that your decision was grounded on research-based knowledge rather than on tradition, routine or myth.

ACCOUNTABILITY – TO WHOM?

There are several lines of accountability within any professional group. The most important one, however, must always be to the client.

Accountability to the patient or client

Since a qualified nurse is expected by society to have a body of knowledge on which she bases her practice, she cannot act in her professional capacity without reference to that body of knowledge. The patient has a right to expect a service from you which maintains the standards laid down by your professional group. Therefore, you should be primarily accountable to your patients for the service which you offer.

Accountability to the profession and the public

The professional representative body for nursing is the United Kingdom Central Council for Nursing, Midwifery and Health Visiting. It was established in response to an Act of Parliament in order to represent the public and safeguard their interests.

One of the major functions of a professional body is to monitor and maintain the professional standards of its members. It also controls a register of members and sets the requirements for entry to that register. It lays down a *code of professional practice*. It also has the right to remove a member from the register if she does not maintain the standards of practice which are required.

As an individual you are accountable to your professional body and, through it, to the public for your nursing actions. You may be called upon to explain and defend them.

Accountability to colleagues

At the clinical level an individual nurse must always be accountable for her own actions. In some instances she may delegate responsibility for a part of patient care to another nurse or an unqualified person, either a nurse learner or a nursing auxiliary. In this situation she is still accountable for the care a patient receives, since she is professionally responsible for ensuring that an individual has the necessary knowledge and skills to be able to complete the work asked of her. If the work is delegated to another qualified nurse with less experience, as might be the case with a ward sister and a newly qualified nurse, the senior nurse is still accountable in that she made the decision to delegate that work. However, the less experienced qualified nurse is also acting in her professional capacity and can be held accountable for her actions since, if she feels unable to fulfil the work asked of her, she has a professional responsibility to state her position. Figure 1.13 shows some of the lines of accountability for all practising nurses.

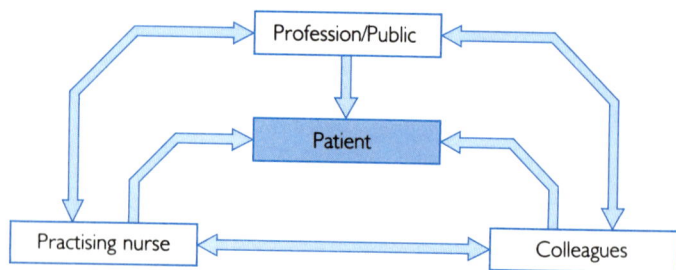

Fig. 1.13 Some lines of accountability

THE NURSING PROCESS AND ACCOUNTABILITY

As we have seen, being accountable means being prepared to disclose the actions you have taken in caring for a patient or client. The nursing process, a systematic problem-oriented approach to nursing, requires that you should identify and record the nursing needs of the patient, the expected outcomes of your actions, the actions you will take and the results of your actions. This approach lends itself to professional accountability. Carrying out care according to predetermined routines removes the mechanism for individual accountability, since the responsibility then lies only in fulfilling a routine and discounts the nurse's freedom and autonomy in meeting the individual needs of a patient. The nurse becomes responsible only for her actions and is not in a position to be accountable to the individual patient or client. This is inappropriate if nurses wish to offer the sort of service patients deserve.

Activity 1.8   Allow 10 minutes

What action would you take?

This activity is designed to help you to translate the concept of accountability into practice.

Bearing in mind the various lines of accountability for nurses described above, briefly outline what actions you would take in the following three situations:

1 It is normal practice to take all temperatures on the paediatric ward at 7 am. A mother has just fed her baby and settled him back to sleep when you arrive to take his temperature. The baby is resting quietly. What action would you take?

2 A doctor asks you to carry out a technical procedure which is usually carried out by nurses, but which you have never performed before. You are the senior nurse on duty in your area. What action would you take?

3 A hospital patient questions the drugs she has been prescribed by the doctor, stating that they are different from the ones she normally takes and which she can identify by name. The drugs do differ. What action would you take?

Authors' comment

There is no single right answer to any of the questions posed above. Your actions will depend on your assessment of the whole situation. However, having thought about your actions in these situations, can you answer the following questions?

1 Has the patient's safety been ensured?
2 Can I justify my actions to the patient?
3 Have I sufficient knowledge and/or skills on which to base my actions?
4 Have I considered all possible courses of action?
5 Do I have enough knowledge about the situation to make an informed judgment of what to do?
6 What are the consequences if I do not take any action?

NURSING IN AN ORGANISATION

Nurses do not work with patients in isolation but as part of a team and within an organisation. The team may include such people as the doctor, the physiotherapist and the dietitian, as well as members of the patient's own family and the patient himself, all of whom have contributions to make towards the patient's total health care. The organisation is made up of many systems, each of which has its special part to play and which are interdependent. These systems include such functions as catering, portering, administration, home helps and transport. They supply the essential resources which are necessary for the smooth running of the service which is offered to patients. Each system, including nursing, has to work within a given budget and nurses must take this into consideration when they are planning care.

THE MULTI-DISCIPLINARY CLINICAL TEAM

The multi-disciplinary clinical team includes all those people who have a direct contribution to make towards a patient's ability to achieve maximum health. Although some aspects of care may be performed by more than one person, each member of that team can justify his membership only if he has something to contribute that cannot be done as well by other members of the team.

In different settings the multi-disciplinary team will have different members. It is important that all members have some idea of the contribution that others make in order that they can work co-operatively, rather than in isolation or even conflict. For instance, although a nurse is dependent upon a doctor for medical prescription of drugs or other forms of treatment, a doctor is often dependent upon a nurse for fulfilment of that prescription. It is therefore important that they understand each other's roles and responsibilities so that expectations are realistic. As the patient is less likely to know what services each member can offer, it is up to the nurse

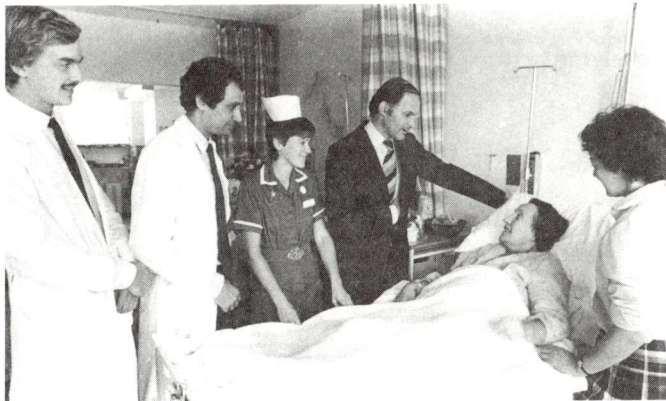

Nurses are members of a multi-disciplinary clinical team

to give him this information and also to discover what resources he, as an individual, has available which can contribute to meeting his needs. Since nursing is the only discipline which offers a continuous service over twenty-four hours every day, one of its major functions is in co-ordinating the contributions of others in the team and giving feed-back to other team members. This emphasises the importance of nurses understanding the roles that others have to play.

Activity 1.9	Allow 15 minutes

Who does what in your team?

This activity asks you to look specifically at working within your own organisation.

Write down the roles of all members of the multi-disciplinary clinical team who work in your area and note what special contributions they have to offer patients.

Authors' comment

Once you have completed this exercise it may be helpful to take a little more time to discuss your answers with the people concerned and ask them for their comments. Alternatively, you may like to ask each member separately to explain to you what they see as their specific contribution to patient care. We hope that this exercise will help you to understand the contribution that other members of the clinical team feel they have to make, rather than what you think it is.

THE ORGANISATION

In order that nurses can work effectively they must also understand how the organisation, that is the hospital or community in which they work, functions. Most organisations have policies which set down the *boundaries of responsibility* for each system. By doing this others can identify what expectations they may have of each service. For instance, a hospital may have a policy stating whether or not housekeeping staff are meant to make beds. If the nurse is familiar with this policy she will not have unrealistic expectations of the housekeeping staff. Similarly policies may exist in social service departments to define what functions or activities home helps can undertake.

Many organisations also have a mechanism whereby each occupational group can bid for money to buy extra resources. Since this budget is not limitless nurses' requests have to stand alongside those submitted by others. An understanding of this mechanism will have clear advantages. Firstly, it will help you as a nurse to consider your requests in the light of the needs of all other groups. If a request is made, you must be able to justify why you require extra resources and to specify the advantages that will be gained, both by patients and by the organisation as a whole. Secondly, it will help you to understand when requests have to be rejected because the needs of another group are greater. However, if requests have been well thought out and can be defended, the likelihood of their being granted is much greater. Using a systematic problem-solving approach when considering requirements can help nurses to present their bids in a clear, concise manner and to justify their value to others.

THE NURSING PROCESS IN CONTEXT

For effective and efficient working, it is essential that good communications are established within an organisation and a multi-disciplinary clinical team. Some members of that team may already use a problem-solving approach to their work. If a similar approach is used in nursing it will help you to clarify your position and enhance your contribution to the work of the team as a whole. Another advantage of using the nursing process within an organisation is the way in which it may be used to help nurses to negotiate. Since we live in a climate where financial resources are limited, managers and administrators are frequently looking for places where cuts can be made. It has always been difficult for nurses to explain how they assess their work-load and therefore how they calculate how many nurses are required to work in specific places. Since the nursing process requires that nurses clearly define which needs they are meeting for the patients and what their goals, actions and evaluations of those actions are, it is an ideal way for nurses to describe what their work entails and to justify claims for resources.

THE REALITY OF THE NURSING PROCESS

The purpose of this first module has been to introduce you to some of the underlying principles which are related to nursing and the nursing process and which are essential to its understanding.

There is no doubt that some aspects of this approach are familiar whilst others are new. Whilst the process itself is problem-oriented, the nursing process as a whole involves:

- using a systematic, rational approach to nursing a patient
- seeing patients as people with individual needs and as part of a family and community
- having an understanding of the role of the nurse
- developing a close partnership relationship between nurse and patient

- basing practice on a model which is meaningful both to individual nurses and the teams in which they work
- accepting accountability for actions
- recognising that nursing is practised within an organisation.

These seven basic points represent the themes of this course, and when the nursing process is referred to in the course, it embraces all of them. In all of the following course work, these themes underly all that is said, and will be referred to frequently.

Group Session 1 will involve some in-depth discussion on your feelings about these themes in relation to your own area of practice.

PREPARING FOR MODULE 2

Module 2, which considers *assessment*, the first step in the nursing process, is somewhat longer than the other modules and contains activities involving about 3½ hours of work. You may wish, therefore, to approach Module 2 in two parts. You will probably find the most appropriate division to be on p. 46, before the section on *Data collection using interviewing skills*.

Before beginning Module 2 you are asked to collect some material from your own work area. This is essential because you will be asked to refer to it as the basis for a number of activities. The material required is as follows:

1 A **blank** specimen of the documentation currently used for nursing assessment in your own work area. This may be a specially designed Nursing Assessment Form, a Nursing History or a system such as Kardex.

2 A specimen of the assessment documentation recently **completed** for a patient on admission or, for community nurses, at first visit. If possible, select a patient who you yourself assessed. Select a patient who is fairly typical of those you are nursing and who interests you. Avoid an unusually complicated case.

You will need to copy the information onto blank forms. It is essential to delete or alter any information by which the patient could be identified (i.e. name, date of birth, address).

Please ensure that you obtain permission from your superior or from another appropriate person to collect the above material. If you need assistance, ask your Group Leader.

You might find it helpful and interesting to pair up with another course member so that two of you 'share' one patient assessment, though you should each obtain your own personal copy of the documentation.

MODULE 2
THE FIRST STEP OF THE NURSING PROCESS ASSESSMENT

Prepared for the Course Team by Alison Tierney

CONTENTS

OBJECTIVES

After studying this module, you should be able to:

1 Describe and critically appraise the way in which you currently approach and undertake nursing assessment.

2 Define 'nursing assessment' and describe its purpose.

3 Understand that nursing assessment should be viewed as a partnership between nurse and patient.

4 Understand why nursing assessment needs an explicit nursing framework (model) and identify a model which is applicable to your practice.

5 Identify and know how to use sources of information available for nursing assessment.

6 Describe the various skills involved in nursing assessment.

7 Undertake the data collection phase of nursing assessment in practice.

8 Record data collected from nursing assessment on appropriate forms.

9 Identify patients' problems (actual and potential) from data collected.

10 Document patients' problems concisely yet precisely.

HOW DO *YOU* ASSESS PATIENTS?

In preparation for this module you were asked to collect from your own work area, one blank and one completed specimen of the documentation which you currently use for nursing assessment. You will be asked to refer to this material, and to comment on it, throughout the module.

You may be wondering why you are being asked to use your own current practice of nursing assessment as a reference point in this module. After all, you are probably hoping to learn how to go about this first step of the nursing process or, at least, to discover new things about assessment. Hopefully, you will learn more about assessment from this module but, equally, we would like to encourage you to review the way in which *you* currently approach assessment in your own area of nursing practice. Even where the nursing process is not being fully implemented, there is obviously still some form of nursing assessment taking place and it would be wrong to ignore this fact. So, whatever stage of development nursing assessment has reached in your own work area, this module should help you to review your current practice and encourage you to see possibilities for innovation, change or improvement.

Activity 2.1   Allow 15 minutes

How do *you* assess patients?

As a first step in working through Module 2, we would like you to review your current approach to nursing assessment.

Consider for a few minutes how *you* assess patients. Then, write a brief description of the way in which you approach and undertake nursing assessment in your own practice. You might find it helpful to imagine you are describing this to a student nurse new to the ward.

Author's comment

You will be asked to review what you have written here later in the module.

SOME 'BASICS' ABOUT ASSESSMENT

Before going on to look at *how* nursing assessment is undertaken in practice, this section of the module considers some of the underlying ideas and issues. Reference is made to the themes identified in Module 1 which underlie the whole of the course, illustrating their direct relevance for the assessment step of the nursing process.

If you have come to this course with little knowledge of the nursing process, this section should be particularly helpful to you in clarifying some 'basics' about assessment. For nurses already involved with the nursing process, much of the material will seem familiar. Nevertheless, working through the section should help you to pull together a variety of ideas and issues in an organised way, and the interspersed activities will encourage you to examine your own ideas and practice critically.

DEFINING 'ASSESSMENT'

For the purpose of this course we are describing the nursing process in four steps: assessment, planning, implementation and evaluation. Even though the first step is commonly called 'assessment', it is probably necessary to clarify how we are interpreting this term here, because it does have various connotations.

Our use of the word 'assessment' describes the first step of the nursing process as a composite of the following activities:

- collecting information (data)
- reviewing the data collected
- identifying the patient's problems from the data.

In other words, using this definition 'assessment' involves more than data collection alone.

You may find some nurses referring to 'data collection' as a separate activity, thereby dividing the nursing process into five steps instead of four. In *A Guide to the Practice of Nursing Using the Nursing Process* (1982), McFarlane and Castledine adopt this division, describing the first two steps of the process as 'data collection' and 'assessment' respectively. Although they refer to the second step as assessment, you may find the term 'nursing diagnosis' being employed instead, as Marks-Maran (1983) advocates.

Pause for a moment and decide which terminology you find most helpful for describing the initial step of the nursing process.

THE PURPOSE OF ASSESSMENT

In Module 1, the nursing process was described as a tool to help nurses to practise *individualised* nursing. If patients are to be considered by nurses as individuals, nurses must obviously have information about each individual patient and that individual's particular problems. Assessment provides the data base for the process of nursing – the basis for an individualised nursing plan and a baseline against which subsequent events can be compared. Each stage of the nursing process is important but this is perhaps especially true of assessment. A nursing plan, and indeed the patient's entire nursing care, can only be as good as the information on which it is based.

Assessment can also be seen to have the purpose of 'getting to know the patient'. It provides the opportunity for establishing rapport between nurse and patient, which is vital in the development of the nurse-patient relationship. The way in which nurses approach patient assessment will not only determine the quality of the information collected but also influence patients' expectations and understanding of nursing. For example, assessment can be approached in a way which encourages patients to express feelings as well as to describe symptoms, to ask as well as to answer questions, to offer information which they themselves consider that it might be relevant for nurses to have. So, assessment provides a starting point for 'partnership', an approach discussed in the section on the *Nurse-patient relationship* in Module 1.

Seeing nursing assessment as a partnership between nurse and patient is, however, a relatively new concept and to succeed in achieving this kind of involvement of patients in the nursing process probably requires some fairly fundamental changes of attitude in nursing. Firstly we need to provide patients with opportunities to express their views – and nurses may well need to assure them that this is both permissible and desirable. We need also to begin to appreciate more the value of patients' own opinions and perceptions of the problems and priorities. And these principles should apply just as much to people who are traditionally considered to be incapable of self-advocacy – the mentally handicapped, for example – as to more educated, articulate and confident patients. If we think along these lines, then assessment can be seen to consist of much more than just data collection and problem identification.

ASSESSMENT IS NOT A ONCE-ONLY PROCEDURE

Describing assessment as a 'step' of the nursing process, or referring to 'an assessment' or 'the assessment procedure' can be misleading because, of course, nursing assessment is never a once-only procedure. When we refer to 'an assessment' we tend to mean such occasions as the planned, systematic assessment undertaken when a patient is either admitted to hospital or has a first contact with out-patient or community services. We also use the term to describe a similarly comprehensive assessment undertaken on a subsequent occasion due to substantially changed circumstances. In reality, assessment is an ongoing activity.

Certainly a continuing review of the patient's condition and reappraisal of the problems is required in any situation which is rapidly changing, for example during labour, in the post-operative period, or when the patient's medical condition changes substantially or medical treatment is altered. In contrast, the condition and problems of a long-stay elderly patient or a psychiatric patient may appear to change much less rapidly and dramatically. Nevertheless, new information is continually being obtained about and from such patients too, and so continuing assessment is as important in long-term care as in more acute situations.

Identifying how frequently patients should be assessed and deciding what new information to report verbally and what to record in writing are skills which draw upon experience and profes-

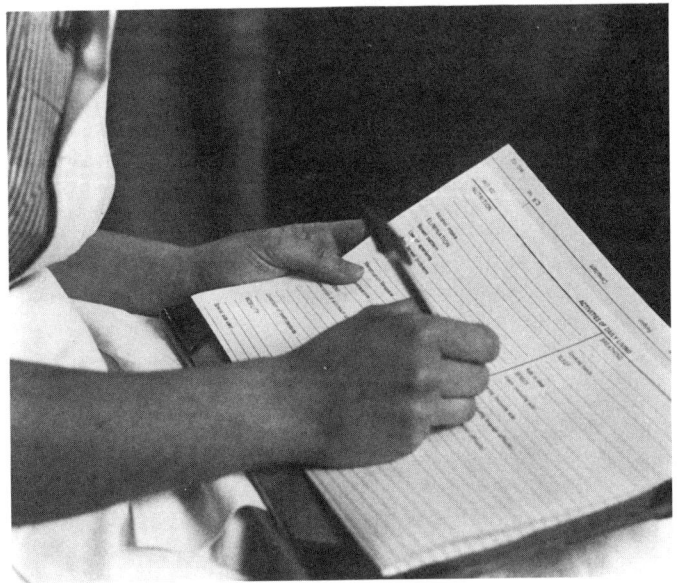

sional judgment. And choosing where to record additional information really depends upon the practice operating in any one clinical area. Small items of information might be added, with the date, to the initial assessment documentation, or to a patient's 'daily record' or 'progress notes' if such documents are maintained. But if a patient's condition changes substantially, it is likely that fresh documents will be needed in order to record a large amount of new information and the problems identified.

There is another reason why assessment should not be regarded as a once-only procedure. It is always necessary to be aware that data collected at the initial assessment may be inaccurate or incomplete. Subsequent assessment, therefore, helps to check the accuracy of data previously collected and guards against the possibility of omissions.

Regarding assessment as an ongoing procedure does help to reinforce the idea of the nursing process as one which is dynamic and ongoing, with closely interrelated steps. In practice, it is sometimes difficult to distinguish whether new information is obtained from assessment or evaluation. Of course, evaluation is undertaken in relation to previously specified goals but if it reveals that the intervention planned has not achieved the desired outcome, then the process begins again – with assessment.

A REALISTIC APPROACH TO ASSESSMENT

A common criticism of the nursing process – and the assessment step in particular – is that it is much too time-consuming and involves too much paperwork. Undertaking and documenting a nursing assessment is viewed as a useful exercise for learners, but often as an unrealistic proposition in practice.

Sometimes this criticism appears to be based on the misunderstanding that an assessment form must be fully completed for every single patient as soon as possible after admission. In any busy ward, or for community nurses with heavy caseloads, this ideal is seldom practicable. If we are to implement the nursing process successfully, we have to take account of the realities of nursing. It is not always necessary nor is it in the real interests of the patient to turn nursing assessment into something exhaustive and time-consuming by nature. For example, with an otherwise well person being admitted to hospital for a minor medical examination it may take only minutes to record essential biographical information, identify the problems requiring nursing intervention and establish that further detailed assessment is not necessary.

To be selective about what information is needed, in what detail and how quickly, requires nurses to exercise professional judgment and to adopt a realistic approach to assessment. For each patient, the circumstances have to be considered and the need for information weighed up against the opportunity to obtain it at the time. Constraints may be caused by patients being too physically ill or tired or confused to participate in a lengthy assessment. Other patients may consider this to be an unnecessary invasion of their privacy. Alternatively, constraints may arise because of inadequate staffing or competing priorities of other patients at the time. More detailed assessment can be carried out later, as appropriate and when time permits.

Even the most ardent enthusiasts of the nursing process must acknowledge that idealism has to be tempered with realism: all we ask is that 'shortage of time' is not used as an excuse. If we accept that a nursing plan – and a patient's nursing care – can only be as good as the information on which it is based, then nursing assessment, appropriate to the circumstances, is a necessity.

Activity 2.2   Allow 15 minutes
A realistic approach?
This activity is designed to help you to evaluate an assessment which has previously been undertaken.
Have a look at the completed patient assessment you collected in preparation for this module. Read through the information recorded about the patient from assessment on admission or at first referral.

Write in your notebook a summary of the information. It might help you to imagine that you have been asked to give a brief verbal summary to another nurse just coming on duty or to the nursing staff at the 'ward report' session or perhaps to a community nurse who will be visiting the patient on your day off.

Now, having written your summary, respond to the following questions:

1 Do you think the information recorded provides a sufficiently comprehensive data base on which to plan the patient's immediate nursing?
(Yes/No)

If you answered 'No', what additional information do you think should have been obtained?

2 Do you consider that all the information is relevant?   (Yes/No)

If you answered 'No', what particular information do you think is superfluous?

3 Weighing up your responses to the questions above, do you think that this patient assessment exemplifies a realistic approach to assessment?
(Yes/No)

Substantiate your response with comments if you wish.

Author's comment
Obviously your responses to the questions above are a matter of personal judgment. However, if you concluded that there appeared to be a realistic approach to assessment (i.e. you answered 'Yes' to Q3) then you probably answered 'Yes' to both Q1 and Q2. If you answered 'No' to Q3, it might have been because you considered there was insufficient information recorded or because there was unnecessarily detailed or irrelevant information. If you yourself completed that patient assessment form, you might have commented on prevailing circumstances which permitted or limited the possibility of an appropriate assessment being undertaken.

WHOSE RESPONSIBILITY IS ASSESSMENT?
There is a tremendous onus of responsibility on the nurse who undertakes the initial assessment of a patient, because it is on the basis of the information collected and the interpretations made that the patient's nursing is planned. Subsequently, this particular nurse is seldom able to assume total responsibility for the patient's nursing except in the case of the one-to-one relationship of health visiting or when primary nursing is practised, in which one nurse assumes overall responsibility for one patient throughout the period of nursing. But more often the reality is of shared responsibility – a necessity to accommodate off-duty periods, holidays, study leave, part-time workers and fluctuating staffing levels. So, one nurse's recorded assessment of a patient will be used by numerous other nurses: it may be read by other members of the health care team; it may ultimately be passed on to staff in another location entirely (e.g. another ward or hospital, or community nursing services); and eventually it may well be consulted as a record to clarify past incidents or perhaps to contribute information to a research project. For all of these reasons, the need for good records is greater nowadays than ever before.

Given, then, that nursing assessment is a very great responsibility, who should do it? Ideally, it ought perhaps to be done by a qualified nurse and indeed some units attempt to ensure that initial assessments are undertaken by the sister or charge nurse. But in any busy ward the trained nurses are unlikely to have time to do all these assessments and the less experienced members of staff and the learners must also have opportunities to practise. Perhaps a good compromise is for a trained nurse to be present, or at least available to review assessment undertaken by learners. And further review

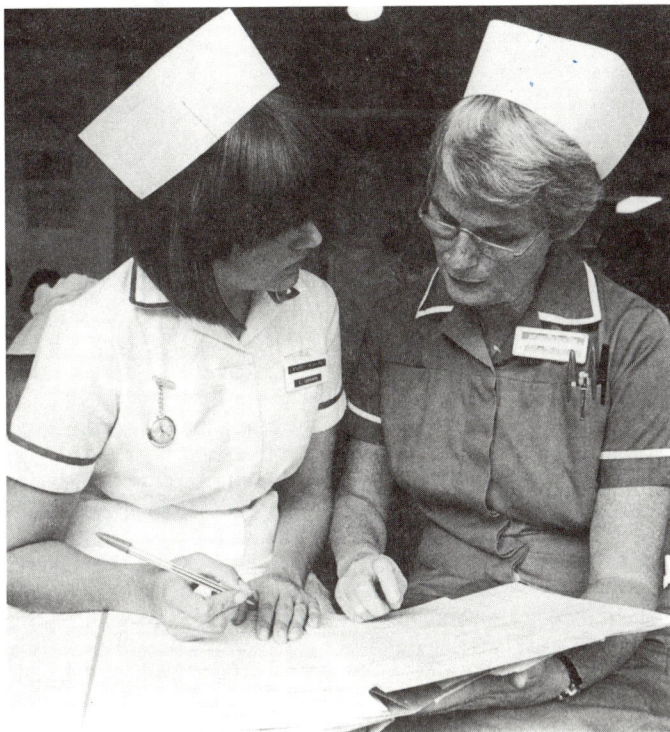

Reviewing a learner's nursing assessment

of the information collected and recorded by one nurse will, of course, occur when the patient's nursing plan is drawn up and when evaluation is carried out. These later steps of the nursing process are more likely to be a collective rather than an individual responsibility although the extent to which responsibility for the process, and assessment in particular, is invested in an individual nurse varies considerably – from the relative autonomy of the health visitor to the collective team approach perhaps most familiar in psychiatric nursing.

Whenever we consider *responsibility* it is relevant to raise the issue of *accountability*, a theme which was discussed in some detail in Module 1. Have a quick look back at that section if you need to, before going on to the next activity.

Activity 2.3   **Allow 15 minutes**

Accountability and nursing assessment

This activity should help you to consider in some depth the issue of accountability.

Look again at the completed patient assessment you collected from your own work area. Would you now feel content to be held accountable for it, were it to be the subject of scrutiny? It is not an easy question. Try to be objective about it; remember, this is just an activity.

The following questions, which point to areas of accountability in the context of nursing assessment, may help you: is the assessment dated and signed (or, in the case of unqualified staff, countersigned)? Is there evidence of the patient's own perceptions of the problems and priorities? Are nursing observations substantiated with appropriate evidence? Have all relevant sources of information been tapped? Is there sufficient information for planning adequate nursing care? Is the information recorded legibly, concisely and unambiguously? Is the assessment complete? If not, is this noted?

1 Would you feel content to be held accountable for the assessment?
   - if so, then note some points to justify this conclusion (bearing in mind the nurse's accountability to the patient as well as to colleagues and in relation to professional standards)
   - if not, identify (with specific examples) the main areas of deficiency.
2 Describe the policy in your work area relating to responsibility for nursing assessment (e.g. the role of qualified staff in relation to learners).
3 Describe what policy you would like to see made explicit in your work area to emphasise accountability in nursing assessment.

Author's comment
The questions in the second paragraph of this activity indicate some of the criteria on which accountability for an assessment might be judged.

THE FOCUS OF ASSESSMENT – THE PATIENT

In Module 1, the development of a close relationship between nurse and patient was described as being a central theme of the nursing process. Such a relationship is more likely to develop if assessment, the first step of the process, is viewed by the nurse as something in which the patient actively participates, rather than as a 'procedure' carried out with the patient in a passive role. However, the approach to participation is as important as the extent of it. Nursing assessment should not focus just on the patient's illness, but also on the patient as an individual and a member of a family. Nurses who have a commitment to the concept of partnership should be able to communicate to patients their interest in them as people and to show a genuine concern about the effects of illness and hospitalisation on their life style, work or schooling, as well as on members of their family.

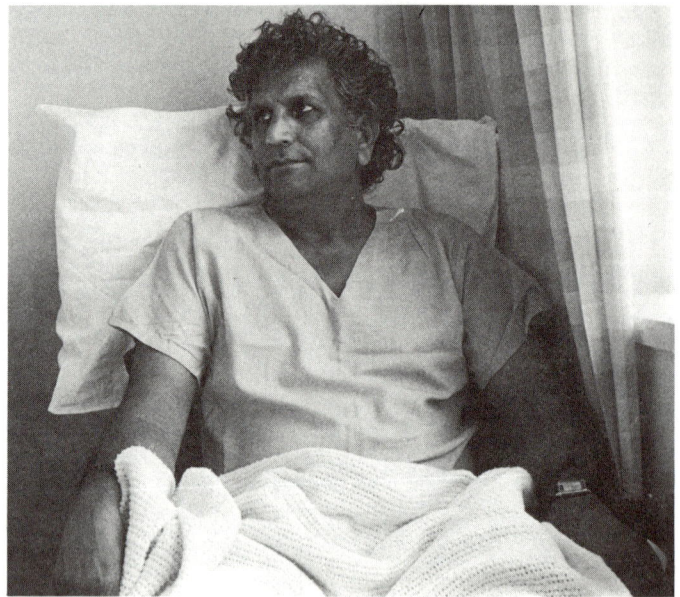

Activity 2.4   Allow 5 minutes

Patients are people

This activity is designed to emphasise the theme of people as patients.

Look again at the completed patient assessment you collected. Do you consider that there is an appropriate balance of information about the various aspects of the person's individuality – a balance of physical, psychological and social factors? Jot down a few examples of information recorded on the form which you think help to portray the patient as an individual.

Author's comment

Examples of physical factors were probably the most easy to find: for example, information about the patient's physical health status, usual diet and sleep problems, elimination and mobility. Almost certainly there would have been some information regarding psychological factors: description of the patient's personality, level of anxiety and current mood, for example. Under social factors, you might have noted the patient's family circumstances, occupation and living conditions. Was there an appropriate balance of information? In the case of a patient with a physical illness and mainly physical problems, there would be more information regarding physical factors than psychological or social factors, whereas the reverse would be appropriate for a patient with a psychiatric disorder.

Topics raised with the patient in the course of nursing assessment are, on the whole, familiar ones – such as eating habits and usual sleep patterns. This is likely to help patients feel at ease and accept opportunities provided by the nurse to indicate important issues and identify their own particular concerns. To a large extent, the partnership approach means that we have to hand over to the patient a measure of control in nursing assessment. Nurses, like other health care workers, have tended to feel that being 'professional' requires assuming control and accepting responsibility for others, but attitudes are changing. Of course, in certain circumstances, a nurse's responsibility is to maintain control of the situation and to protect the patient. But, more often, the truly professional approach is to respect the freedom and autonomy of the person, balancing the rights of the patient and the interests of other parties.

So although nursing assessment as practised in any particular setting will to some extent adopt a standardised approach, it is its adaptation to each individual patient which will ensure that the nursing process achieves the goal of individualised nursing. Usually, before meeting patients for the first time, nurses may know little more than their name, age and medical diagnosis. But to the perceptive nurse, a patient's individuality makes itself apparent within a few moments.

Here is an example. Two patients, both with a previous myocardial infarction and recently suffering from angina, are admitted to the ward. Asked by the nurse why he thinks he is being admitted, one patient replies "I have been having angina . . . I had a heart attack a year ago . . . the G.P. referred me here for tests". The nurse, immediately realising that the patient knows his diagnosis, would approach his assessment in a manner quite different (particularly in her choice of words and questions) from that used with the other patient, who tells her "I've had the heartburn again and I need something done about it so I can get back to work as quickly as possible".

No two patients are alike. Each has a unique personality, each lives in different circumstances, and each holds a particular view and understanding of the meaning of his illness and its implications. Hence the nurse's approach to assessment must differ for each individual patient.

NURSING ASSESSMENT NEEDS A FRAMEWORK

Having just emphasised the importance of adapting assessment to individual patients, it may now seem contradictory to say that "nursing assessment needs a framework". But it does. Each assessment *is* different, but a nurse does not approach every one with her mind blank or with a different set of objectives on each occasion. Assessment needs to be approached within some sort of predetermined structure, a framework.

The theme of *models for practice* was discussed in Module I and a model was described as a framework or pattern that we follow, reflecting and giving direction to the way we act. It was emphasised that the nursing process is meaningless in practice without an explicit framework. The nursing process itself really only provides a logical way of thinking, a method.

Assessment, planning, implementation and evaluation are steps used in all disciplines, not just in nursing. The process only becomes a process of nursing when it is used with an explicit framework unique to nursing, in other words, a nursing model. Three different nursing models were described in Module I (pp. 16–21). A short summary of these is given below, followed by a brief outline of how they serve as frameworks for nursing assessment.

I **Roper, Logan and Tierney's Activities of Living Model:** this is based on a model of living which has as its focus twelve activities of living. Nursing is viewed as helping the patient/client to solve, alleviate, cope with, or prevent problems related to activities of living.

2 **Orem's Self-Care Model:** this is grounded in the belief that self-care is a fundamental requirement for effective living. The goal of nursing is to assist patients with self-care deficits.

3 **Saxton and Hyland's Stress-Adaptation Model:** this is based on an appreciation of the process of stress and of adaptive responses that an individual makes to that stress. Nursing aims to assist the individual's adaptations in pursuit of effective functioning.

Each of these models can serve as a framework for nursing assessment:

I **The Activities of Living Model:** the twelve activities of living provide the framework for assessment of patients. Data are collected in terms of the physical, psychological, sociocultural and economic aspects of each activity of living in order to discover:
- what the patient can do for himself
- what the patient cannot do for himself
- problems (actual/potential) and previous coping mechanisms.

2 **The Self-Care Model:** information is collected about the influences on self-care ability and performance in relation to meeting the common requirements for effective living – the *developmental influences* and *influences related to health state*. The objective is to identify an individual's self-care deficits.

3 **The Stress-Adaptation Model:** using a problem-solving approach, information is collected about the patient's current stress level (physical, chemical, microbiological, physiological, developmental, emotional) and the adaptive processes adopted (anatomical, physiological, psychological).

One interesting point about how these three models can serve as a framework for nursing assessment is that, although the terminology is different, they all share certain components. For example, the 'requirements for effective living' which are central to Orem's model are very similar to the group of 'activities of living' in the Roper, Logan and Tierney model. This, in turn, although not employing the term 'self-care', does utilise this concept by emphasising the person's independence. Its concern with 'previous coping mechanisms' is akin to the 'adaptation' dimension of the stress-adaptation model of Saxton and Hyland. So, the differences are mainly ones of emphasis.

In relation to assessment, the differences in these models are reflected in the approach to data collection, depending upon whether information is collected and reviewed with a view to identifying 'problems with activities of living' (Roper, Logan & Tierney), 'self-care deficits' (Orem) or 'stressors' (Saxton & Hyland).

Activity 2.5   Allow 10 minutes

Your framework for the nursing process

A word of encouragement. This activity may not seem inspiring, especially if you have found the discussion of models a bit dull or even confusing. But have a go at it – it may help you to appreciate the relevance of this theme.

Look back to Activity 2.1 on p. 28. In your description of how *you* approach nursing assessment, did you refer to an underlying framework? If you *did*, identify which, if any, of the three models discussed above it uses, or to which it is closely related.

If you did *not* identify a framework for your nursing assessment – and this is more likely – look at the *blank* specimen of assessment documentation collected from your own work area. Even if you did describe a framework in Activity 2.1, you would probably still find it useful to do this.

Does the way in which the documentation is organised, and the topics included, suggest an organising framework? For example, are the topics described in terms of activities of living, self-care deficits or stressors? If you can identify an organising framework, outline it and note aspects of any of the three models discussed above it uses, or to which it is closely related.

Author's comment

If you have found it difficult (or impossible) to identify and describe the framework used for nursing assessment in your own work area, you might like to discuss this with some of your colleagues. They may know why your form was designed as it is and they may be interested to discuss how the underlying framework could be made more explicit or be adapted, or whether a different one might be more appropriate.

SOURCES OF INFORMATION AND SKILLS INVOLVED IN NURSING ASSESSMENT

SOURCES OF INFORMATION

There are five main sources from which information can be collected for nursing assessment of patients: the patient; members of the patient's family; nursing colleagues; other members of the health care team; and records.

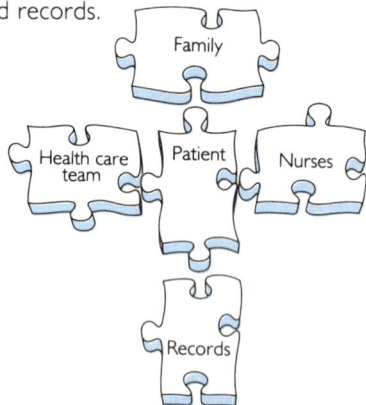

Fig. 2.1   Sources of information for assessment

The patient: in most cases, the patient is the primary source of information and other sources are tapped to add to, clarify or verify that information. However, there are instances when the other sources must be depended upon for much of the information: for example, when a patient is unconscious or otherwise unable to communicate adequately, perhaps because of confusion or severe mental handicap. But remember that, even if he is unable to speak coherently or communicate verbally at all, a great deal of information can be obtained by observation of the patient.

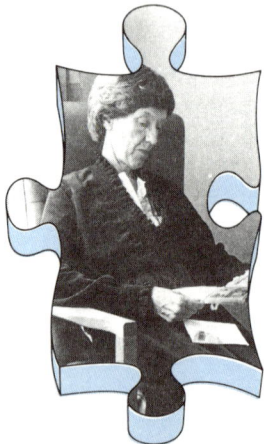

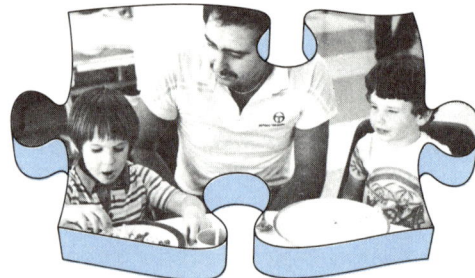

The patient's family: close relatives, or others in a significant relationship with the patient (e.g. friends) should be viewed as a valuable source of information. This is especially true if the patient is unable to participate actively in assessment, where it is particularly important to consider the family's wishes (for instance, when the patient is a child or has a fatal illness), or when members of the family themselves are to be actively involved in the patient's nursing (at home or in a long-stay hospital, for example). Of course, some patients – especially those who are old – may have no relatives or close friends. In such instances the assistance of other people, such as a minister or home help, could be sought.

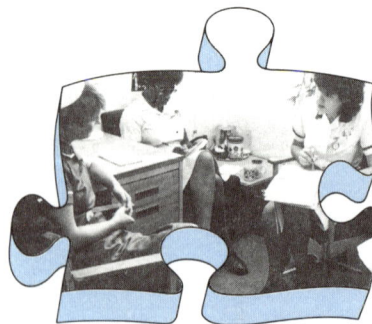

Nursing colleagues: it hardly needs to be said that other nurses provide an important source of information about the patient, even when one nurse assumes responsibility for the initial assessment and documentation. Most patients in hospital are nursed by a large number of nurses, those on night duty as well as those on day shifts. Every nurse in contact with a patient is a potential source of information, especially in relation to ongoing assessment. Hospital nurses and community nurses should also view each other as vital sources of information, particularly at such times as the patient's admission to hospital or discharge home.

Other members of the health care team: nurses, as members of a multi-disciplinary team (a point developed in Module I in the section *Nursing in an organisation*), can obtain much information of relevance to nursing assessment from their colleagues. Details about the patient's medical diagnosis, investigations and treatment which have direct implications for the patient's nursing, can be obtained from

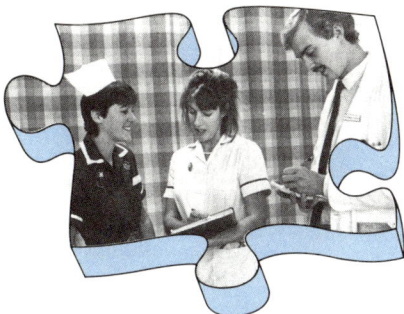

members of the medical team. Indeed, because in most instances nurses and doctors work so closely together – and because some of a patient's nursing care is derived directly from medical prescription – continual exchange of information about patients is absolutely essential between nurses and doctors.

Similarly, information from other members of the health care team contributes to nursing assessment. For example, the physiotherapist can provide details of a patient's mobility problems and physiotherapy regime; or, in a mental handicap hospital, the school teacher may be asked by the nurse about a child's behaviour in the different environment of the classroom. Likewise, in a psychiatric setting, the occupational therapist will be able to contribute information about a patient's behaviour and problems off the ward.

Records: a great deal of relevant information can often be obtained from existing records; in particular, details of the patient's medical history, diagnosis, investigations and treatment can be ascertained from the medical notes. If the patient has been admitted previously, information about past problems and nursing intervention (and its outcome) can be obtained from nursing records on file. Similarly, a midwife or health visitor can learn about a woman's previous

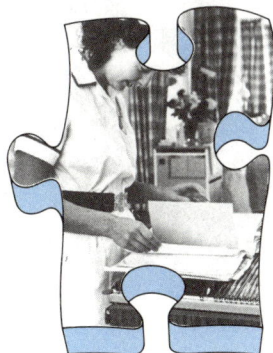

obstetric history and her other children from existing records and this is likely to be useful on subsequent occasions.

Consulting existing records can save nurses' time and is also a useful means of corroborating or supplementing information provided by patients themselves. Although the accuracy and relevance to the present obviously needs to be checked, obtaining information from records does help to avoid asking patients to repeat the same information over and over again. If a nurse shows that she is already conversant with existing information this is likely to convey to the patient that there is good communication among members of the health care team. Of course, confidentiality of records must be respected and the nurse should check which records she is entitled to consult.

Activity 2.6   Allow 5 minutes

Sources of information

In this activity, you can review how much use you yourself have made of various sources of information.

Look at the completed patient assessment you collected from your own work area. Select examples of information collected from each of the sources discussed above:

- the patient
- the patient's family or friends
- nursing colleagues
- other members of the health care team
- records.

Author's comment
You may not have found an example for all five possible sources – and that doesn't matter. Did you find it easy to identify the sources of different pieces of information? If not, do you think it is important that nurses do record the source of information? Certainly there would seem to be instances when doing so is necessary: for example, when the patient is unable to act as the primary source of information or if information from different sources (e.g. the patient/family members) appears contradictory.

SKILLS INVOLVED IN ASSESSMENT

In this section we are going to consider briefly the different skills utilised in data collection: observing, measuring and interviewing.

Observing: every nurse is aware of the crucial importance of astute and accurate observation. Florence Nightingale wrote in *Notes on Nursing* (1859): "The most important practical lesson that can be given to nurses is to teach them what to observe – how to observe – what symptoms indicate improvement – what the reverse – which are of importance – which are of none – which are the evidence of neglect – and of what kind of neglect". And she goes on to conclude that ". . . if you cannot get the habit of observation one way or other, you had better give up being a nurse, for it is not your calling, however kind and anxious you may be". As ever, Nightingale's writing is stern stuff but the basic message is as apt today as it was in her time: accurate observation is an important means of collecting information about patients.

Even though we may not realise that we have begun 'to assess', as nurses we make observations about patients from the very moment we set eyes upon them. We might register that the patient being admitted is on a trolley or in a wheelchair or, if walking, is using a stick or has a limp or an unsteady gait. If the patient is in a seriously ill condition on admission, we would automatically observe details such as facial colour, any respiratory difficulty, the presence of an intravenous infusion . . . and so on. Observations are made not only of the patient's physical condition but of indicators of his psychological and emotional state too: for example, signs of anxiety or distress, and evidence of confusion or disorientation. And an important point to stress is that observation depends not just on the sense of sight, but also uses the senses of hearing, touch and smell.

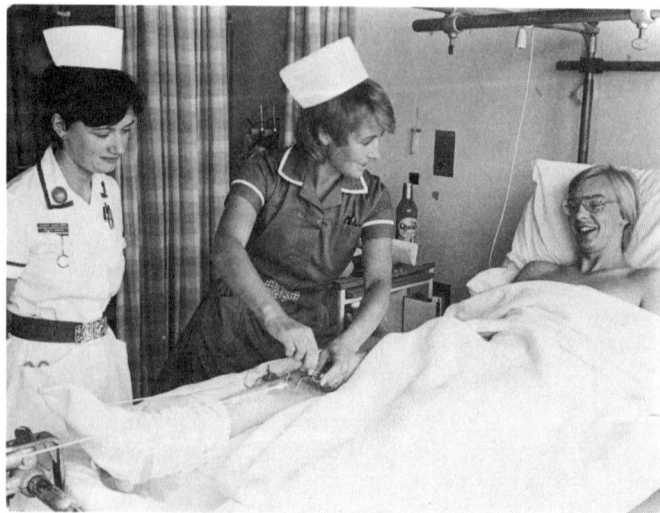

There is no need here to labour the point which, quite simply, is to remind nurses that their initial observations about patients contribute substantially to nursing assessment. To a large extent these observations will direct the nurse's subsequent, more systematic, approach to data collection and this will include further observation of specific factors.

Measuring: this term refers to data which are measurable, and hence more objective, than either observation or interviewing can be. Obvious examples of measurements in data collection are of the patient's temperature, pulse, blood pressure, height, weight, urine output and fluid intake. In many instances, measuring may be carried out to substantiate information obtained from observing or questioning the patient. For example, the nurse may observe that a

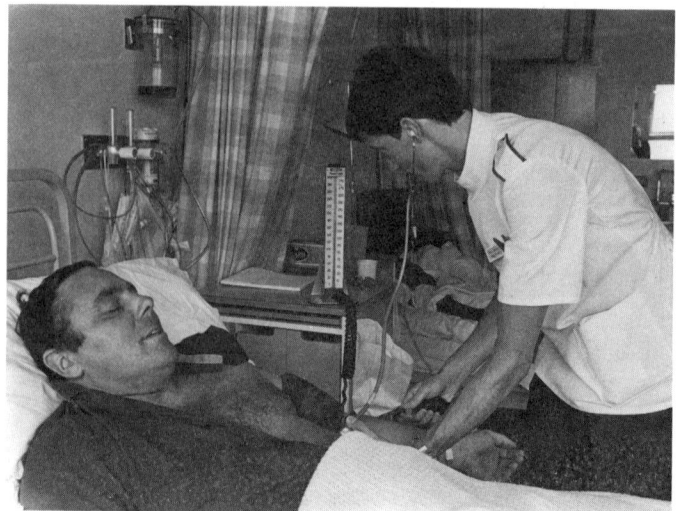

Observing

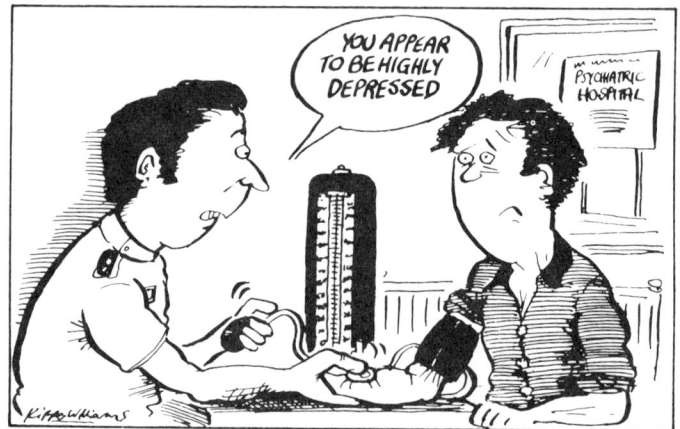

Measuring

person looks 'overweight' and can ascertain this fact more objectively and precisely by weighing the person and comparing the weight with height in relation to age and sex. Then, having obtained a precise measure, any subsequent change in weight (gain or loss) can be accurately compared against the baseline. This example relates to a physical factor but, increasingly, measurement instruments are being devised for psychological or emotional factors too. Further examples of such instruments are given later in the module.

Interviewing: observational skills also play a part in interviewing because information is forthcoming from patients' 'non-verbal communication', in addition to what they actually say. And whether or not the non-verbal cues appear to support or contradict the verbal communication may be of importance. For example, a mother in the post-natal ward might say to the midwife "Yes, I'm coping fine with breast-feeding" but, at the same time, be showing obvious signs of anxiety or uncertainty about breast-feeding technique.

Despite having mentioned observational skills first, we should not underestimate the importance of skilled verbal communication in interviewing. A great deal of information about patients is collected by nurses using skills of interviewing. The admission of a patient usually commences with an interview and it is from this structured discussion (which may also involve relatives) that a great deal of crucial information is obtained. This topic is raised again in more detail, later in the module.

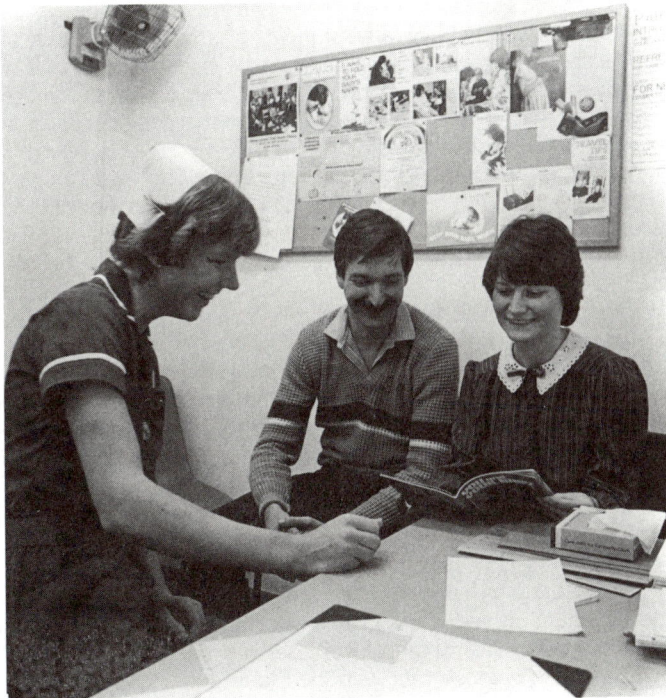

Interviewing

Activity 2.7 — Allow 5 minutes

Observing, measuring and interviewing

The purpose of this activity is to encourage you to think about the way in which you use the skills of observing, measuring and interviewing and how you record the information thus collected.

Using the completed patient assessment you collected from your own work area, note examples of information collected by:

- observing
- measuring
- interviewing.

Author's comment

You will have found this easy to do if you, or the nurse who recorded the assessment data, differentiated between an observation (e.g. "looks depressed") and information elicited from interviewing (i.e. "says she is depressed"). If this was not evident, you might like to consider whether it would be useful to indicate in the documentation how a particular piece of information was obtained. In the examples you wrote down, you may well have included a particular item of information in more than one category, because the different skills are often employed jointly.

Activity 2.8 — Allow 2 minutes

Temperature estimation

This activity illustrates how the different skills of observing, measuring and interviewing are often used together.

When collecting information relevant to estimation of a patient's body temperature, note:

1 What you might *observe*
2 What you would *measure*
3 What you might *ask/be told* by the patient.

Author's comment

You probably do not need any feedback on this activity, but we will be returning to the topic of temperature measurement later.

In this section we have looked at skills employed in the data collection phase of assessment: observing, measuring and interviewing. In the ensuing phases of nursing assessment – reviewing the data and identifying patients' problems – different skills come into play. Here the nurse uses intellectual skills to draw upon knowledge, in order to make sense of the information obtained about a particular patient. The specific information is considered in the context of an understanding of normal human function, deviation from the range of normal, and what constitutes (or may cause) a problem amenable to nursing intervention. More is said about this phase of nursing assessment later in the module.

DATA COLLECTION IN PRACTICE

DATA COLLECTION IN STAGES

Earlier in the module it was pointed out that assessment is seldom a once-only procedure, even though the most comprehensive assessment of the patient is usually undertaken following admission or at first referral. But even this initial phase of data collection is usually undertaken in stages. In *A Guide to the Practice of Nursing Using the Nursing Process* (1982), McFarlane and Castledine suggest that, in their experience, the gathering of information about patients is best undertaken in two stages.

The *first stage* nursing history (their terminology) is completed shortly after the patient's admission to hospital. The purpose at this point is to obtain sufficient information for the nurse to begin nursing the patient. Information is collected by means of:

- a brief interview with the patient and/or relative
- a systematic head-to-toe examination of the patient (to identify any problems such as difficulty in breathing or deficient skin condition)
- an assessment of the patient's risk of developing pressure sores, and the recording of temperature, pulse, blood pressure and weight.

This information is recorded on a first stage nursing history form.

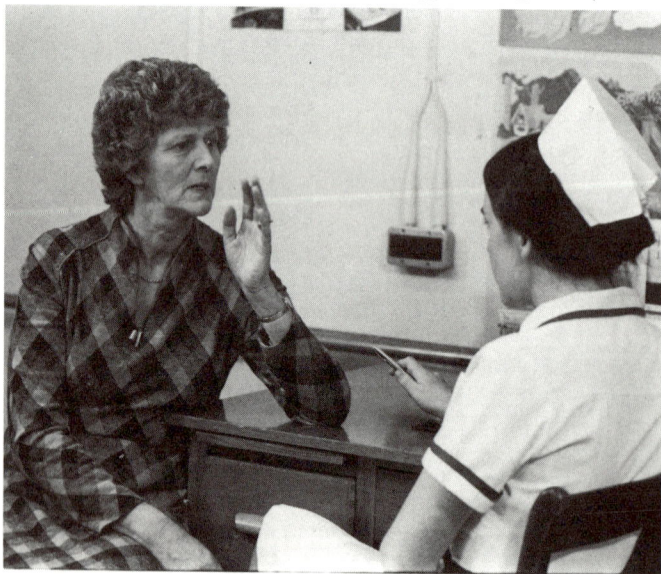

Obtaining information from a relative as part of assessment.

The *second stage* nursing history entails a more detailed physical and psychological examination. This may be carried out at the same time or shortly after the first stage and is repeated for regular updating and reassessment of the patient's condition and problems. The second stage nursing history form (Figure 2.2) covers eight basic physiological factors and six aspects of emotional state. Information is entered in two columns: *history or usual condition* and *present condition/behaviour*. You will see from the prompts entered in the first column the kinds of information which would be collected under these headings.

PROFORMA FOR DATA COLLECTION

The nursing history form at which you have just looked is an example of a proforma for data collection in nursing assessment. As you will be aware, many different kinds of proforma are in use by nurses throughout the country, in the various branches of nursing and often even in different wards of one hospital. Nurses have sometimes devoted a great deal of time to selecting or designing a form for nursing assessment. A good form is a useful guide in data collection as well as being a helpful way of achieving a degree of standardisation in how data are recorded by different nurses in any particular work area. But a form can only be an aid. What is much more important is for nurses who work together to agree upon an explicit *framework* for assessment.

Earlier in this module, the need for a framework was emphasised. You were asked to identify the framework underlying nursing assessment in your own work area and to consider how well this framework was reflected in the organisation of the documentation used for assessment.

Designing a proforma for data collection which reflects a particular framework need not result in a complicated document. Indeed, it should help in achieving something very simple because, if nurses are familiar with the framework, the form need only act as an aide-memoire. Figure 2.3 overleaf serves to illustrate this point.

This simple Patient Assessment Form was designed by Roper, Logan and Tierney (1980) to reflect their model for nursing, one of the three nursing models which have already been discussed. The left-hand side of the form is for the collection of *biographical and health data;* the right-hand side for recording *assessment of Activities of Living* (ALs), which provide the framework for the assessment of the patient. You will notice that the form does not contain any specific questions or prompts because, in order to use it, nurses need to be fully conversant with the model and, in particular, the

History or Usual Condition	Present Condition/Behaviour

(I) *Basic Physiological Factors*

(a) *Activity/Movement*
Use of aid, e.g. frame, walking stick, gait.
Ability to move in bed/chair.

(b) *Rest/Sleep*
Length, time, sedation.

(c) *Nutrition*
Appetite.
Eating habits – frequency, amount, variety.
Likes/dislikes.
Difficulties – dysphagia, anorexia.
Nausea/vomiting.
Malnutrition.
Weight.

(d) *Elimination/Continent State*
Bowels/bladder.
Difficulties – frequency.
Remedies.
Routine urine test.

(e) *Fluids and Electrolytes*
Amount, type, frequency.
Likes, dislikes.
Dehydration.
Condition of mouth and teeth.

(f) *Breathing and Circulatory State*
Respiratory difficulties, cyanosis, hypoxia, number of pillows needed, peripheral circulation.

(g)(1) Pain – degree, usual method of coping with this.
(2) Sensory disturbances.
(3) Speech.
(4) Hearing – aids.
(5) Vision – aids – spectacles.
(6) Temperature of skin.
(7) Smell.

(h) *Skin Condition*
Wounds, cuts, abrasions, ulcers, pressure area lesions, size, colour, location, quality of hair.

History or Usual Condition

(II) *Emotional State*

(a) *Perception of Health*
Patient's insight into his health state and illness.
Any awareness of imminent death, chronic illness or body image disturbance.

(b) *Conversational Ability*
Alert, orientated to time, place and person. Able to express and communicate his feelings and wishes. Vague, unwilling to communicate. Short term or long term memory loss.

(c) *Reaction to being a Patient* (in hospital) and being too dependent upon others. Level of interdependence.
Too dependent?
Too independent?
Knows when to seek nursing aid.

(d) *Significant Non-verbal Gestures*
Looks away, watches carefully, agitated, frowns, fumbles, bites nails, sits quietly, ruminates.

(e) *Usual Reactions to Stressful Events*
Ways of coping with problems in lifetime.
Usual physical and emotional reactions to situations such as loss, pressure at work, pressure and stress at home, financial problems, injuries and past illnesses.

(f) *Observable Behaviour and Mood Swings*
Is the patient's behaviour appropriate to situation:
Co-operative   Anxious
Withdrawn   Calm
Irritable   Confused
Aggressive

Present Condition/Behaviour

Fig. 2.2 *The second stage nursing history form (McFarlane and Castledine, 1982)*

Patient Assessment Form: Biographical and health data

Date of admission _____ Date of assessment _____ Nurse's signature _____

Male ☐   Age ☐   Surname _____   Forenames _____

Female ☐   Date of birth _____   Prefers to be addressed as _____

Single/Married/Widowed/Other

Address of usual residence _____

Type of accommodation
(incl. mode of entry
if relevant) _____

Family/Others at this residence _____

Next of kin   Name _____   Address _____

Relationship _____   Tel. no. _____

Significant others
(incl. relatives/dependents
visitors/helpers
neighbours)

Support services _____

Occupation _____

Religious beliefs and relevant practices _____

Significant life crises _____

Patient's perception of current health status _____

Family's perception of patient's health status _____

Reason for admission _____

Medical information (e.g. diagnosis, past history, allergies) _____

GP Address Tel. no. _____   Consultant Address Tel. no. _____

Plans for discharge _____

Fig. 2.3 Patient Assessment Form (Roper, Logan and Tierney, 1983)

40

Assessment of Activities of Living

AL	Usual routines: what he/she can and cannot do independently	Patient's problems (actual/potential) (p)= potential
● Maintaining a safe environment		
● Communicating		
● Breathing		
● Eating and drinking		
● Eliminating		
● Personal cleansing and dressing		
● Controlling body temperature		
● Mobilising		
● Working and playing		
● Expressing sexuality		
● Sleeping		
● Dying		

● Communicating	Wears glasses at all times. She is a pleasant lady who is very open and easy to talk to. Generally anxious about coming into hospital and leaving her mentally handicapped son. He is being cared for by her sister.	● Anxiety about her son
● Breathing	Smokes 20 cigarettes a day. Has a "wheeze" and becomes breathless on exertion. Has a slight cough.	● (P) Chest infection
● Eating and drinking	Unable to eat a full meal or fatty foods. Recently she has been "picking" at her food. She occasionally suffers from dyspepsia after eating but refuses to consider medication and copes with the problem by taking small meals. Overweight and is concerned about this. Wt. 81.2 kg. Ht. 1.626m.	● Overweight
● Eliminating	No problem with micturition. Urinalysis good. Bowels move regularly each day. No aperients taken.	
● Personal	Personal cleanliness good. Smart well groomed lady.	

Fig. 2.4 An example of information from assessment of Activities of Living recorded on the Patient Assessment Form (Roper, Logan and Tierney, 1983)

twelve ALs and guidelines for assessment offered by the authors (Roper, Logan and Tierney, 1980 and 1981). Figure 2.4 gives an example of the kind of information which might be recorded in assessment.

Despite being very simple, this form appears to be an adequate one. It was used by a group of nurses who participated in a project to test out the Roper, Logan and Tierney model for nursing in practice. The nurses carried out patient studies in nine different settings: a diabetic unit, health visiting, district nursing, midwifery and in surgical, geriatric, medical, psychiatric and neurosurgical wards. In commenting on their studies, all said that they found that the activities of living framework provided a relevant and manageable approach to nursing assessment, and some commented that the framework alerted them to consider the patient's abilities as well as difficulties. Others liked the focus on the person rather than on the illness or on body systems, and in several studies nurses mentioned the patients' own positive reactions to the assessment focusing on activities of living (Roper, Logan and Tierney, 1983).

However, following these comments, it seems appropriate to say a few words about 'disease'. Deliberately, in the creation of models for nursing, there has been a loosening of nursing's traditional attachment to the 'medical model' in which, though changing, the emphasis has been firmly upon disease.

The focus of the nursing models is firmly upon the individual and they concern the unique contribution of nursing to that person's health care.

Perhaps in striving to shift the focus, the creators of nursing models have failed to pay sufficient attention to the continuing relevance of the patient's disease condition and the essential interdependence of nursing and other disciplines, particularly medicine.

As a member of the Roper, Logan and Tierney trio, I can say that we have certainly been giving considerable thought to this issue. Our model, intentionally, is concerned mainly with the nurse-initiated component of nursing – the part of a patient's care which is uniquely the role of the nurse. Therefore, our Patient Assessment Form which you have just been considering is a reflection of that. However, we have become aware of the need to make more explicit the relationship between this and the other component of nursing – the intervention which involves collaboration with, or in fact is determined by, doctors and other members of the health care team.

In the most recent book about our model Using a Model for Nursing (Roper, Logan and Tierney, 1983), we have discussed this issue and we have added a Nursing Plan to the Patient Assessment Form. The plan has provision for nursing interventions related to activities of living (i.e. the focus of assessment) and, in another section, for nursing interventions derived from medical or other prescription. A mere alteration in documentation does not, of course, tackle all the complexities of this issue. However, we do need to consider how, in all steps of the nursing process and in their documentation, we can retain a focus on the individual without neglecting to make explicit the relevance of the patient's disease condition and of medical or other care.

Reviewing your documentation

Now that you have read the section on proforma for data collection and have looked at some examples, this activity will give you an opportunity to look critically at your current documentation.

Have a look at the blank specimen of documentation for assessment which you collected from your own work area.

1　Look at the part of the proforma designed for collection of factual biographical and health data and compare it with the left-hand side of the Roper, Logan and Tierney Patient Assessment Form (Figure 2.3). Probably many of the headings are very similar. Note any headings on *your* form which are not on the Roper, Logan and Tierney form and which you consider are useful.

　　Also note any additional headings on the Roper, Logan and Tierney form which you think would be useful to include on your form.

2　The remainder of your documentation may have headings which are similar to activities of living or to the categories on the McFarlane and Castledine form (Figure 2.2) which reflect Orem's model, or may use headings in Saxton and Hyland's terminology. Note anything which you feel you might like to rethink about this part of your documentation.

Author's comment
You might like to take the opportunity to discuss the notes you have made about your documentation with colleagues in your own work area. This would be a logical extension of a discussion about frameworks, which was suggested to you in Activity 2.5.

USE OF SPECIAL DATA COLLECTION INSTRUMENTS

Appropriate *special data collection instruments,* which were briefly referred to earlier in the section on *measuring,* are important adjuncts to specially-designed proforma for data collection in nursing assessment.

　　Such instruments are useful because they have been developed through research and their reliability and validity have been subjected to empirical testing. They therefore allow for direct comparison of a phenomenon among different patients, or in the same patient at intervals over a period of time. They provide a more objective means of backing up a patient's description of a specific condition or the nurse's own observation. Because the measurement is objective, it reduces the subjectivity inherent in the interpretation of data, a problem in nursing when so many different nurses are involved in the care of any one patient. Four examples are given below of special data collection instruments with direct relevance for nursing.

The Norton Scoring System for assessing patients' risk of developing pressure sores. Identification of patients at risk of incurring pressure damage is the critical factor in deciding on a policy of selective, preventive nursing intervention. To achieve this it is obvious that a quantitative measure is preferable to a qualitative judgment. Even experienced nurses who consider that they are able to recognise predisposing factors can be aided by routine use of an instrument which will detect patients at risk at a stage early enough for preventive measures to be effective. Doreen Norton devised her scoring system for research purposes some twenty years ago (Norton, McLaren and Exton-Smith, 1962). However, it is only relatively recently that knowledge of the scoring system has become widespread, partly as a result of an article published in the *Nursing Mirror* (Norton, 1975) and also because in 1979 the *Nursing Times* produced for its readers a pocket-size *Pressure Sore Risk Calculator.*

Fig. 2.5 The Pressure Sore Risk Calculator (Nursing Times, 1979), based on the Norton Scoring System

Pressure Sore Risk Calculator

Instructions for use

1. Identify the most appropriate description of the patient (4, 3, 2, 1) under each of the five headings (A to E) and total the result.

2. Record the 'score' with its date in the patient's notes or on a chart.

3. Assess weekly and whenever any change in the patient's condition and/or circumstances of care.

A 'score' of 14 and below denotes need for intensive care, i.e. 1-2 hourly changes of posture and the use of pressure-relieving aids.

Note: When oedema of the sacral area has been present a rise of score above 14 does not indicate less risk of a lesion.

Scoring system
Key: Total score of 14 and below = 'At Risk'

A Physical condition		B Mental condition		C Activity		D Mobility		E Incontinent	
Good	4	Alert	4	Ambulant	4	Full	4	Not	4
Fair	3	Apathetic	3	Walk/ Help	3	Slightly limited	3	Occasionally	3
Poor	2	Confused	2	Chair-bound	2	Very limited	2	Usually/ Urine	2
Very bad	1	Stuporous	1	Bedfast	1	Immobile	1	Doubly	1

Using Norton's system, the calculation of pressure sore risk takes less than a minute. The application of preventive measures has been shown to be most effective if begun when the score is at or below 14. By monitoring a patient in this way and recording the scores in the nursing documents, a concise record of the patient's condition in terms of pressure sore status is provided. If you are not familiar with this instrument and are nursing patients who are susceptible to pressure sores, you may find it useful to try it out.

The Glasgow Coma Scale. Patients with impaired brain function as a result of head injury, subarachnoid haemorrhage, stroke, drug overdose or various metabolic disorders are common in all general hospitals. Level of responsiveness is an important parameter to monitor in all such patients and any change may be an alert to emergencies such as pulmonary embolus, haemorrhage, myocardial infarction or metabolic imbalance. Traditionally, nurses have referred to 'level of consciousness', using terms such as 'alert', 'semicomatosed' and 'stuporous'. However the meaning of these terms is vague and subject to differing interpretations by observers and thus it becomes impossible for any exact comparison of observations to be made at intervals of time.

The Glasgow Coma Scale provides a means of describing a patient's level of responsiveness more precisely and objectively. It was developed at the Institute of Neurological Sciences in Glasgow (Teasdale and Jennett, 1974) and was described in the *Nursing Times* by Teasdale (1975) and Teasdale, Galbraith and Clarke (1975).

Fig. 2.7 *The pain thermometer (Hayward, 1979)*

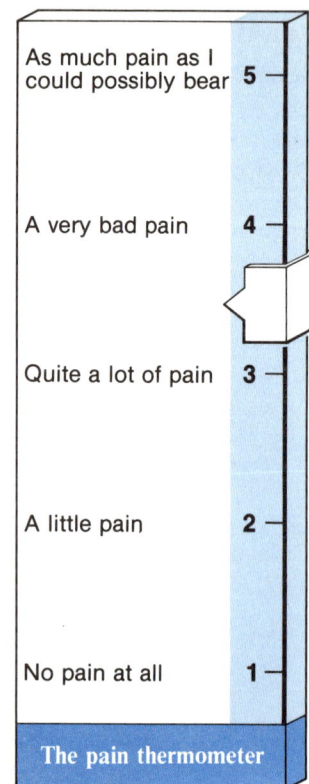

As much pain as I could possibly bear	5
A very bad pain	4
Quite a lot of pain	3
A little pain	2
No pain at all	1

The pain thermometer

Fig. 2.6 *The Glasgow Coma Scale (Teasdale, Galbraith and Clarke, 1975)*

INSTITUTE OF NEUROLOGICAL SCIENCES, GLASGOW
OBSERVATION CHART

NAME

RECORD No.

DATE

TIME

C O M A S C A L E	Eyes open	Spontaneously
		To speech
		To pain
		None
	Best verbal response	Orientated
		Confused
		Inappropriate words
		Incomprehensible sounds
		None
	Best motor response	Obey commands
		Localise pain
		Flexion to pain
		Extension to pain
		None

Eyes closed by swelling = C

Endotracheal tube or tracheostomy = T

Usually record the best arm response

The scale, which is shown in Figure 2.6 and is part of a larger observation chart, consists of three parts – assessment of eye opening, verbal response and motor response – each with a scale describing levels of responsiveness. The scale has been subjected to extensive reliability tests and has been shown to be a quick, accurate and simple tool for assessing neurological status.

The Pain Thermometer. Various approaches have been explored in the search for a reliable means of recognising and measuring pain. Although a truly objective or mechanical method might seem the ideal answer, even this would need to take account of the patient's verbal, subjective description of pain. Various scales have been designed to try to put a measure of objectivity on subjective verbal reporting. For example, a patient is asked to rate the severity of pain on a simple three-point scale (high-medium-low). The 'pain thermometer' (Figure 2.7) or, more accurately, 'painometer' is a development of this idea and was first described by Professor Jack Hayward (1979), a nurse who has undertaken research into pain. This simple device indicates five levels of pain, described colloquially by a sample of patients, and a sliding pointer which the patient sets at the present level of pain. The useful thing about this instrument, although it may be regarded in some situations as too simplistic to be of any real value, is that it at least offers a way of obtaining a measure and some possibility therefore, of comparison at subsequent assessments.

The Hospital Anxiety and Depression Scale. This is a self-assessment scale for detecting clinically significant states of depression and anxiety in patients undergoing investigation and treatment in non-psychiatric hospital out-patient clinics. In the introduction to their paper on the scale, (see Figure 2.8), the authors (Zigmond and Snaith, 1983) comment that the prevalence of psychiatric disorder in general hospital out-patient clinics is known to be high. Although physicians and surgeons are usually aware of the emotional components of physical illness, they are often too busy to investigate this adequately. It is suggested that this scale, which has been developed and tested, offers a reliable and quick means of assisting screening for states of depression and anxiety in medical and surgical out-patients departments.

Figure 2.8 shows the items included in the questionnaire. Patients are asked to underline the reply which comes closest to how they have been feeling in the past week. Details of scoring are included in the paper referenced.

Of particular interest to nurses is the authors' comment that "The scale was found to be very acceptable to the patients who had no difficulty in understanding its purpose and completing it. Nurses who issued the scale said that patients showed considerable interest and frequently commented that doctors should take more account of emotional disorder".

These, then, are just a few examples of special data collection instruments which are used, or could be considered for use, in

I feel tense or 'wound up':
Most of the time / A lot of the time / From time to time, occasionally / Not at all

I still enjoy the things I used to enjoy:
Definitely as much / Not quite so much / Only a little / Hardly at all

I get a sort of frightened feeling as if something awful is about to happen:
Very definitely and quite badly / Yes, but not too badly / A little, but it doesn't worry me / Not at all

I can laugh and see the funny side of things:
As much as I always could / Not quite so much now / Definitely not so much now / Not at all

Worrying thoughts go through my mind:
A great deal of the time / A lot of the time / From time to time but not too often / Only occasionally

I feel cheerful:
Not at all / Not often / Sometimes / Most of the time

I can sit at ease and feel relaxed:
Definitely / Usually / Not often / Not at all

I feel as if I am slowed down:
Nearly all the time / Very often / Sometimes / Not at all

I get a sort of frightened feeling like 'butterflies' in the stomach:
Not at all / Occasionally / Quite often / Very often

I have lost interest in my appearance:
Definitely / I don't take so much care as I should / I may not take quite as much care / I take just as much care as ever

I feel restless as if I have to be on the move:
Very much indeed / Quite a lot / Not very much / Not at all

I look forward with enjoyment to things:
As much as ever I did / Rather less than I used to / Definitely less than I used to / Hardly at all

I get sudden feelings of panic:
Very often indeed / Quite often / Not very often / Not at all

I can enjoy a good book or radio or TV programme:
Often / Sometimes / Not often / Very seldom

Fig. 2.8 Questions from the Hospital Anxiety and Depression Scale (Zigmond and Snaith, 1983)

nursing assessment. All have been developed through research and tried out in practice. One important point is that they allow for collection of comparable data at intervals of time, thus reinforcing the ongoing nature of assessment. If any of the instruments mentioned above are unfamiliar to you, try to find time to look at the literature and, if necessary, ask your librarian to help you to obtain the references.

You may feel that certain aspects of nursing assessment would benefit from the development of validated instruments. If so, look up a bibliography in the library under the subject (e.g. 'incontinence, assessment of'), or ask your nursing officer or in-service education officer if they know of any relevant literature.

DATA COLLECTION USING INTERVIEWING SKILLS

Earlier in this module, we discussed the skills employed in data collection: observing, measuring and interviewing. In this section, some further comments are made regarding *interviewing skills* in preparation for the assessment which you will hear on the audiotape. Even though a great deal of information can be collected through observation and measurement, data collection in nursing assessment relies heavily upon the nurse's skill at interviewing patients. Perhaps talking with patients and their relatives is a simpler way to describe this, even though the initial discussion is commonly referred to as an 'admission interview'. It does sound rather formal to use the term 'interview', and it may possibly be intimidating to patients. On the other hand, however, it may be a helpful way of encouraging nurses to appreciate the need to acquire a good 'interviewing technique'.

In an article discussing the importance of interpersonal communication in nursing, Faulkner (1981) writes: "Assessment of the patient's needs may be made on the basis of a nursing history. For this, not only must the nurse be able to communicate generally, but she must also be skilled in interviewing techniques. This is another new area for nurse training and an important one". And she continues "Basically, the nurse needs to learn to ask the right questions, to know how to encourage the patient to give information, and, perhaps most important, to recognise clues given by the patient".

So, interviewing is much more complex than simply bombarding patients with questions. This point is made well by Norton (1981), writing about 'the nursing process in action':

An individual's complex of needs and problems are personal, sensitive issues and therefore cannot be identified successfully by formalised interrogation. . . History-taking is tending to take on the characteristics of a procedure – a formalised question-and-answer session – with the emphasis on physical/clinical aspects . . . [and] a lack of discretional flexibility in its application. . . The most pertinent questions that nurses should continually ask must surely be addressed to themselves. 'What is the purpose of conducting the interview?' 'What do I need to know about *this* patient in *these circumstances* in order to identify and assess needs and decide an appropriate plan of care?'

AN EXAMPLE OF AN ADMISSION INTERVIEW

You will need to allocate approximately 45 minutes to complete this section of the module, which focuses on the first part of nursing assessment – assessment on admission. Although it has been divided into separate activities, the whole section needs to be completed at one time.

One of the activities involves listening to the first part of the audiotape, so set up the tape now, even though you do not need to play it until you have completed Activity 2.10. You will also need your notebook and the audio notes for Mrs Finnegan which you will find in Part II of the *Case Files*.

Background to the admission interview
The patient's name is Mrs Finnegan. She is 61 years old and is being admitted to hospital from the waiting list for investigation of indigestion which has troubled her over the past eighteen months.

Activity 2.10	Allow 10 minutes

Preparing for and beginning an admission interview
This is an activity centred on a particular patient, Mrs Finnegan, which focuses on the preparatory stages of an admission interview.

PHOTO A
Here you see the nurse getting ready for the interview with Mrs Finnegan. Note briefly what needs to be done in preparation for an admission interview.

PHOTO B
Here you see the nurse greeting Mrs Finnegan on arrival to the ward. Write down the points you think are important about greeting patients on admission.

PHOTO C
Here you see the setting in which this interview is to be conducted. Note any features about this which strike you as satisfactory or unsatisfactory.

PHOTO D
And here is a close-up of Mrs Finnegan. Note down all the points about her which you observe at first sight.

PHOTO E
Now the interview is beginning. Write down how, if you were the nurse here, you would open this interview with Mrs Finnegan.

Author's comment
You will have an opportunity to compare your responses with those of other course members at Group Session 2.

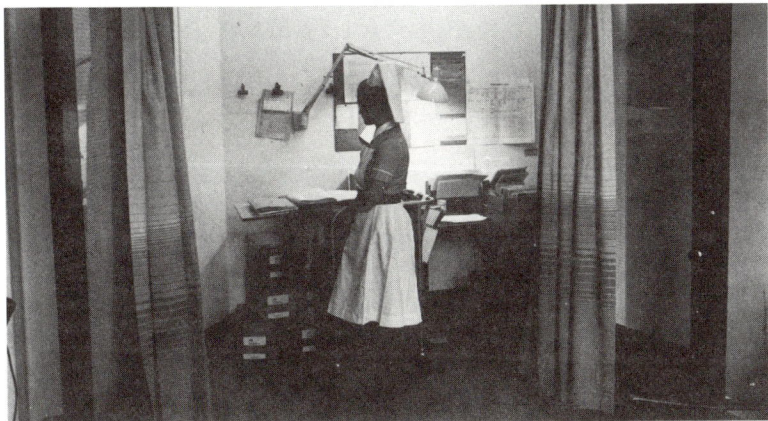
PHOTO A

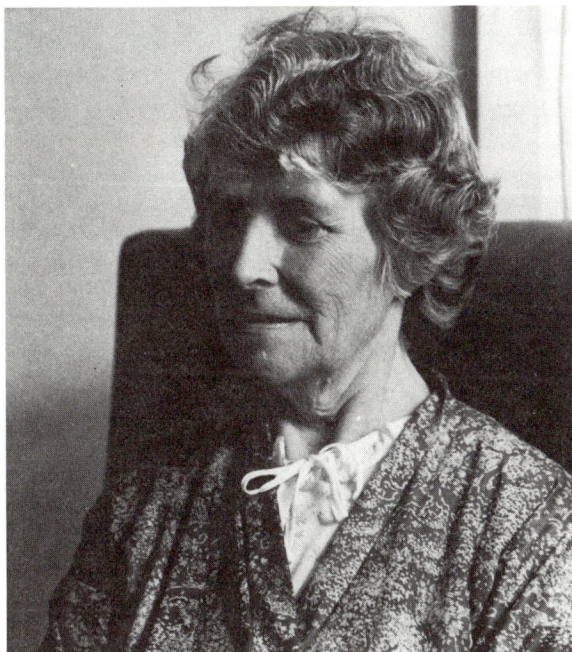
PHOTO B

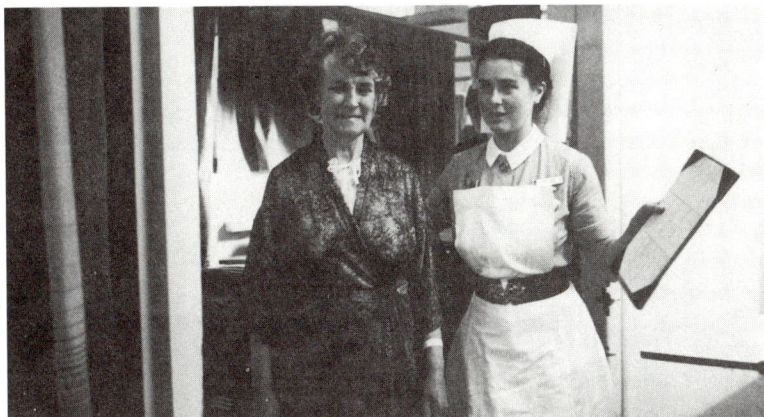
PHOTO C

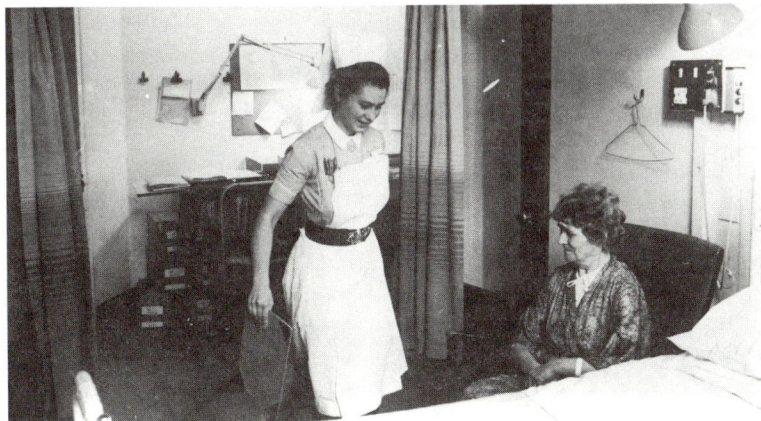
PHOTO D

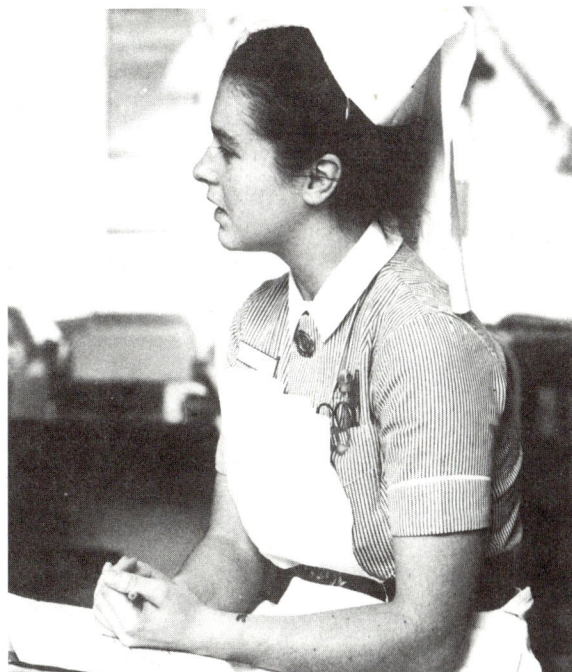
PHOTO E

Activity 2.11 — Allow 35 minutes

An admission interview: audiotape

This activity gives you an opportunity to listen to an actual admission interview and to comment critically on the way in which it is conducted.

This activity involves listening to the nurse-patient interview on the first part of the audiotape and answering questions about it. The interview lasts about eight minutes. We want you to concentrate on the verbal communication between the nurse and the patient, Mrs Finnegan, on the nurse's approach to the patient and how the patient responds to the nurse, and to think about the nurse's interviewing technique. Read your audio notes in the *Case Files* and then play the tape.

Author's comment

You will have an opportunity to compare your responses with those of other course members at Group Session 2.

In the next section of the module you will be studying the nurse's documentation of her interview with Mrs Finnegan. In the group session following this module you will be trying to agree a statement of Mrs Finnegan's problems and will also see a videotape of the nurse commenting on the interview and outlining her perception of the patient's problems.

So, by way of the admission interview and ending in the group session with identification of the patient's problems, you will be working through all the stages of nursing assessment with this patient.

RECORDING DATA COLLECTED

In Part I of the *Case Files*, you will find data from the interview with Mrs Finnegan recorded on the assessment form used in that ward by the nurse who admitted her. You will notice that some additional information is included, which was collected after the interview to complete the assessment, but for the following activity, concentrate on data available from the interview itself.

Activity 2.12 — Allow 15 minutes

Recording data from assessment

In this activity, you are asked to evaluate data recorded from the interview and to judge how clear and useful it is.

How adequately do you think the nurse has recorded the data collected at the interview with Mrs Finnegan? Answer this in the following questions:

1 Has all relevant data available from the interview been recorded? (Yes/No)

   If not, what would you have added?

2 On the whole, is the information written concisely? (Yes/No)

   If not, give an example of what seems to you an unnecessarily lengthy entry.

3 Is there anything recorded incorrectly or in an ambiguous way? (Yes/No)

   If so, note an example.

4 Is the information recorded in a way which would be meaningful to others who will consult the form but were not present at the interview? (Yes/No)

   If not, give an example of something which is incomplete or confusing.

Author's comment

If you have any difficulty with any of the questions, discuss them with another course member or, if necessary, make a note to raise the difficulty at Group Session 2 when you will be studying this documentation further.

Recording information from nursing assessment in a succinct yet meaningful way is a skilled activity, but one which improves and becomes quicker with practice.

Activity 2.13 — Allow 5 minutes

Recording data in your work area

You now have an opportunity to review your own documentation again, in the light of what you learned from completing the previous activity.

Having looked fairly closely at the documentation of Mrs Finnegan's assessment, now take another quick look at the completed form which you collected from your own work area. Note any positive or negative features which strike you about the way the data from the assessment have been recorded.

Author's comment

Positive features might have included attributes such as the relevance, conciseness, clarity, legibility and usefulness of data recorded. Negative features could have related to apparent irrelevance, repetitiveness, use of uncommon abbreviations, unclear meaning, illegible writing and incompleteness of data recorded.

SELF-RECORDING BY THE PATIENT

A useful way of obtaining information from patients, although not yet much used in nursing, is to ask the *patient* to record information, perhaps on a specially designed proforma. Here are some examples of when this might be done:

- a woman could be asked to bring to the ante-natal booking clinic notes concerning her previous pregnancies/deliveries, details of her menstrual cycle, information about her past medical history, details of her usual diet, a list of questions which she would like to ask the midwife and her own 'birth plan'
- a health visitor, who has been asked by a mother for help with her baby who is "constantly crying and won't sleep", could ask the mother to keep a diary for a week to record the baby's pattern of crying and sleep and related events
- a person attending a psychiatric out-patient department for treatment of a phobic condition could be asked by the nurse therapist to record episodes of the phobia over a certain time period.

Perhaps on a more widespread basis, patients could be asked to complete a proforma, covering specific aspects of the initial nursing assessment, to bring with them on admission. This idea was tested in a North American research project (Aspinall, 1975). A group of thirty patients was asked to complete a questionnaire, following which they were also given the routine admission interview. Information written by the patients and information obtained by the nurses was compared. It was found that, in 25 of the 30 cases, the nurses made more errors of omission in the interviews than the patients did in the questionnaires. In addition, the average time of interview was 11½ minutes, compared with the 54 seconds needed on average to explain the questionnaire to patients. The results of the study are discussed as a means of providing accurate data and saving nurses' time.

Activity 2.14   **Allow 5 minutes**

Your views on self-recording

If the idea of self-recording is new to you, this activity should help you to decide on its value in your area of work.

1. Do you think that it might be useful to try out self-recording by patients in your work area?   (Yes/No)
2. Saving nurses' time is one argument in favour of introducing self-recording by patients. Can you think of:
   - other advantages to nurses?
   - disadvantages from the nurse's point of view?
3. One advantage it might offer to *patients* is that it might encourage them to put forward their own viewpoints on what information it is important for nurses to have. What other advantages might it offer to patients?
4. There can, of course, be disadvantages too. For example, some patients may feel compelled to write down what they think is expected. Are there any other disadvantages?
5. In some areas, patients are encouraged to participate in the recording of ongoing assessment data: completion of fluid balance charts or blood testing by diabetic patients, for example. Would you encourage this? Can you think of any other examples?

Author's comment

This is another topic related to nursing assessment which you might be interested to discuss with colleagues in your own work area.

REVIEWING THE DATA COLLECTED AND IDENTIFYING THE PATIENT'S PROBLEMS

REVIEWING THE DATA COLLECTED

Once information has been obtained, the next stage of nursing assessment is to review the data. Firstly, attention should be paid to possible omissions and to any inconsistencies which appear to exist: for example, a discrepancy between what the patient has described and the nurse has observed. In the course of collecting the data, the meaning and significance of the information will already have been considered. The nurse has in fact been making judgments of this kind in deciding what information to seek and, of that, what to record and in how much detail.

Making sense of the data collected, and then accurately identifying the patient's problems, requires considerable intellectual skill. It demands an appreciation of the interrelationship between separate pieces of information about the patient: is there a link between the reported recent difficulty in getting off to sleep and the patient's manifest, though denied, anxiety about the impending operation? What is the significance of the information obtained concerning the patient's usual bowel habits? The frequency of once every three or four days is usual for that patient, but how does that compare with our knowledge of the range of normal? Is there a link between the patient's bowel habits and diet? Interpreting the meaning and significance of data collected about a particular patient in the course of nursing assessment is a complex and vital, yet little understood, part of the nursing process.

Let us return to the simple example of body temperature, which was the topic of Activity 2.8, to illustrate the complexity. The most accurate method of obtaining information about a person's body temperature is by measuring, using a thermometer. First we need to be certain that the person's temperature is taken very accurately – which requires attention to the type of instrument, placement site, time in site and influencing factors such as the temperature of the environment and the previous activity of the patient. Suppose this reveals the patient's temperature to be 38.5°C. What is the significance of this information?

The immediate interpretation would be that the patient is pyrexial, based on the knowledge that normal body temperature for adults is within the range 36–37.5°C. However, the real significance of this information would need to be interpreted in the light of other information which may influence such a conclusion. One factor to consider would be the patient's usual body temperature, because obviously a rise from 36°C to 38.5°C is of greater concern than a rise from a usual temperature of around 37°C. As important a consideration would be whether or not the patient's recorded temperature of 38.5°C represents a decrease on a previous recording (which would be interpreted as a positive improvement) or, in contrast, a sudden increase in temperature. If the latter occurs in the case of a patient who has undergone surgery, the information would suggest the presence of infection. The nurse may well have observed other indicators of the increased body temperature: for example, flushed skin, excessive perspiration or lethargy. The patient may complain of feeling hot and perhaps even indicate the cause of the pyrexia by reporting, for example, discomfort at the site of the wound.

So, even this apparently simple piece of information – raised body temperature – requires careful consideration, if a correct interpretation of its significance is to be made by the nurse. Of course, what seems on paper a laborious and rather obvious mental exercise is in practice executed quickly and easily. But perhaps it is worthwhile, from time to time, to analyse how we do make judgments about the data collected from nursing assessment. At the very least, this would help us to help student nurses to learn about the nursing process.

IDENTIFYING THE PATIENT'S PROBLEMS

In reviewing the data from assessment, the question we are asking is: what is the significance of the information collected for the patient's nursing? As mentioned earlier, deciding about this is described by some as *making a nursing diagnosis*. We are adopting a more commonly used term – *identifying the patient's problems*.

McFarlane and Castledine (1982) describe this review process as comparing what is 'normal' for the individual with his present condition i.e. comparing the information in the two columns of the second stage history form (Figure 2.2). By making this comparison the nurse is able to form a judgment about whether any aspect of daily living presents a *problem* to the patient. Figure 2.9 provides an example of how the right-hand column displays the patient's problems.

Usual condition/behaviour (or normal self-care behaviour)	Present condition/behaviour (or disabilities in self-care)
able to dress himself	Unable to make fine adjustments in clothing (do/undo back zips fully, tie shoe-laces etc.)
able to maintain personal hygiene	Unable to wash 'good' arm because of immobilisation of one arm in plaster

Fig. 2.9 An example of problem identification (McFarlane and Castledine, 1982)

Figure 2.9 also serves as an example of how Orem's self-care model (used by McFarlane and Castledine) provides a framework for identifying patients' problems. As you will see, the columns are sub-titled to equate *usual condition/behaviour* with *normal self-care behaviour* and *present condition/behaviour* with *disabilities in self-care*.

'PROBLEMS' RATHER THAN 'NEEDS'

A few words about the use of the term 'problems'. Some nurses dislike using this term, preferring to refer to the patient's *needs*. However, *all* people have needs such as the physiological need for food and the psychological need for love. It is when people are unable to continue to meet their needs independently – in other words, when they are experiencing *problems* – that they require nursing assistance. The problems are the manifestation of the person's inability to continue to meet human needs.

There is another reason why some nurses seem to dislike the word 'problems' and this is related to describing the nursing process as a problem-*solving* approach rather than as a problem-*oriented* approach. Writing about the nursing process Virginia Henderson expresses concern, asking "whether problem-solving is all there is to nursing?" (Henderson, 1982). The answer must be 'yes' if the nursing process is viewed as being synonymous with problem solving, although not if a wider concept of problem orientation is adopted. Roper, Logan and Tierney (1980), who do advocate use of the term 'problems' in the application of their model for nursing, take care to describe nursing as helping patients to "*solve, alleviate, cope with* or *prevent* problems with their activities of living".

Problems or needs . . . what do *you* think?

'ACTUAL' AND 'POTENTIAL' PROBLEMS

The fact that nurses are not only concerned with solving problems but also with their prevention is reflected by the increasing use in practice of the terms 'actual problems' and 'potential problems'.

An *actual problem* is a problem which exists. We know it exists because the patient tells us about it or because we can observe the problem. A patient might for example report having pain – this is an actual problem and the exact nature of the problem can be clarified by the patient's description (the pain's location, duration, severity, onset etc.) and through nurses' observations (for example, of distress, raised pulse rate or limitation of associated movement).

A *potential problem* is a problem which *may* occur. A common example is the potential problem of the risk of developing pressure sores. We would identify this as a potential problem for a particular patient on the basis of information pointing to the specific circumstances known to contribute to the development of pressure sores. In fact, we can identify patients at risk quite accurately by using available assessment tools, such as the Norton Scoring System, mentioned earlier.

The concept of potential problems is a very useful one in nursing assessment because it directs nurses to review the data collected, with a view to identifying problems which could occur (which often, like pressure sores, might be prevented by appropriate intervention) as well as those which actually exist. Some nurses, for example health visitors, are in fact mainly concerned with the prevention of potential problems such as accidents in the home, risks of childhood infections, child abuse or the over-feeding of babies. No health visitor would need help in identifying potential problems, although she may have difficulty in deciding priorities among them, which ones to list and for which to make specific plans. And that is a difficulty for nurses in any setting – the list of potential problems for almost every patient could be endless. The notion of establishing the *priority* of problems (both actual and potential) will be dealt with in detail in Module 3.

WHOSE PROBLEMS ARE THEY?

The problems are the *patient's* problems. It is, therefore, important for nurses to become skilled at describing problems *as they are experienced by the patient*. Indeed it is often helpful to describe a problem in the patient's own words. For example, a nurse may record as "depression" what the patient has described as "feeling low, can't sleep, can't concentrate on work, don't feel hungry, feel irritable with the children". Using the patient's description is likely to encourage nurses to make a nursing diagnosis and to result in more appropriate intervention being planned. It will almost certainly make it easier for the nurse to communicate with the patient about the nature of the problem.

Although problems should focus on the patient, sometimes the problems (or different/additional ones) are in fact the *family's*. For example, a nursing assessment of a child with leukaemia will result in identification of problems pertaining to the parents, and possibly siblings or other close relatives, as well as the child.

WHAT PROBLEMS CONCERN NURSES?

Although it may seem obvious, it may be useful to remind ourselves that nursing assessment is concerned with identifying problems which are amenable to *nursing* intervention. So, what problems concern nurses?

In Module 1 you will remember that in discussing *the role of the nurse*, the components of nursing were categorised as comprising:

- the *unique* role of the nurse: i.e. those aspects of care, largely related to everyday living activities, which the special skills of nurses enable them to perform and which other professionals are unlikely to carry out
- the *collaborative* role of the nurse: i.e. those nursing activities which are dependent upon the role of other professionals (for example, the nurse's responsibility for implementing some aspects of medical treatment), or which are carried out in conjunction with others (for example, nurses and physiotherapists co-operating in assisting patients with problems relating to mobility).

So, patient problems which concern nurses include not only those generally accepted as the specific domain of nursing, but also those arising from medical prescription (for example, problems arising from the doctor's prescription of 'total bedrest', for which the patient requires nursing assistance), as well as those which are the joint concern of nurses and other members of the health care team. Interdependence within the team also enables nurses to refer problems which, although identified from nursing assessment, cannot be dealt with within the limits of nursing expertise. For example, returning to the case of a child with leukaemia, it may emerge that the parents are unable to afford the cost of frequent visits to the hospital: this problem could be referred by the nurse to the social worker as in the case of Peter O. (see Part I of the *Case Files*). Or the nurse may discover that the parents feel confused about their child's treatment regime: this problem would be referred by the nurse to the doctor.

In some units, particularly in the field of psychiatry, a multi-disciplinary approach to problem identification and goal planning is adopted. This, of course, takes the idea of interdependence further than the system of 'referral of problems' described above. You will be considering such a team approach in relation to goal planning in Module 3.

or physically exhausted. But in these cases a relative, or parents if the patient is a child, might be willing and able to participate on the patient's behalf.

It is quite likely that the way in which we, as nurses, view the problems will change as we discover how patients themselves perceive the problems and priorities. Patients may identify problems not perceived by nurses. On the other hand, nurses will realise that some things they tend to regard as problems are not appreciated as such by patients. Some patients may need to be helped to recognise the existence of a problem, and their very blindness to such a problem would itself properly be identified as a problem. And sometimes nurses may need to be helped by patients to avoid creating problems which don't actually exist or are not considered important. There are many things which we might ascertain from nursing assessment which are not problems as such. We will only begin to become skilled at problem identification when we begin to listen to the person with the problem – the patient.

The greater the extent to which nurses and patients have reached agreement about the problems by the end of the assessment step of the nursing process, the more likely it is that effective, individualised nursing will be planned and implemented for patients.

CONFIRMING THE EXISTENCE OF PROBLEMS

Some patient problems will be very easily identified from the data collected by the nurse. But sometimes, if there is doubt, additional information may be needed to confirm the existence and precise nature of a problem. This may be collected through further observation, by asking the patient additional questions or perhaps by using a special data collection instrument.

If at all possible, nurses should discuss their views of the problems with patients themselves, so that the act of confirming the existence of problems, and deciding the priorities among them, becomes an exercise in partnership. This might take place after the assessment following admission or at first referral, once the nurse has taken time to record and study the information collected, or it could coincide with a goal-planning session. In either event, the nurse could explain it as follows: "I've now had an opportunity to look carefully at all the information we have about you. I have made a note of what I see as the problems which the nursing staff can help with. Before we decide how to deal with them, I'd like to discuss my ideas with you so that we can reach agreement on what the problems are and which are the most urgent to consider".

Obviously, there are some circumstances when this would not be possible or appropriate. In such cases, nurses must rely entirely on their own judgment concerning problem identification. An unconscious patient or a very confused old person would be unable to participate. And it might not be in the best interests of some other patients, for example if they are seriously ill, emotionally distressed

LISTING THE PROBLEMS

Once identified, the patient's or family's problems must be listed. The list of problems is likely to be more meaningful if put alongside the data recorded from assessment, although current practice more commonly involves a separate 'problem list'. Wherever it is recorded, the written statement of problems must be precise yet concise. Wherever possible, the statement of a problem should include an indication of its cause, because this is relevant when setting goals and deciding upon the required intervention. As an example, consider nappy rash, a problem frequently referred to health visitors by mothers. The nature of the problem, and the intervention appropriate, would differ in the case of "nappy rash due to teething" (perhaps the mother's perception of the problem) from that of "nappy rash due to inadequate washing and drying of the peri-urethral area" (perhaps the health visitor's perception of the cause).

Below are some examples to illustrate ways in which problems can be listed. The first three examples relate to the three nursing models which we are illustrating throughout the course.

Example 1

As mentioned earlier, McFarlane and Castledine (1982) illustrate the use of Orem's self-care model for the nursing process. Figure 2.10 provides another example, this time relating to rest/sleep, to show how data collected from assessment are recorded. The left-hand column (*usual condition*) concerns normal self-care behaviour and the right-hand one (*present condition*) focuses on deficits in self-care.

Usual condition	Present condition
Rest/Sleep	
Usually went to bed at 10 pm and read until midnight. Woke once during the night, usually to micturate. Got up at 6.30 am; washed, and breakfasted at 7.30 approx. Dozed in chair for about an hour in afternoon.	Having difficulty in sleeping more than 2-4 hours; finds he wakes at 4am and unable to get back to sleep. Afternoon naps are shorter than he would like.

Fig. 2.10 *An example of a written statement of problems (McFarlane and Castledine, 1982)*

The authors suggest that to make a precise statement of the problem – preserving the normal sleep pattern – the cause should be included. The problem could, for example, be listed as "disturbed sleep pattern due to change of environment and anxiety about admission".

Example 2

The Roper, Logan and Tierney model for nursing is reflected in their Patient Assessment Form (Figure 2.3). On the form, the patient's problems are listed alongside data collected from assessment of the activities of living (ALs). The statement of problems can be brief because background information (for example, the cause of the problem) is adjacent. This system of documentation also encourages goal setting to take account of the patient's abilities as well as problems. A potential problem is distinguished from an actual problem in the list by the symbol (*p*). Figure 2.11 illustrates some examples.

Example 3

Using the Saxton and Hyland stress-adaptation model, information is recorded about past and present stresses which are affecting an individual. Each stress is classified according to its type and adaptations which have been made to cope with the stress are identified. The statements of 'adaptation' are indicators of need which provide the rationale for planning nursing intervention. This part of the information recorded from assessment is, therefore, equivalent to

(a) AL of communicating: an elderly lady suffering from senile dementia

AL	Data from assessment	Patient's problems
Communicating	Speaks clearly, and responds appropriately to simple instructions but conversation often confused and rambling. Frequently disorientated (time/place/person) during evening and night. Poor concentration and short-term memory. Hearing good. Sight poor.	Confusion Disorientation (pm) Poor concentration/memory Poor sight

(b) AL of breathing: middle-aged man with acute bronchitis

AL	Data from assessment	Patient's problems
Breathing	Severe dyspnoea on admission; breathing wheezy and gasping - relief obtained from O₂ therapy. Perpetual morning cough with sputum. Breathless on exertion. Smokes 20 cigarettes a day.	Severe difficulty in breathing (p) Exacerbation of bronchitis due to smoking.

(c) AL of eating and drinking: middle-aged woman admitted for cholecystectomy

AL	Data from assessment	Patient's problems
Eating and drinking	Appetite unaffected by epigastric pain and other discomforts (waterbrash, "flatulence"). Varied diet, though has cut down on fats. Overweight for height by 10 Kg.	Gastrointestinal discomforts Overweight.

Fig. 2.11 *Listing problems: an example using the activities of living model*

the statement of 'patient's problems' in the Roper, Logan and Tierney model, illustrated in example 2.

Figure 2.12 illustrates some of the stresses experienced by a patient with a neoplasm of the large bowel.

Stress	Type	Adaptation
Neoplasm of large bowel	Physiological	Pressure on surrounding tissue. New growth of tissue
Narrowing of large bowel	Physical	Slow passage of digestive waste products. Distention above level of partial obstruction
Frequent liquid stool movement	Physical	Digestive waste products unable to pass obstruction freely. Excess peristalsis
Fear of diagnosis, prognosis and management	Emotional	Unable to rest. Cannot remember information given
Deprived of liberty through hospital admission	Emotional	Depressed, withdrawn, dislikes proximity of other patients and staff

Fig. 2.12 Stresses experienced by a patient with large bowel neoplasm: an example using the stress-adaptation model of Saxton and Hyland (1979)

Example 4

Finally, here is a miscellaneous list of problems. Because we are concentrating here on problem *statements*, we have not included the background data from assessment as in the above examples. Remember that a problem statement is only truly meaningful in the light of those data. The comment accompanying each of the problems listed below is to remind you of some of the points we have been considering about identifying the patient's problems, in this section of the module.

PROBLEM STATEMENT	COMMENT
Unable to stand without support of two nurses.	A simple example of a patient's problem. Expressed as a problem rather than a need ("needs help to stand").
Risk of chest infection due to anaesthesia and immobility.	A potential problem. Note that the cause is included.
Says she "feels utterly terrified" about her impending operation.	A statement which includes the patient's own description of feelings.

PROBLEM STATEMENT	COMMENT
Mother seems unaware of her child's poor prognosis.	Example of a problem which is the parent's rather than the patient's.
Does not accept that smoking is a serious threat to his health.	Example of a problem which is in fact the patient's denial of a problem.
Six-month history of epigastric pain following meals.	Useful inclusion of the duration of the problem here.
Embarrassed about bed-wetting at night.	A more meaningful and precise statement than the more frequently used general expression of "nocturnal incontinence of urine".
Becomes constipated without bran for breakfast.	A potential problem. Stated so precisely that preventive nursing action is self-evident.
Severely nauseated following cytotoxic therapy.	Example of a problem resulting from medical management which has implications for nursing.
Anxiety about financial implications of absence from work.	Example of a problem which has been identified and which would be referred, by the nurse to social worker in this instance.

Activity 2.15 — Allow 15 minutes

Listing the problems

In this activity you have an opportunity to practise the formulation of problem statements in relation to your own assessment.

Again look at the completed assessment you obtained from your own work area. Study the information recorded and then write a list of the patient's problems. Bear in mind issues we have been considering in this section of the module: describing problems as experienced by the patient; the family's as well as the patient's problems; problems arising from medical or other prescription; differentiation between actual and potential – use the symbols (a) and (p); stating the cause of the problem; writing problems precisely yet concisely.

Author's comment
In reviewing what you have written, check carefully that you have included all the issues identified in the activity.

PREPARING FOR GROUP SESSION 2

Group Session 2 will focus on the assessment of Mrs Finnegan which you heard on the audiotape and studied in the *Case Files*. Activity 2.16 will remind you of this patient and assist you to prepare for the session.

Activity 2.16   Allow 30 minutes

Mrs Finnegan's problems

This activity is designed to help you to apply what has been said about listing problems to the case of Mrs Finnegan.

Re-read Mrs Finnegan's documentation in the *Case Files* and make a list of her problems. When your list is complete, decide on an order of priority and number the problems accordingly.

Activity 2.17   Allow 10 minutes

Reviewing assessment

Having worked through the module, you now have an opportunity to review what you have learned and consider how you may want to adapt your own approach to assessment.

At the beginning of this module you were asked to write a description of the way in which *you* assess patients (Activity 2.1). Look back at what you wrote. Having now given considerable thought to your own approach through activities utilising the patient assessment collected from your work area, and having worked through the module, is there anything you have learned which you would like to incorporate into your future nursing assessment?

Author's comment
Here are just some of the topics which have been discussed which you might have mentioned:

- *adopting a more patient-oriented approach – a partnership*
- *developing a more explicit policy regarding accountability for assessment*
- *giving consideration to an underlying framework/selecting a model for nursing*
- *improving assessment documents – by making the underlying framework more explicit, recording the source of information, amending/extending the form or designing/adopting a new one*
- *improving interviewing technique*
- *considering the use of special data collection instruments*
- *considering how to increase self-recording by patients*
- *refining the way in which patients' problems are stated and listed.*

Author's comment
You will have an opportunity at the group session to discuss all your responses to the activities related to Mrs Finnegan. You may find it useful to re-read your answers to Activities 2.10, 2.11 and 2.12 and the related notes in the Case Files.

The group session will also give you a chance to comment on the module as a whole and to seek clarification on any specific points you may wish to raise.

PREPARING FOR MODULE 3

The next module, Module 3, is about the planning step of the nursing process. This involves three activities – deciding aims of care for individual patients, deciding what nursing activities would assist patients to achieve them and communicating the plan of care to others involved in patient care.

A number of short activities are included in the module to provide you with some practice in writing aims and goals for patients and developing nursing care plans. In order to complete these activities it is necessary to have:

1 A list of patient problems. You have already completed some work on identifying and testing patients' problems at the end of Module 2. You may wish to use the problems for the patient that you selected to work on for Activity 2.15, or those for a different patient. In any case, it is best if you select documentation for a patient with whom you are familiar.

2 It is also useful to have a set of goals or aims of care for this patient and the nursing orders of prescribed care associated with them. Your current form of patient documentation may not be set out in this way. If not, it does not matter as long as you obtain or construct a problem list and have some knowledge of the care being given to the patient.

Remember to omit all details by which the patient might be identified. If it is not possible for you to obtain information about a patient, you will be able to use the documentation on Peter O. in the *Case Files*, but it is infinitely preferable to base your activities on information about a known patient.

Because the module is quite long, you may wish to organise your study time into two sessions. The bulk of activities and reading are in the sections related to writing patient goals. A major activity also comes at the end of the module, for which you will need to use the audiotape. It is important to complete this activity *before* you attend Group Session 3.

MODULE 3
THE SECOND STEP OF THE NURSING PROCESS PLANNING

Prepared for the Course Team by Senga Bond

CONTENTS

CONTENTS

OBJECTIVES

After studying this module, you should be able to:

1 Explain the importance of the planning of care in the process of nursing.

2 Write clear goal statements.

3 Distinguish between long and short-term goals.

4 Involve patients/clients and their families in goal setting.

5 Determine goal priorities.

6 Identify how personal and professional values and beliefs, and models of nursing influence goal setting.

7 Decide appropriate nursing intervention to help patients reach identified goals.

8 Write a clear nursing care plan.

9 Involve other relevant disciplines in the planning of nursing care.

10 Describe the contribution of standard care plans to individualised care.

INTRODUCTION

This module deals with the planning step of the process of nursing. Three major stages are involved in planning. The first stage is the setting of goals for patients – deciding, with them, the aims of their nursing care and, more specifically, what they will be able to do. The second stage is the identification of the most appropriate nursing interventions to meet these goals – carrying out actions on behalf of patients, or assisting them to undertake their own care. The final stage in planning is the communication of the goals and associated nursing activities to others involved in patient care. This often involves the use of written nursing care plans.

Module 3 examines each of these stages in some detail and provides some practice in planning care. Writing good goal statements is of critical importance and you are advised to practise this as the basis for good care planning. To become proficient may take a long time, so do not be disheartened should you feel that there is still room for improvement by the time you reach the end of the module.

Bear in mind that we are dealing here with *nursing* as one component of a patient's total care. The major reason for nurses to assume a goal-directed approach to care is to achieve good quality. In using this approach, the underlying rationale for each nursing action is made known. This is why it is important to state clearly not only what patients' problems are, but also *what* nursing is aiming to achieve, and *how* these aims will be met.

By producing a comprehensive plan of care the scope of nursing responsibilities is acknowledged, as are those specific actions for which nurses are prepared to hold themselves accountable and responsible.

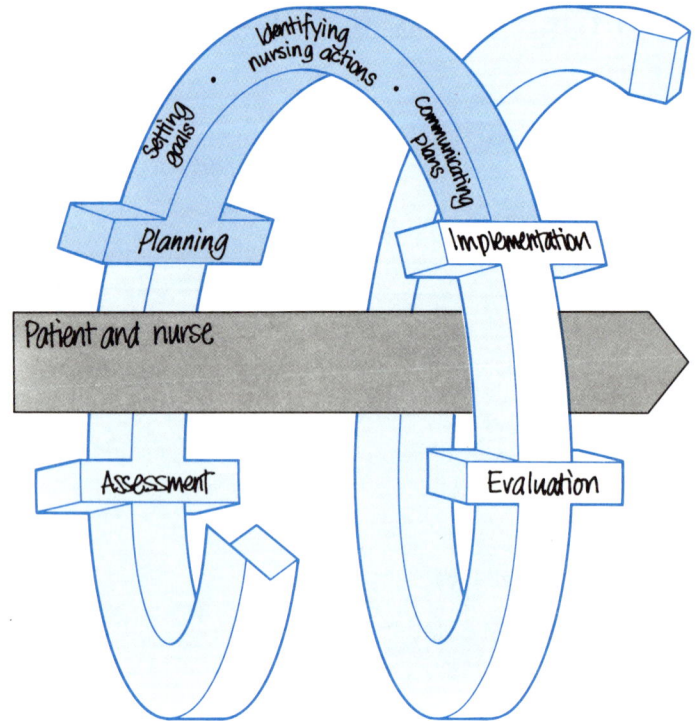

Fig. 3.1 The planning stage expanded

A GOAL-DIRECTED APPROACH

In a goal-directed approach, the plan of care for a patient is based on goals which have been formulated in response to identified patient problems. Goal planning takes place after patients have been assessed, but before nursing interventions to deal with actual or potential problems are actually carried out. It can be instantaneous, as in an emergency when someone is choking and the aim is to assist the patient to breathe by removing the obstruction. It may involve a more protracted process, for example, in working out a series of goals for a rehabilitation programme for a handicapped person. Sometimes, the emphasis may be on the prevention of problems; certainly this is the case in ante-natal care and health visiting. While these are very different situations, the goal-directed approach has the following common features:

- a recognition that the current or potential state of affairs is not satisfactory, either to the patient or to the nurse

- a desire by at least one of them for a different outcome
- the setting of specific goals or outcomes to be achieved.

THE NATURE OF GOALS

Goals are sometimes referred to as 'aims of nursing'. They can also be termed 'objectives', 'desired end results' or 'expected outcomes of care'. Patients may describe them as 'hopes', 'wishes' or 'aspirations'. Some authors attach more specific meanings to terms, using 'outcomes', for example, to refer to the *final* point that the patient is expected to reach, and 'goals' to indicate intermediate steps along the way. It does not matter which term is preferred, but it is important to agree locally on a standard terminology to be adopted. All these terms imply some desirable future state of affairs.

Little and Carnevali (1976) describe a nurse-client goal as "a statement of a desired, achievable outcome to be attained within a predicted period of time, given the presenting situation and resources".

To be useful, goals need to be stated in such a way that they are clear and precise. One way of achieving this is to state them in *behavioural* terms – what you would expect to observe, hear or see demonstrated if the goal is achieved. This broad definition of behaviour implies gaining information, through our own *observation*, about the patient's current status. Observable behaviour can include:

physiological signs: temperature, skin texture, the smell of urine or breath

physical behaviour: walking, micturating in the toilet

verbal behaviour: describing the symptoms of insulin reaction, expressing feelings of anxiety.

In other words, you set a *measurable* response which you would expect *from the person for whom the goal is set*, and subsequently observe whether it has been achieved. You would carry out your 'measurements' in ways appropriate to the specified behaviour: by taking physiological measurements, by smelling a patient's urine, by counting the number of times a patient reports pain or smokes a cigarette, by observing a patient get on to a bus, by listening to him telling you his feelings about losing his leg, or how he feels about his spouse or the patient in the next bed. It is important that we take an interest in what is going on *inside* people's heads or 'hearts' – what they are thinking and feeling. This is something which we have to infer from what they do, and so there is an emphasis on observable actions. If, as nurses, we were not concerned with producing change we would not need to look at behaviour, but that is a responsibility which we do have.

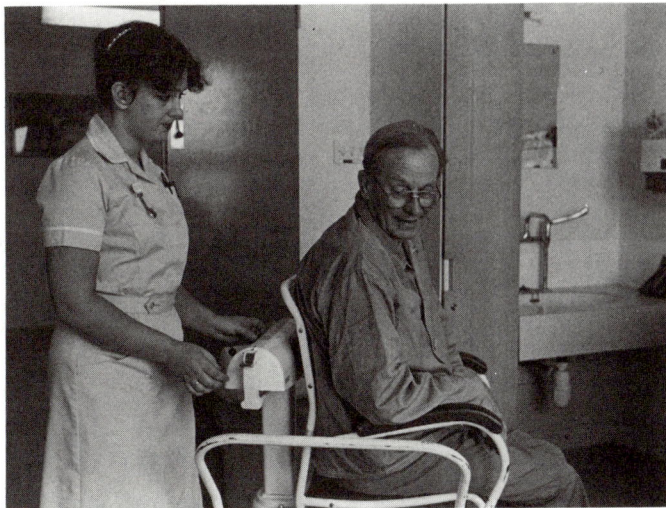

Obtaining a measurable response

WRITING BEHAVIOURAL GOALS

Statements of behavioural goals should contain the following five elements:

1 **Who** is to demonstrate the desired behaviour: i.e. the patient.

2 The **actual behaviour** which will demonstrate that the goal has been achieved: for example, reporting less anxiety, passing urine, touching, walking.

3 The **relevant conditions** under which the behaviour will be performed, such as the level of assistance needed from other people or aids (e.g. "walks alone or with a stick"), or where the behaviour will take place (e.g. "on the level" or "on stairs").

4 The **standard** that will be used to evaluate the behaviour. This entails specifying the criterion of success, which may relate to the frequency of the behaviour demonstrated (e.g. "voids in the toilet *on each occasion*"), or to a time limit (e.g. "completes dressing *in 20 minutes*").

5 By what **time** it is expected that the behaviour will be achieved. This may be almost immediately, as in a life-saving emergency. Alternatively, a specific time interval may be appropriate; for example, a patient may be required to learn some behaviour pre-operatively that is relevant to his post-operative recovery, and this goal should be achieved the day before surgery and certainly before the pre-med. is given. At other times, more long-term goals may be involved, such as increasing a person's ability to initiate interpersonal contact, or to increase self-care activities over a number of weeks.

These are the elements you would expect to see in any well-written goal statement. Each of these components is identified, by number, in the following goal statements:

1 2
John / will carry the supper to other patients at his table /
3 4 5
unaided, / and without spilling it, / every evening this week.

1 4 2
Mr Bain / will make no more than three / self-deprecating
3
remarks / in a half-hour conversation with Nurse Wilson, /
5
within seven days.

1 2
Miss Hagel / will be able to cleanse her colostomy / using bland
3 4 5
soap and water, / without prompting or supervision, / by Friday.

1 2 5
Mr Jones / will bring Jason to the child health centre / for each
4 3
birthday check / without being reminded.
(In this goal statement, the time element is *each* birthday.)

Activity 3.1   Allow 5 minutes

Goal components

This activity gives you practice in identifying goal components, before you actually write your own goals.

Examine the following two goal statements:

1 After breakfast and before going to bed, Joan will carry out her knee exercises for five minutes, with the assistance of her mother.
2 Mr Grey will report no more than two episodes of giggling in public, when he comes to the clinic next week.

Now, as in the examples given above, try to identify by number each of the following five components:

1 Who will perform the desired behaviour
2 The actual behaviour to be performed
3 The relevant conditions under which the behaviour will take place
4 The standard used to evaluate the behaviour
5 The expected time frame within which the behaviour will have been achieved.

Author's comment
See p. 81.

While all the examples of goals given so far have indicated behaviour to be performed by patients, goals may sometimes relate to the patient's state or condition. It may be appropriate, for example, to set goals linked to 'good hydration' or 'normal temperature', but to achieve them the patient is still likely to have to carry out certain behaviours – for example, to drink 3 litres of fluid in 24 hours. This can then be written as a behavioural goal:

The patient will drink 3 litres of the fluid of his choice over 24 hours.

Initial attempts to identify and write goals often result in the use of non-behavioural terms and what Mager (1972) calls "fuzzy" language, as well as the setting of goals for nurses rather than for patients. This is unhelpful in assisting us to know exactly what is being aimed for, and whether it has been achieved.

An example of a "fuzzy" goal for Mrs Jones might be: "will improve eating". This goal might have been agreed with Mrs Jones, but it tells us nothing about what "improvement" entails or how it will be achieved. A better way of writing it would be:

Mrs Jones will eat 8000 KJ in three well-balanced meals a day, in the company of other patients.

Writing it in this way allows anyone to check whether Mrs Jones is eating three meals, of what and how much they consist, and under what conditions they are being eaten.

This way of writing goal statements may look presumptive and dogmatic. However, the goal should have been set in agreement with the patient, and a major emphasis in writing goals must be economy of language, as well as precision.

Activity 3.2   Allow 10 minutes

Writing goal statements

This activity will give you practice in writing goal statements from identified patient problems.

Look at the problems identified in the completed patient assessment which you have collected in preparation for this module. If you do not have your own patient assessment documentation, use the problems listed in the case notes on Peter O. in Part 1 of the *Case Files*, but do not yet look at the goals stated there.

Select two patient problems. Then, for each problem, write goal statements which include each of the five components which we have just discussed. It does not matter which of the patient's problems you select.

Author's comment
Now check that the goals you set refer to patient behaviour and not to nurse behaviour, that the behaviour or state is observable, that any conditions to be met in achieving the goal are clearly identified and that the desired degree of success and the time by which you would expect the goal to be achieved are indicated.

Writing goals in this way requires you to specify a *measurable* response that you would expect from the patient, which will indicate that the goal has been achieved. Knowing how to check that they have been achieved is fundamental to writing clear goals.

Activity 3.3   Allow 10 minutes

Getting rid of "fuzzies"

If goal statements are to be useful, they must be explicit. This activity helps you to test your ability to recognise clear and "fuzzy" goals.

Here is a list of goal statements. Read them through and tick those which are *clear* i.e. those which you would be able to measure. Put an F beside those which present measurement problems – the "fuzzy" ones. Comment why you have come to each decision.

Goal statement	Clear or fuzzy	Comments
1 Increase mobility		
2 Drink at least 6 cups of fluid between 7 am and 8 pm		
3 Sleep 6 hours uninterrupted each night		
4 Accept her illness		
5 Make one or no self-deprecating remarks during follow-up interview		
6 Communicate verbally and non-verbally.		

Author's comment
See p. 81.

DIFFERENT LEVELS OF GOALS

Nurses deal with a vast range of patient problems. Accordingly, the goals set for patients will cover an equally broad range of behaviours, relate to different time-spans and have varying degrees of specificity. On one level, we can consider broad principles related to the overall nursing objectives for a unit – encouraging independence among chronically ill patients, for example. On another level, goals may relate to tiny segments of behaviour, such as a patient being able to grasp a hair brush, as one step towards being able to manage his own hygiene.

BROAD AIMS OF CARE

There is a danger that goals which refer to very broad content areas may be written in such a way that they become nothing more than platitudes. Statements such as "Mr Wilson will die with dignity", "Mrs Turnbull will accept her diagnosis" or "Mr Welsh will be successfully integrated into the community" are not very helpful as goals, because they are far too inexplicit and unmeasurable. A number of interpretations could be placed on what constitutes "dying with dignity", "accepting a diagnosis" or "successful integration" into this nebulous thing "the community".

Rather than goals, such statements are better thought of as broad aims of care, stating what may be desirable for patients. They are likely to evolve from patients' own concerns, as well as from nurses' hopes of what may be desirable and achievable. They should take account of patients' desired life styles and their own major health-related goals. Some examples are:

- live with maximum independence, on discharge from hospital to group home
- manage all self-care activities
- play physical games, once adjusted to artificial leg
- while continuing home dialysis, as far as possible adopt the same life style as before the illness.

To be useful, such broad aims must be related to a perceived problem – to the prevention of additional problems or the relief of present ones. Setting broad aims lays a foundation for identifying more specific target behaviours for a patient to achieve. For example, if a young amputee who is a keen footballer desperately wants to continue to play football, would it then be more appropriate for *him* to attempt football again, rather than to take up snooker or archery? Positive achievement in this field is likely to overcome some of the negative features of loss associated with amputation. Because negative consequences of this kind of surgery are predictable, we can begin to assist him to overcome them at an early stage in his care. In this way, there are often preventive components in the setting of broad aims of care.

Activity 3.4   Allow 10 minutes

From broad aims to goals

This activity is designed to give you practice in refining broad aims of care for patients and in translating them into clear goals, which subsequently can be evaluated.

Mr Wallace is a 74 year-old man who is going to be discharged home to live by himself after suffering a cerebrovascular accident. He can walk slowly with the aid of a Zimmer frame, dress himself with adapted clothing and his speech is unimpaired. However, he has problems of right-sided weakness and urinary incontinence, and he is showing some signs of memory impairment. He prefers to live at home, even though he is alone.

A general aim of nursing for Mr Wallace is "to maintain maximum independence while living alone at home".

Select two of Mr Wallace's problems and write more specific goals for his care, in relation to each problem.

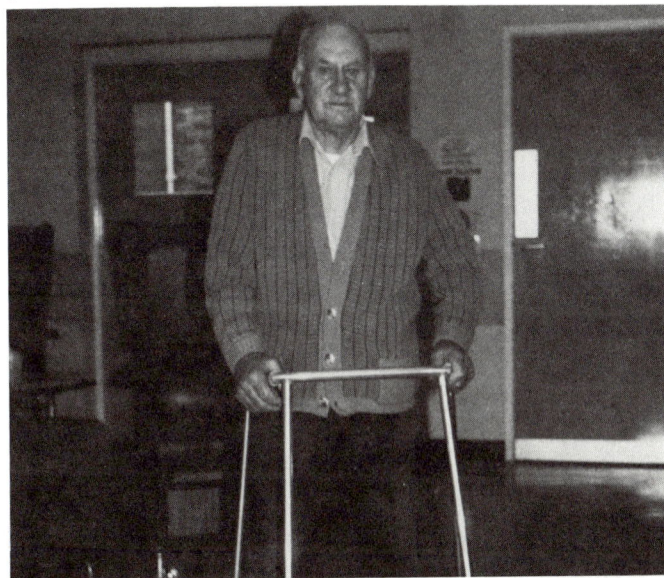

Mr Wallace

Author's comment
You may have identified goals such as:
Mr Wallace will be able to:

- *manage his pouch incontinence appliance independently by 14/7*
- *make simple meals with his adapted kitchen aids, before discharge home*
- *take a shower by himself every morning, by Friday.*

This activity shows the importance of working from problems identified for patients. Had you simply taken the general aim of care for Mr Wallace you could, from a nursing perspective, have set goals in all the activities of living described in the Roper, Logan and Tierney model. However, even if you focused on activities where problems have been identified, you are still likely to have felt some uncertainty about predicting what might actually be achieved by such a patient. Will he want and be able, for example, to cook or to keep his skin in good condition? In setting goals, a major feature must be that they are realistic as targets for that patient. As a patient's status changes, appropriate goals will need to be re-established. Mr Wallace may have some loss of fine finger movement, as well as weakness. Appropriate goals for him in relation to cooking and dressing himself are likely to require adjustment as his physical condition changes, since it may not improve to anticipated levels. It would also be important to set goals with him that attempt to maintain his physical and mental state, or to prevent further deterioration – goals associated with problems due to limited ambulation, incontinence and memory loss.

SPECIFIC GOALS

Broad aims of care give direction to specific goals identified for patients, which can themselves be regarded as steps on the way to more general, ultimate desirable outcomes. Because goals are more limited, in the sense of being more directly related to specific problems, they require a more refined level of analysis. As a result, these kinds of goals represent more clearly achievable targets than do broad aims of care. If you think of your own patients or turn to the case notes on Peter O. in the *Case Files,* you will observe that, in fact, most goals are at this level. They are of the type identified for Mr Wallace in the comments on Activity 3.4 and as a final goal for Avril, in her health visitor's goal planning record form (Figure 3.3).

GOAL STEPS

It is sometimes appropriate to analyse goals into even smaller steps, so that resources can be organised most effectively to achieve each of these steps – and ultimately, the final goal. In this case, the stages would involve:

1 Setting a clear positive goal or goals

2 Breaking down each goal into small goal steps

3 Setting target dates to achieve each goal step

4 Spelling out each person's tasks in helping to achieve each goal step.

If we think of Mr Wallace, we had as a broad aim of care: "to maintain maximum independence while living alone at home". We then identified a number of possible goals associated with this aim, including that Mr Wallace will be able to manage his pouch incontinence appliance independently by 14/7. In order to be able to accomplish this goal, a number of subsidiary goals or goal steps have to be achieved. They are illustrated in Figure 3.2.

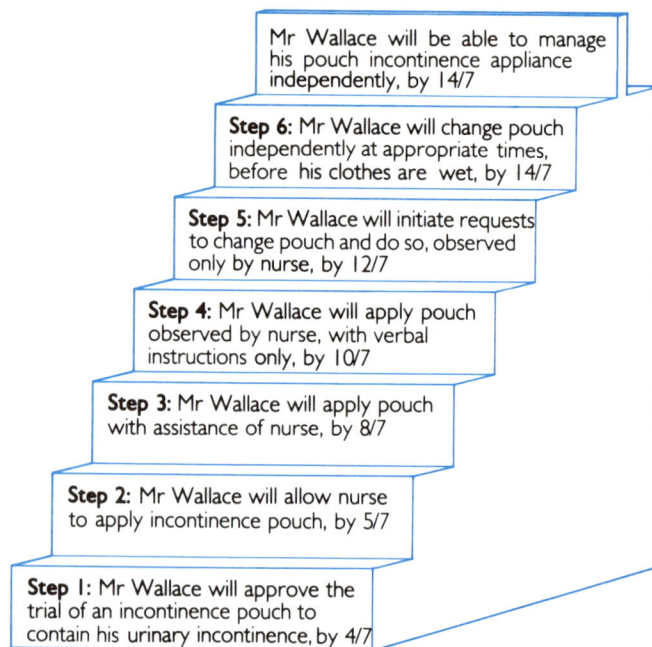

Fig. 3.2 Goal steps for Mr Wallace

The purpose of what may seem to be a very protracted and complicated exercise is gradually to build up all the component behaviours which are necessary to achieve the goal. This kind of approach has proved to be extremely useful in helping people with a wide range of social, educational and psychiatric problems. Reproduced in Figure 3.3 is a health visitor's goal planning record form, developed within a project where health visitors worked with mentally handicapped people in their own homes, to develop appropriate skills (Revill and Blunden, 1980).

The final goal for Avril was for her to make and pour a cup of tea for herself and her mother, unaided, every tea-time. Note that the patient's current abilities and strengths are identified, since they can be crucial in setting the ultimate goal and the goal steps.

Activity 3.5   Allow 10 minutes

Goal steps

Goals can usually be broken down into a number of intermediate steps. This activity provides practice in identifying and writing some steps.

Select a patient goal and then write some appropriate goal steps, adding some realistic target dates.

You may wish to work on a goal for a patient problem with which you are very familiar. Or, if you prefer, write the goal steps and target dates for a hemiparetic patient, such as Mr Wallace, whose goal is to walk a few steps after a cerebrovascular accident.

Author's comment
See p. 82.

HEALTH VISITOR'S GOAL PLANNING RECORD FORM

Name of Goal Planner: MRS DAVIS   Date: 1-6-79

Name of Client: AVRIL THOMAS

Present Client Behaviour (and strengths used in plan): AVRIL CAN WASH, FEED AND DRESS HERSELF. SHE CAN GO ON A BUS TO THE ADULT TRAINING CENTRE AND SOCIALISE WHEN SHE GETS THERE. SHE KNOWS 10p, 50p AND £1 NOTES. SHE BATHS AND TOILETS HERSELF, DUSTS, LAYS TABLE AND IRONS TEA TOWELS.

Final Goal: AVRIL WILL MAKE A POT OF TEA AND POUR A CUP OF TEA FOR HERSELF AND HER MOTHER WITHOUT AID EVERY TEA-TIME.

Goal Step (What client will be doing when each step is reached. Use as many or as few steps as you need.)	Target Date	Method (Staff and/or family responsibilities.)	Achievement Date
1ST STEP: AVRIL WILL FILL THE ELECTRIC KETTLE AND THEN SWITCH ON THE ELECTRICITY, WITHOUT AID, WHEN MOTHER HAS PLUGGED IN KETTLE, ONCE A DAY.	8-6-79	MOTHER WILL COMPLETE TEA-MAKING AND WILL GIVE AVRIL VERBAL PROMPTS WHEN NECESSARY AND PLENTY OF PRAISE.	6-6-79
2ND STEP: AVRIL WILL FILL THE ELECTRIC KETTLE, PLUG IT IN AND SWITCH IT ON, WITHOUT AID, ONCE A DAY.	15-6-79	"	11-6-79
3RD STEP: AVRIL WILL FILL THE ELECTRIC KETTLE, PLUG IT IN, SWITCH IT ON AND SWITCH IT OFF WHEN BOILING, WITHOUT AID, ONCE A DAY.	22-6-79	"	22-6-79
4TH STEP: AVRIL WILL BOIL A KETTLE OF WATER, PUT TEA IN TEAPOT AND FILL TEAPOT HALF FULL OF WATER, WITHOUT AID, ONCE A DAY.	29-6-79	"	26-6-79
5TH STEP: AVRIL WILL MAKE A POT OF TEA AND POUR A CUP OF TEA FOR HERSELF AND HER MOTHER, WITHOUT AID, EVERY TEA-TIME.	6-7-79	MOTHER WILL GIVE VERBAL PROMPTS WHEN NECESSARY AND SHE AND OTHER MEMBERS OF THE FAMILY WILL GIVE AVRIL PLENTY OF PRAISE.	4-7-79

Fig. 3.3 Health visitor's goal planning record form (Revill and Blunden, 1980)

One view of this kind of activity is that it is too lengthy to be really feasible within the constraints of the work situation. If, however, we are to use goal planning and to develop realistic ways of achieving goals, then we must acquire the appropriate skills. Some of what is included in goal steps may remain implicit but, if this is the case, it will hinder different members of staff from knowing how far patients have progressed, and hence may impede effective caring for them. It also lessens the chances of inexperienced nurses extending their knowledge of the appropriate sequence and timing of behaviour to attain specific goals. Should there be a problem in achieving a particular goal step, then this should immediately alert everyone involved to the advisability of not going any further, since later steps are likely to be impossible if earlier ones have not yet been achieved.

This method has been used successfully by health visitors with mentally handicapped people. It would be useful to test it in the rehabilitation field and in other settings in which goal steps can be clearly defined.

The other major reason for analysing goals into goal steps is to *motivate* nurses and patients. Theoretically, we know that we learn best by being rewarded for appropriate behaviour. To achieve progress – and to be seen to be achieving progress – is highly rewarding for nurses and patients. Analysing behaviour into several goal steps provides a number of opportunities for rewards, during the often very lengthy progress to achieving a final goal. Thus, as Revill and Blunden have shown, goal steps have a motivating quality.

THE TIMING OF GOALS

We have already indicated that an important component of goals is the time-span within which they should be achieved. The relevant time-span for goals will, however, vary according to different care settings, the nature of patients' problems, their abilities and resources.

SHORT-TERM GOALS

Most patients in acute settings are likely to have some short-term goals – to be achieved now, today, or in the space of a day or two. Many goal steps could be seen as short-term goals, for instance, that the patient will:

- drink 2000 mls. of fluid in 24 hours
- go to the shop by himself today
- report gains in insight, in response to his wife's visit on Tuesday
- feed her baby on demand with breast milk from 6 am.

There are some other examples of short-term goals in the case notes on Peter O. in the *Case Files*. Because short-term goals are so precise, they are of major importance to the evaluation stage of the process of nursing (described in Module 5). Using them can also influence the pace at which nursing activities progress, by permitting care to move on to the accomplishment of the next goal step as quickly as possible. In this way, they can increase efficiency.

GOALS IN SHORT-TERM CARE

Some of the nurses who have expressed most difficulty in adopting a problem-oriented approach work in short-term care settings – in theatre, out-patient and family planning clinics, and day-surgery units. In these settings, goals must invariably be very short-term and may even have to be achieved in a single nurse-patient encounter – for example, a man learning to use a new type of colostomy appliance in a single visit to a stoma therapist, or a woman learning

how to insert a diaphragm. In short-term care, it is important to decide realistically what goals can be achieved in the available time.

When emergencies occur, such as antepartum haemorrhage or some of the cardiac problems which occur in intensive care and coronary care units, then there must, of course, be immediate action. This does not mean that goal planning is irrelevant, only that it happens quickly, that goals are not written down and are unlikely to be based on a mutual agreement with the patient. These crises are examples of the process of nursing being adapted to the setting in which it is being practised, and demonstrate the need for flexibility in its application.

LONG-TERM GOALS

Long-term goals have a much longer time-span, usually of weeks to months. They may relate to the development of a complex skill such as speech, or to conditions which may take a long time to resolve, losing weight, for example. Alternatively, they may apply to the maintenance of a condition, such as keeping a job for six months or carrying out an exercise programme.

Some goals may not have a specified time-span, either because they are enduring and will cease only when the patient dies, or because they are there as a source of direction, but are of a kind where it is hard to attach a specific attainment date. Without long-term goals, however, it could be difficult to determine in which direction to develop activities and where to place the major emphasis of care.

Activity 3.6   **Allow 15 minutes**

Short or long-term goals?

This activity tests your professional knowledge about the time it is likely to take a patient to meet identified goals and goal steps.

1 For Activity 3.2 (p. 60) you wrote two patient goal statements.

Look at these again and identify appropriate time limits for these goals. Note whether each one is short or long-term.

2 Now try to break down each one into goal steps and identify an appropriate time by which the patient might achieve each step.

Author's comment
Check that your goal steps each contain the appropriate elements of a goal statement. In practice, you are likely to find that you have to adjust timings according to patient capabilities, the resources available to *achieve the goals in terms of equipment and personnel, and your own developing skills in deciding what is feasible. The rate at which goals are achieved can be a useful measure of the efficiency and effectiveness of care and, in this respect, could serve as a component of evaluation.*

Being able to write a clear goal statement is a necessary first step, but is not sufficient in itself to ensure a goal-directed approach to nursing. It is necessary also to be able to identify *appropriate* goals with patients and to decide their *priority*.

SELECTING GOALS

APPROPRIATE GOALS

Professional knowledge is necessary to identify the appropriate behaviour which will be indicative of a goal being met. We learn the signs of good hydration and normal temperature but more sophisticated behaviours, like mother-infant bonding or self-assertiveness, are more difficult to measure. It is also difficult to identify external behaviour indicative of internal emotional states such as anxiety, or cognitive states like confusion. It is often hard, for example, to decide if an old person is confused or deaf. In such instances, there is a growing use of standardised assessment instruments such as the Hospital Anxiety and Depression Scale, referred to in Module 2 (p. 45). A goal could be to aim for a particular score on a standardised scale over a defined period.

The appropriate level of goal for which to aim will depend on what the patient assessment has told you about the patient and how much he is likely to achieve. However, we need to be wary of setting goals that are well-nigh impossible to attain or those which do not permit the patient to achieve optimally, and this requires skill.

ESTABLISHING GOAL PRIORITIES

Most patients have complex problems which necessitate setting a variety of goals. It is unlikely to be possible to work on all goals simultaneously.

The most important goals, and those which should be met first, can be determined by working out goal priorities, in conjunction with patients. These will depend on the *urgency* of problems, with those which are life-threatening being afforded the highest priority, and it can be assumed, in most instances, that these will be agreed by patients and their families. This cannot, however, be taken for granted. Members of some religious sects, for example, would refuse a blood transfusion. Some patients may prefer not to receive cytotoxic therapy, changing their goals from cure to the alleviation of their symptoms, by means other than cytotoxic drugs. Some patients may have the welfare of others as a first priority, rather than their own welfare.

A crude way of ranking goals could be to correlate them with the different levels described in Maslow's *hierarchy of needs* (Figure 1.3, p. 10). However, even within a single level, such as that relating to physiological needs, there could be a range of goals. In addition, problems at one level may become manifest in others. Depression, for example, might result in both a lack of self-esteem and an indifference to physiological needs, with reduced eating and exercise and a disregard for personal safety. This brings us back to the question of which goals should have the highest priority.

Activity 3.7   **Allow 5 minutes**

Selecting priorities
This activity provides an example of possible differences in perspective in identifying priorities for action.

Look at the following list of broad goals identified for a mentally handicapped eight year-old boy and his parents.

1 Take on the perspective of **parent** and put a tick beside the two to which you, as a parent, would give highest priority and a cross beside the two to which you would give least priority.

	Parent	Nurse
• increase social activity		
• control violent movements		
• stop dribbling		
• dress unaided		
• be continent of urine		
• be continent of faeces		
• feed himself		
• reduce aggressive behaviour		
• stop screaming when left alone		
• minimise feelings of personal failure.		

2 Now do the same activity from the perspective of a **nurse** who is caring for the child.

You may want to compare your views with other group members.

There are no right answers to this activity and you will discover that views are likely to differ, according to whether you are a nurse or a parent. In reality, views will also differ between parents and between nurses. You may think of some potential problems of this child which might be more stressful for you than those listed above. In order to support patients and their families, we have to find out first what they regard as problems and what produces stress for them. Efforts can then be focused initially on goals which relate to the most pressing problems of the individuals and families concerned.

We cannot assume either that there will necessarily be agreement between what health workers regard as priorities, or indeed as appropriate goals. Remember that the two district nurses whom you saw talking with Flo in the videotape shown in Group Session 1, held different views on the importance of Flo losing weight. The general practitioner's opinion that this should have high priority was also mentioned. In the future, Flo may decide that her skin and weight problems are sufficiently severe to justify reconsidering her priorities, in which case the district nurse would revise goals with her and with her general practitioner.

RE-ORDERING PRIORITIES

At different times, problems will assume different priorities as some become worse, some are resolved and new ones emerge. The re-ordering of priorities may also result from the patient wishing to make changes, or from different resources becoming available to facilitate meeting a goal.

A patient with severe walking difficulties, who lives in an upstairs flat, will obtain a different outlook on life and change his problem priority list if he is rehoused on the ground floor and can use a wheelchair. Patients with alcohol problems are likely to re-order their priorities once they have brought their drinking under control. New mothers will be little concerned with play until they have managed to establish a sleep routine for themselves and their babies and are more confident in handling and feeding them. While goals may remain the same, priorities about which goals to attain first will vary according to circumstances.

A re-assessment of goals is also required when new and different problems present themselves. Mr Wallace, referred to earlier, may be regaining mobility quite well and be walking 25 metres, three times a day. Should a severe respiratory tract infection occur, then new goals will have to be set in response to the new problems which have arisen. These are likely to give high priority to dealing with his chest problems and his next goal plan – for walking up and down stairs – will have to be put aside until his breathing improves and his temperature is lowered.

A patient in severe pain will usually give relief of pain a high priority. However, if the measures required to achieve this prevent him from doing something important, he may be prepared, at times, to endure pain in order to achieve other goals. Patients who are terminally ill may choose to meet important life goals (such as making a journey to a special place or going to a wedding or christening),

preferring to tolerate pain or to accept some adjustment to their pain control regime, in order to achieve what is their most important goal at that time.

POSITIVE GOALS

The priority given to a goal could also be related to what patients are likely to be able to attain *most easily*. One danger to be avoided in using a problem-oriented approach is to focus on problems as things which patients are unable to do or which they lack, thus minimising and underestimating their capacity for change. The other side of the equation is what patients *are* able to do, what motivates them, what their strengths are and what adaptive behaviours are within their capabilities. Note that the health visitor working with Avril (Figure 3.3) capitalised on her patient's strengths, while helping her to develop new behaviour.

Recently, greater emphasis has been placed on increasing the range of possible behaviours, rather than on trying to eliminate what is regarded as problem behaviour. Fleming, Barrowclough and Whitmore (1983) describe how they improved the behaviour of elderly demented patients by making the kind of activities associated with problem behaviour purposeful, rather than by trying to eradicate the 'problem' behaviour itself. One patient's problem, as perceived by the nurses, was his tendency to 'wander' round the busy psychogeriatric ward. An increase in activity, by involving him in doing things in a structured way, alleviated the 'problem'. Of course, the real problem could have been one of boredom and inactivity which manifested as wandering. This 'constructional' approach, which was developed by Goldiamond (1976) is positive, focusing on the growth of appropriate behaviour, rather than on a reduction in the frequency of 'problems'.

A tendency to focus either on eradicating problem behaviour, or on what patients *cannot* do for themselves, may reflect a belief by nurses that their role is primarily to do things for patients, thus justifying nursing intervention to assist them. While this is most obvious in long-term care for mentally ill, handicapped and elderly people, it is equally relevant in other settings. A problem may be identified that "since her operation, Mrs Bailey does not take as much interest in other people as she used to. She seems to be more introverted and keeps to her own room for much of the time".

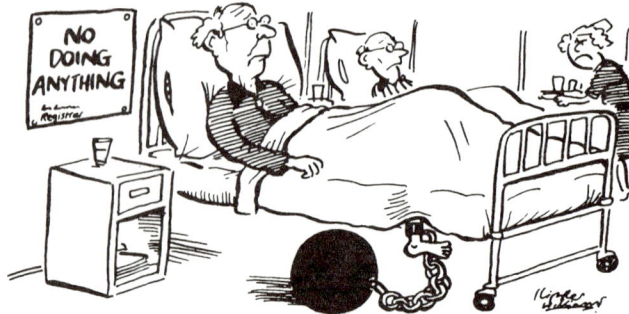

Here, the problem is stated negatively. However, it could be stated in a positive way: "Mrs Bailey will be offered opportunities to help her to mix with other people". This kind of positive statement can then give rise to positively-stated goals:

Mrs Bailey will have coffee in the lounge with other residents, every morning. Nurses will assist her to attain this goal by offering her the opportunity to do so.

Mrs Bailey will help her favourite nursing assistant to take the tea round to other residents, tomorrow afternoon.

When defining problems and constructing goals, we need to overcome a tendency to regard problems always in a negative way, or to minimise patients' positive strengths.

Activity 3.8   Allow 10 minutes

Stating goals positively

This activity provides practice in framing goals in a positive way.

Rewrite each of the following negatively-stated problems, indicating (a) an example of positive behaviour appropriate to each one and (b) a goal statement to assist in achieving this behaviour:

1 Mr Tate is constipated. His diet is without roughage and he takes no exercise.

2 Miss Miles has had two abortions and two unplanned pregnancies, and she cannot remember to take her contraceptive pills regularly.

3 Fred gets his tablets mixed up.

Author's comment
See p. 82.

Orientation towards those activities which patients *can* do is found in the nursing models discussed in earlier modules. Roper, Logan and Tierney's model, which includes a dependence/independence continuum (Figure 1.6), can be used to structure problems and goals to provide a means of assessing the patient's level of independence in each of the activities of living. Orem is even more emphatic, since her model is based on the belief that self-maintenance and self-regulation are crucial factors in determining how well individuals function. If a goal of nursing is to assist individuals to meet their own self-care needs, then self-care must be a central principle in setting goals. However, Orem's life change factors, shown in Figure 1.8, do emphasise negative influences on self-care. Perhaps more attention should be given to known positive influences in promoting self-development. Saxton and Hyland also refer to a major goal of nursing as being to assist patients to make healthy adaptations to stress, which will lead to development. Sometimes, however, goals for patients have to be framed in terms of maintenance, or of slowing down deterioration, especially among the very elderly and chronically sick. In all settings, goals should emphasise and capitalise on what patients *can* do.

MUTUAL GOAL SETTING

INVOLVING PATIENTS

Helping patients to assume greater responsibility for their own health is an important focus of activity for *all* nurses. All too often the emphasis is on attempting to gain patients' *compliance* with goals, with the methods to attain them being determined by others – nurses, as well as other members of the health team. Apart from the ethical issue of patients' rights to be involved in making decisions about their own health and well-being, research evidence suggests that patient participation in goal setting can result in more effective achievement and greater satisfaction for those providing health care.

British studies in this field are lacking, but a study was conducted in the United States by Hefferin (1979) in medical-surgical and psychiatric in-patient units and in out-patient departments. Patients were assisted by trained nurses to identify health goals for themselves, to set target dates for their achievement and to write statements on how to achieve these goals. A control group did not participate in their own goal setting. The findings showed that better progress was achieved by those patients who actively participated in goal setting and that they took fewer days to attain goals. The nurses, who had received some training in setting goals with patients, also reported more satisfaction with their work.

This study is important because it was undertaken with patients in general hospital wards and out-patients, as well as with psychiatric patients. In Britain, the practice of developing goal contracts with patients is well established in some mental handicap and psychiatric settings, including day hospitals, but it is used to a far lesser extent elsewhere.

Willer and Miller (1976) and Galano (1977) have shown the importance of direct participation of clients in all stages of the identification and planning of goals. The approach is not so effective if only part of this procedure is included – if patients have goals set *for* them, or are only involved in deciding responsibilities for achieving them or in receiving feedback about their attainments. These studies show that a fully collaborative approach led to both more effective therapy and greater client commitment to therapy. Equally important was the finding that when clients were fully involved in goal setting, it did *not* result in goals that were any less or more difficult or useful than when clients were not involved.

What the American studies suggest then, is that using a goal-directed approach, which fully involves patients who are coherent and able to discuss their health goals, is not only rational and ethical but also produces better results for patients and adds to nurses' job satisfaction.

It would be useful to replicate this work in the United Kingdom to find out how patients here respond to being invited to become *full* partners in their care, and to establish whether there are any culturally specific factors which might influence the effectiveness of this approach.

Of course, not all patients are able to make decisions for themselves nor to be full partners in setting goals. Patients who are unconscious, severely confused or mentally handicapped are obvious examples. In these cases, it would fall to relatives or friends to become involved in establishing appropriate goals with nurses.

CONFLICTING GOALS

It would be naive to assume that patient goals will always correspond with those of health care professionals – be they doctors, nurses or other members of the health care team – or that professionals will always agree on what is most appropriate.

CONFLICTS WITH PATIENTS

This module has stressed that goals which nurses set should derive from *identified patient problems* and that the chances of obtaining agreement between nurses and patients about goals are increased if they are worked out in partnership.

It would be a great waste of effort for a nurse caring for a depressed patient who is unconcerned about her appearance, to set goals for the patient to apply cosmetics and style her hair, if she has never done so and has no future intention of ever doing so. Similarly, before appropriate goals can be established for dealing with potential problems associated with either breast or bottle-feeding, it needs to be established how a prospective mother plans to feed her baby. Even though a patient has sought help for some health problem, he may set goals which are quite different from those planned by health care workers. This is not surprising given our differences in value systems and perspectives on life, as well as knowledge about health matters.

Flo, the overweight lady with rheumatic problems shown in the videotape for Group Session 1, had a very different view of what she wanted from life than had her general practitioner and one of the nurses. Losing weight was not on her agenda.

There is no absolute right or wrong in this kind of situation; it is a matter of different perspectives. A patient with cardiac problems may prefer to continue to "burn the candle at both ends", despite

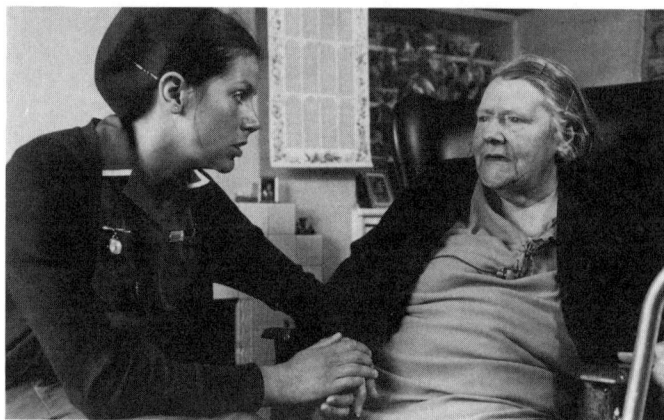

Whose priority is dieting?

being warned of the potential consequences. This is his choice and reflects a goal which can differ from that of the nurse, who is trying to encourage him to adopt a life style likely to prevent a recurrence of his cardiac problems.

Sometimes, conflicts are more about means than ends. Patients are often detained in hospital to die or to give birth, because *health staff* consider this to be most appropriate. Both patients and staff, and perhaps families, may aspire to the same goals but they believe that there are very different methods of attaining them. Obtaining an understanding of the patient's point of view could help to avoid or resolve a conflict, without detriment to meeting the goal and perhaps positively increasing the chances of accomplishing it.

There are many possible reasons for differences of opinion, including social and cultural factors, and perhaps previous unpleasant experiences. However, the woman who seeks a very short stay in hospital after having a baby is not necessarily making a negative comment on the care she received last time in hospital; she may simply prefer to return to her family as soon as possible and regard this as the best way of integrating the new baby into it.

At times, there may be a tendency to misinterpret what are really differences in goals between patients and nurses and to label them 'personality clashes', because the patient is seen to resist or not to comply. Perhaps, from the patients' perspective, the same could be said of nurses.

Nevertheless, labels such as 'demanding' and 'unco-operative' are not infrequently applied to patients. Rather than simply slotting him into the 'problem patient' category, it would be more helpful to find out *why* the patient is behaving in this way, and to examine whether the problems identified and the goals set for the patient are really ones which he regards as either appropriate or important.

Patients may respond to conflict by withdrawing – becoming apathetic, refusing to participate, avoiding nurses or missing appointments. They may become more hostile in their response to suggestions and become aggressive. Similar behaviour towards patients can sometimes be observed on the part of nurses, when patients refuse to meet nurses' goals. Nurses may manifest this by provoking fear, shame or guilt in their patients, in order to try to achieve compliance.

Of course, some goal differences result from nurses having greater technical knowledge, for example about the importance of women having cervical smears, or the possibly negative consequences of too rapid a return to work after major surgery or radiotherapy. However, it is not always a case of nurses knowing best; often, in fact, the patient knows better what is right for him. Arriving at an agreed list of goals is not only a matter of listening to each other – but sometimes of teaching and learning from each other.

But what of those occasions when agreement cannot be reached? When it is important that a paraplegic patient is moved regularly to avoid pressure and possible skin breakdown, but he refuses to have his sleep interrupted just to be turned and does not want to go on "one of those fancy beds", the patient's goal is uninterrupted sleep. This taxes nurses' ingenuity to find a way of relieving pressure regularly, without always having to wake the patient up to do it. They are part way there, however, by acknowledging that there is a difference in goals, at least during the night. How much control should patients have to determine what will happen to them?

Do you, for instance, believe:

- that patients should always co-operate readily with the plan of care, because it is drawn up by nurses who are educated to know what is best for them?

- that patients should make their own decisions whenever they are able, after being informed of the options and probable outcomes?

At times, the notion of *clients* rather than patients is helpful. Clients seek the advice and help of professionals; they are not under the power of professionals. Ultimately, clients can take or reject the advice given them and are, in the end, responsible for this decision. Apart from those unable to assume this responsibility, patients are, in the final analysis, responsible – but may sometimes require help, guidance, advice, information and support to be able to assume this role.

Activity 3.9   Allow 10 minutes
Goals in partnership

This activity provides an opportunity for you to consider the extent to which patients and their families could be involved in goal planning.

Turn back to the goals you set for your patient in Activity 3.2 on p. 60.

1 Look at each goal and decide to what extent it was, or could have been, set in partnership with the patient. Then consider whether, in each case, priorities about goals could be agreed with the patient or his family.

2 Had it been another patient with the same problems, might the goals or their priority have been different? Might the goals have been different if you or one of your family had been the patient? Use your imagination and write down some different goals for the same problem.

Author's comment
The types of goals that take account of individual variations are generally those which are not related to basic physiological states. There tends to be more similarity than difference between patients' physiological functioning, although this will of course depend on the patient's metabolism and level of functioning.

Once physiological needs are satisfied, then problems and appropriate goals in other spheres are likely to be much more varied. The amount of weight loss, the degree of mobility, the quality of manipulative skills, the extent of social integration to be achieved, or the number of cigarettes to be smoked will all vary according to the status, the ability, the attitude and wishes of the patient involved.

DIFFERENCES AMONG PROFESSIONALS

On occasion, different professionals may set different goals for patients. One, for example, may wish to resuscitate a patient who has collapsed, with the goal of restoring life; another may wish the patient to die peacefully and to avoid the risk of brain damage. A patient may have problems of liver damage and a major goal would be to rest the liver. However, to do so may result in withholding analgesia when severe pain is being experienced. Another goal for this patient would be associated with the relieving of pain. Again, there is conflict between two goals, this time over which should have priority.

Sometimes, there may be conflicting opinions about the means used to achieve goals, rather than about the goals themselves. For example, a psychiatrist's method of assisting a very anxious patient with advanced cancer who is referred to him, could be to confront him with the reality of his illness and the possibility of death. Unknown to the psychiatrist, the radiotherapist and the nurses involved in his care may be using tactics which deny the real nature of the illness and the possibility of it being fatal. Both approaches are concerned with the problem of anxiety and its alleviation, but the means of doing so are in opposition and the patient suffers.

Differences in orientation between professionals may result from different definitions of illness. When haemoglobin reaches a certain low level, the patient is judged as anaemic and corrective therapy advised. One very elderly lady, aged 101 years, who still enjoyed going out for drives in her son's car, was thought pale by her district nurse. A blood test showed that her haemoglobin level was less than half the desirable level. Her general practitioner urged her to go into hospital for a blood transfusion. The district nurse's view was that she was not really 'ill', to the extent that she needed to go into hospital to have a blood transfusion, but that she might benefit from an oral iron preparation and improved diet. The woman herself felt neither ill nor incapacitated and wanted nothing to do with transfusions or medicines. These different interpretations of the problem by those involved influenced what were regarded as appropriate goals and ways of achieving them.

Clearly, it is important for there to be an attempt to reach agreement about goals and their priorities, both among professionals and with patients. Ideally, consensus is achieved through discussion at team or ward meetings, with the interests of the patient being the central focus. On occasion, it will not be possible to achieve consensus, in which case someone will be responsible for making the final decision about which goals to set and their priority. In practice, when goals are set by a number of professionals, the recommendation of the senior member is most likely to be adopted. Others in the team may not fully approve or agree, but for the patient it is important that all professionals work toward the same rather than opposing goals.

DIFFERENCES AMONG NURSES

In Module 2, we suggested that your views of nursing will influence your initial identification of problems. In the same way, your views will influence the goals which you consider to be appropriate. If a physically handicapped patient expresses a problem of sexual frustration, nurses might set goals associated with the patient meeting his sexual needs or with denying that he has any, depending on their views. When such radical differences can and do occur, the importance of establishing a *shared perspective* among all those involved in the care of a patient is obvious.

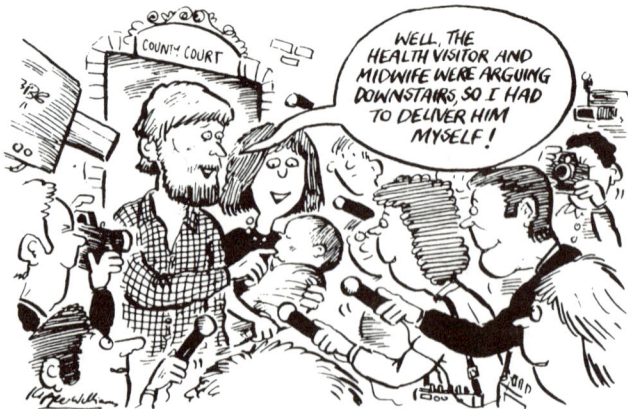

WELL, THE HEALTH VISITOR AND MIDWIFE WERE ARGUING DOWNSTAIRS, SO I HAD TO DELIVER HIM MYSELF!

An overall aim of nursing may be agreed to be helping patients or clients to participate in living as effectively as possible. This does not specify what aspects of living, nor how much responsibility lies with nurses for promoting independence. Matters like these will be influenced by your own, often implicit, model of nursing as well as by the organisation in which you work. To avoid conflict, open discussion and the attainment of agreement about goals need to be a regular feature of ward or primary care team conferences.

Activity 3.10   **Allow 10 minutes**

Collaboration in goal setting
You have now covered a great deal of ground and this activity gives you an opportunity to reflect on what you have learned, by re-examining the goals which you set at the beginning of this module. It also asks you to consider the issue of collaboration in goal setting.

1 Look carefully at the goals which you set for a patient in Activity 3.2 (p. 60). You may feel that you have now learned more about goals and want to refine them, making sure that they are patient-centred.
2 Suggest whether collaboration between nurses and other health care workers would be required in setting and helping the patient to meet any of these goals and, if so, identify which other professionals would be involved.

Author's comment
Depending on the particular patient, there may be problems and associated goals with which several different professions are dealing simultaneously, each bringing their own knowledge to bear. Goals associated with pain relief, reducing weight, expectorating are obvious examples. In some instances, such as assisting a patient to talk again, the speech therapist may be the person primarily involved in setting goals, but nurses can assist the patient to attain them by using the same approach as the therapist, in her absence.

The occupational therapist may be promoting self-care goals by teaching a patient how to feed and dress himself as well as how to manage the toilet. The nurses, however, may find it easier to feed and dress the patient themselves and to manage his incontinence garments for him. It is important to clarify how both sets of professionals can work together for the patient's benefit.

Because of the nature of nursing, it is possible that nursing-related goals will encompass a wider range of patient behaviour than do those of any other single profession, for example, goals associated with personal hygiene, keeping occupied or adjusting to chronic illness. This will depend on the breadth of your own perspective on nursing in relation to assisting patients to develop and live to their maximum potential.

This completes the first section of the module on setting goals. Throughout, it has been emphasised that goals should be patient-centred. This means that they should be statements about what will be achieved by the patient or client, although involving assistance from nurses, other professionals, family or friends. Nevertheless, they refer to behaviour that patients will achieve, rather than that which nurses will carry out. Once you have managed to overcome the tendency to write goals as nursing actions, you will be able to develop your skills in setting goals more fully.

Always bear in mind that goals should be set in terms of *observable* patient behaviour or states.

PLANNING HOW TO ATTAIN GOALS

In the previous sections on goal planning, you have learned about:

- collaborating with patients and other professionals to decide appropriate patient goals
- stating these goals in behavioural terms
- analysing goals into a number of steps
- setting priorities among goals.

Now you need to be able to specify means of achieving goals. Consideration of means will have entered into decisions about priorities, because goals which are easy to attain, as well as those which are related to high risk, are likely to feature prominently. The means of attaining goals will also take account of patients' particular strengths or resources, which you will have identified during the assessment step of the process of nursing. We have discussed how important it is to capitalise on patients' strengths in goal setting.

STATING NURSING PRESCRIPTIONS FOR CARE

Statements about how to attain goals are *nursing prescriptions for care*. They will draw on your professional knowledge, but will be decided, wherever possible, in consultation with patients as well as with colleagues. The feasibility of putting your ideas into practice – the resources available to you in terms of skills, staff, time and equipment – will be an important feature in decision making. The aim will be to individualise care and to make it appropriate to solving the problems of patients and their families.

Various terms are used to describe statements about nursing actions to meet goals: nursing orders, nursing prescriptions, nursing activities, nursing interventions or nursing plans. In essence, they tell us what nurses will do to, with and for patients and are written in the care plan section of the patient's nursing notes.

COMPONENTS OF NURSING PRESCRIPTIONS

Like goal statements, nursing prescriptions need to contain a number of specific components. These are likely to include some or all of those shown in Figure 3.4.

1 Date: including a date enables you to check when the order was introduced so that when it comes to be reviewed, its duration is known. The time intervals for reviewing prescribed care will vary of course, depending on whether a short, medium or long-term goal is involved. A review will probably lead to modifications – deleting activities associated with goals which have been achieved, amending them to make them more effective or adding new ones. It is closely linked to evaluation of whether the action prescribed is appropriate to the attainment of the specified goal, as shown by progress towards the goal.

1 Date	14th April
2 Which nurse	S/N Crump
3 What a nurse will do to, with and for the patient	Observe only
4 What the patient will do	Ascend and descend 20 stairs
5 How and where the patient, nurse or both will do it	Without assistance on the stairs between wards O–P
6 Time element	Once daily just before lunch.
7 Signature	Jean Crump.

Fig. 3.4 Components of a nursing prescription for care

2 Which nurse: this may not actually be specified since it will sometimes depend on staff availability, according to shifts and the demands of other patients. Sometimes, however, a specific nurse will be identified because she has developed a particular relationship with the patient, or because she has some special skill and will therefore be the person most able to assist him to meet the goal: for example, a clinical nurse specialist such as a stoma or ostomy nurse, a nurse therapist in psychiatry, or simply a nurse in the ward team who is well suited to the patient and the care he requires. It is important to indicate when more than one nurse should be involved. This can be especially important when lifting and moving heavy patients to avoid injury to either nurse or patient, or when difficult dressings have to be changed.

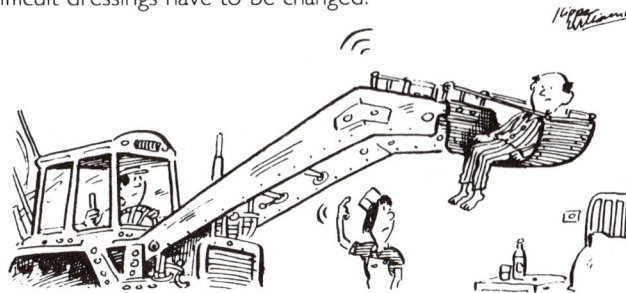

3 What the nurse(s) will do: this might refer to nurses providing resources to help patients to be as fully independent as possible, such as aids to assist eating or modified clothing. Nurses themselves may carry out activities; they may feed, dress or inject the patient. At other times, it might be more appropriate to refer on to others who can assist with a particular goal – another professional or parent, for instance. The nurse's role may be merely to remind the patient to carry out an activity or to check that he has done so.

Specificity is important so that no doubt is left about *which* nurse is involved and *what* the nurse carrying out the prescription is to do. On reflection, I wonder what I meant when I told nurses to "keep an eye on" a patient feeling suicidal in a Radiotherapy Ward – to stay in the patient's room all the time and observe, to talk to the patient every few minutes, to try to ascertain the likelihood of a suicide attempt and plan further on the basis of that? To be able to make a clear statement about *what* to do demands knowledge about effective nursing strategies to resolve problems, yet it is here that nurses' language is often most imprecise.

Activity 3.11   Allow 5 minutes

How clear are our prescriptions?

This activity should help you to think critically about the precision of your own prescriptions for care.

A commonly used prescription in nursing is to "reassure" the patient. Write down all the different ways you can think of to reassure patients.

Author's comment
You are likely to have included such behaviour as:

Tell him not to worry	*Tell him this is normal*
Stay with him	*Tell him what to expect*
Hold his hand	*Stay away to indicate you know he can manage by himself*
Listen to his fears	*Touch him*
Tell him how well he is doing	*Introduce him to others who have managed to overcome the same stress.*

For different patients, and for the same patient at different times, the most appropriate approach will vary.

We regularly use words like 'teach', 'mobilise', 'push' (as in fluids), 'counsel' and 'help', all of which are imprecise. Each nursing activity is likely to contain some elaboration of 'where' and 'what': "teach how to give insulin", "mobilise the affected knee joints", "counsel about the stillbirth". It is important that prescriptions contain more than this, however. Teaching someone how to give insulin can involve description, demonstration and practice of the skills of drawing up the injection as well as carrying it out, calculating the dosage and maintaining a healthy injection site. "Mobilising joints" may involve only certain joints and both active and passive movements. Again, being specific is of major importance.

Saxton and Hyland's stress-adaptation model is useful here, because it specifies that nursing interventions are directed toward preventing, limiting or reducing stress. It also indicates the appropr-

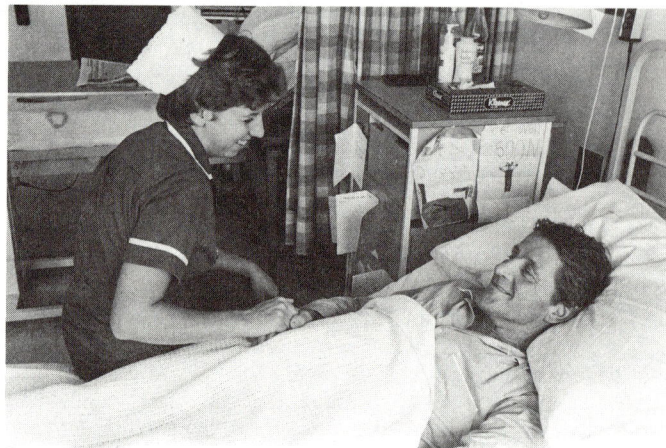

Reassuring a patient?

riate *level* of intervention to assist the individual's adaptations: supporting, limiting, altering, interrupting or supplementing the patient's own responses. While models cannot prescribe the actual care to be given, this one focuses attention on the most appropriate level of intervention.

Of course, one goal may be reached by several different interventions. An intake of 2000 mls. fluid may be by intravenous infusion, orally or intraperitoneally. Increasing parenting skills may involve different forms of teaching, group discussions, watching videos or films, actually handling babies or reading appropriate literature. The different possibilities need to be taken into account to decide what is feasible, most acceptable and most likely to produce the best results. In other words, that the means achieve the ends we seek.

4 What the patient will do: Orem's self-care model of nursing lays particular emphasis on the agent of care – whether the patient himself, the nurse or some other person. Since *self-care* is the major feature of this model, and indeed may be a goal to which nurses and patients aspire, the patient's part in care must be clearly indicated. Anyone who has children, or has tried to teach a skill to another person, knows that it is often easier and quicker just to do the task oneself. However, this could be detrimental to the other person's interests and could increase nurses' work. For example, incontinence is often 'contained', rather than efforts being made to train or retrain patients to be continent. A clear definition of what the patient will do not only makes for a more useful prescription of care, but also promotes awareness that patients have an important – and often the major – role to play in achieving goals.

Of course, not all patients can actively participate in all or perhaps any of their care, if they are comatose, for example, but we can try to give patients as much responsibility as possible. In psychiatric hospitals, removing responsibilities from patients has often resulted in major problems in their eventual rehabilitation. Equally, in other forms of long-stay care, it can make nurses' lives easier in the short term to do things for patients – cutting their toe nails, for instance, but it may not always be the most positive approach. In shorter-stay settings the same holds true. Hospital policy may prevent patients being responsible for their own medication; however, once they are discharged home they are left to manage and have a better chance of succeeding if they have already been able to take on as much responsibility for their own care as possible.

Obviously, what is to be done by the patient and what by the nurse may change over time. A patient may have needed assistance from a nurse yesterday to walk up and down stairs, whereas today it is only necessary for her to observe him.

A gradual increase in responsibility for self-care would be motivating for most patients. For those patients whose self-care activities have *had* to be assumed by nurses, great sensitivity is demanded so as not to reduce their own self-respect.

5 Conditions: prescribing nursing care is not only a question of who does what, but also of the conditions under which it will be performed. In the example shown in Figure 3.4 (p. 71), the conditions related to how and where the patient would manage stairs. Conditions could also relate to whether a specific piece of equipment is to be used, for example to take a patient to the bath, or to the kinds of rewards available to patients when specific behaviours are achieved – praise, or something it is known that the patient enjoys, such as being stroked. By specifying conditions, those carrying out the care are then relieved of having to make their own interpretation of what is required and how they are to go about doing it. The possibility of error is reduced and the likelihood of a more consistent pattern of care is increased.

6 The time element: the time element refers to when, how often and for how long nursing actions should take place. When different people are involved it may be appropriate to state time by the clock, as we do with medication prescriptions, rather than in terms of how often. However, the times at which specific nursing activities take place can often be adjusted to meet a patient's preferred activity patterns. For instance, if visitors always come in the afternoon, it would be a pity if a patient on a regular turning schedule was always lying prone at that time.

Patient behaviour may be specified, when nursing activity is dependent on it. Some nursing intervention could be warranted "each time he goes to the toilet by himself", "when she is breathless", "if she reports feeling suicidal", or "when she reports pain".

The other important time element is duration. This is often specified in relation to the time allowed for visitors to see particular patients, such as those in intensive care. It is also relevant to oxygen therapy and inhalations, to exercise regimes and is sometimes specified for early breast-feeding.

It may be important, in some instances, to make explicit how long nurses should remain with patients. Bond (1978) observed that nurses in a general hospital rarely spent as long as three minutes with patients not requiring physical care, and Altschul (1972) observed the same phenomenon in psychiatric wards.

When goals require that nurses spend time with patients who do not require physical care – perhaps to assist them to understand the implications of their illness, or how to manage some symptom – then it may be helpful to specify a time period for just talking and to make the *purpose* of the talking clear. On the other hand, some patients, such as those in coronary care units where they should be resting, can be so bombarded with interruptions that it may be in their interests to specify a time interval when they will *not* be disturbed, in order that they can rest.

Nursing activity statements are, however, sometimes poorly defined in relation to time, if specified at all. Lelean (1973) observed how variable were such statements as "up for short periods" and "up for long periods", which made them of little value in guiding appropriate care. When a time element is included as a component of a nursing prescription then, like all the other components, it must be unambiguous.

7 Signature: the final element in a written nursing prescription is the signature of the prescriber. We are very careful that the doctor who prescribes medication signs the prescription. The same rule should apply in nursing, for the major reason that the nurse is accountable for care prescribed. This is important for professional reasons, that is that the care prescribed should adhere to professionally acceptable standards. It may also be necessary for legal reasons, in that the person responsible for prescribing an action may be required to defend it in a court of law.

Accountability for making nursing prescriptions lies with a nurse, that is, with a professionally qualified person. In practice, a nursing prescription is sometimes delegated to a nursing student or pupil, or to a nursing assistant or auxiliary. This may be to provide an educational or training opportunity, in which case the student would require supervision and assessment. It may be that the unqualified person is more familiar with, or knowledgeable about, a patient and so it is more appropriate that she prescribes care. It may be that there are no nurses with sufficient time or knowledge about a patient to write a prescription for his care and so an unqualified staff member must write it. Irrespective of who actually writes and signs the order, the fact remains that accountability rests with the *nurse* in charge of the patient's care. Therefore it is prudent, even though not required by law, to have any nursing order which bears the signature of a professionally unqualified person countersigned by a nurse with the authority to do so.

The second reason that a signature is required is simply that it is necessary to know who prescribed care so that, if necessary, clarification can be sought and the prescription reviewed with her. Often problem identification, goal planning and the choice of appropriate interventions will be carried out by the same person, especially if patient allocation or primary nursing methods of work organisation are involved. This will assist the cohesiveness of patient care planning.

Activity 3.12   Allow 5 minutes

Writing nursing prescriptions

This activity will help you to assess whether your written prescriptions for nursing care are as explicit as they might be.

You should now have a good idea of how to specify nursing actions for inclusion in a care plan. Look at the care plan which you have collected.

Does each prescribed nursing action include the following components: date, which nurse, what the nurse will do, what the patient will do, under what conditions, within what time frame, signature?

If not, re-write two nursing activities or prescriptions and include as many of these components as are relevant. If these nursing actions were complete or if you have no care plan, write two actions relevant to goals for Mr Wallace, the patient with the cerebrovascular accident (Activity 3.4, p. 61), or for one of your own patient's goals.

Author's comment

Achieving specificity may seem laborious, but how else can we ensure that there is a uniformity of approach and that appropriate care will be prescribed, to be given at the right time? Being this specific about nursing plans means that the prescription for care must be appropriate. If it is less than satisfactory the patient could suffer since, if all nurses strictly adhere to the nursing prescription, there will be no chance opportunity of alternative and perhaps better care being given. It is for this reason that the soundness of nursing actions is so important and writing them down really exposes our activities for the rest of the world to see. This may seem threatening, especially if there are uncertainties about knowing what is best in a particular situation, or if there are conflicts about appropriate means to attain goals. Often there is no one answer to a problem. However, attempting to make care explicit raises opportunities for discussion and agreement about what to do in this case and, of course, paves the way for sound evaluation of what is achieved and how it has been achieved. This process is as relevant to deciding how best to manage incontinence for an elderly patient as it is to the kind of catheter to use, when long-term catheterisation has become the final answer.

SELECTING NURSING PRESCRIPTIONS FOR CARE

SELECTING FROM ALTERNATIVES

You have learned something about how to state a nursing prescription, but can you be sure that the care which you are prescribing is the *best possible* within the resources available to you? When more than one form of care is possible, how do you decide, for example, whether to retrain a patient to continence or to contain the incon-

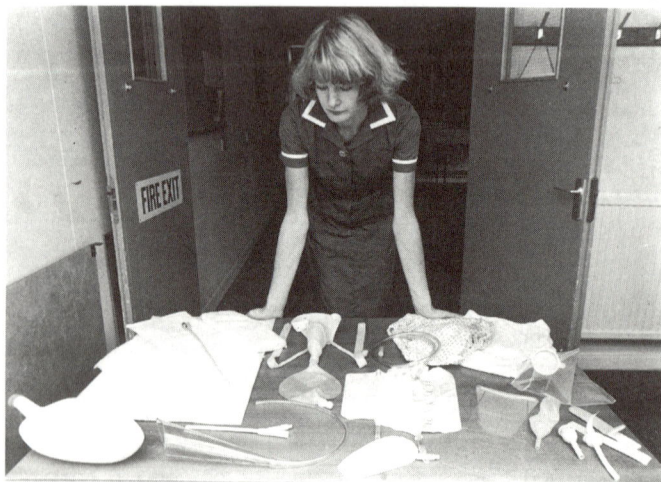

Spoiled for choice

tinence? Answers to these questions are grounded in your own and your colleagues' available nursing knowledge and the way in which it is used.

To take another example, if a patient has a problem of dehydration, how do you deal with it? The first level answer would be to increase the amount of fluid he takes in and/or to reduce the amount of fluid he puts out, although the most effective action will depend on knowing the *cause* of the problem. However, the *effects* of the problem, such as constipation and the danger of damage to the patient's skin and mouth, must also be considered. How will you deal with a dry or possibly dirty mouth? Correcting the dehydration will help, but should you also stimulate the naturally moistening and cleansing process of salivation? If so, how? – by asking the patient to imagine he is sucking a lemon, by giving him some diluted lemon juice or by cleansing with chemical substances? Once you really examine nursing, it is not always as simple as it may seem and there is certainly nothing routine about it.

PREVENTING PROBLEMS

Nursing prescriptions do not only apply to ways of achieving goals which deal with actual problems; they also apply to goals concerned with the prevention of problems. As an example, a major concern should be the prevention of hospital-acquired infection. Every year thousands of patients enter hospital infection-free, yet acquire some form of infection. Patients with indwelling urinary catheters are most at risk. Prescribed nursing care for all patients who have an indwelling urinary catheter should be monitored to prevent infection. Avoidance of urinary tract infection would be a specific goal, as discussed by Horsley (1982) and Bond and Hagel (1982). As a broad level of activity, we are learning better ways of helping an old person to maintain a sense of awareness and orientation, as exemplified in the work carried out by Holden and Sinebruchow (1978) and Hanley et al (1981). This approach, which has generally come to be known as 'reality orientation', requires very careful and controlled implementation in order to be effective. The work of Parkes (1979) has been useful in assisting us to identify and help those at most risk of suffering problems after bereavement.

This knowledge tells us how to carry out some aspects of patient care, but decisions about what to do will, to a large extent, ultimately rely on what nurses regard as the boundaries of nursing and what is relevant and appropriate for each patient.

RESEARCH-BASED PRACTICE

Many nursing interventions are decided on the basis of nursing ideology, past experience, routine or tradition. There is a growing concern however, that nursing practices should be based on sound research evidence, whilst not losing the vocational aspect of nursing. This is a difficult, but not impossible, challenge. Some nurses are earnestly searching for research evidence to guide their actions and have formed clinical care groups, to review such evidence in peer groups. A research base for nursing prescriptions provides part of the answer about what to include, but there still remains a large element of clinical judgment and experience to be used in deciding what is best for any individual patient. The approach to goal planning used by the health visitors working to develop the skills of mentally handicapped people (p. 62), was prompted by research evidence. However, the final decisions about which skills to develop and how to do so in analysing behaviour into smaller steps, depended on the health visitors' knowledge of their clients, on what was important and feasible in the settings involved and on their capacity to involve the patients and their parents in the scheme.

Activity 3.13	Allow 5 minutes

The basis of your practice

This activity asks you to examine the knowledge base of your practice.

Turn to the nursing prescriptions you wrote for Activity 3.12. Look at each one and decide the basis for each nursing action prescribed: is it routine, tradition, order from another authority, experience, intuition or research? More than one of these may be involved.

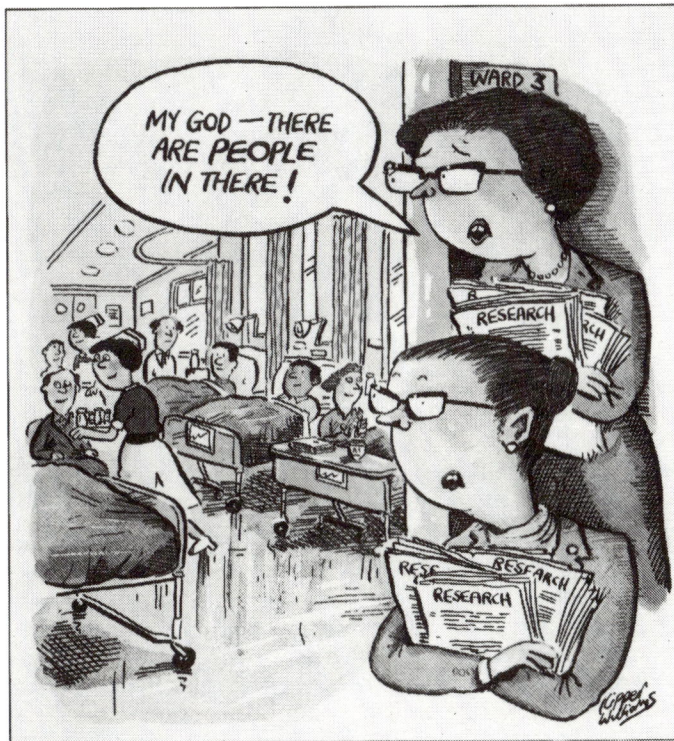

Author's comment
It is sometimes difficult to remember why a particular form of care has evolved, and who is responsible for having introduced it. Over time, particular forms of care become accepted practice. Shaving skin pre-operatively is one such example yet, when we examine why this is done, there is no evidence that it prevents infection – on the contrary, it can be harmful. There may be an assumption that it is a medical directive but on checking, this sometimes turns out not to be the case. It is important that 'accepted practice' is reviewed regularly, so that there is always good practice which, where possible, is based on sound evidence. For if it is not, have we any basis for talking about professional standards of care?

COMMUNICATING NURSING PLANS

AN ORAL TRADITION

Traditionally, in hospital, nursing orders have been discussed and passed on verbally at change of shift reports. While notes are kept, the passing on of information often relies heavily on oral communication. This tends to come more from the person in charge of the ward than from the person dealing with, and having more intimate knowledge of, the care of the patients being discussed. Some orders are generally written down, especially those which are medically derived; rather less often are those related to nursing interventions recorded in writing. There are widely-reported difficulties in communication between different care settings about patients but a health visitor, for example, needs full information about a new mother and baby, as does a district nurse about an elderly patient being discharged from hospital.

Attention to communicating *nursing* activities should influence the quality of communication between nurses themselves, and with other professionals. We have advocated using a very precise definition of goals and nursing prescriptions, and these must be communicated in the most manageable way, whilst remaining unambiguous, up-to-date and accessible. Emphasis is now placed on written communication, because of its availability to different members of staff.

WRITTEN CARE PLANS

The question is, in what format and where should written information be provided? This is not an issue that relates only to this step of the nursing process; it is relevant to all steps. Since we are trying to develop more systematic approaches to nursing care, its content needs to be placed into a total, logical communication system, which can be extended to encompass the total care given to patients by *all* health professionals.

The use of proforma for data collection has been discussed in Module 2. It is equally important to have well-organised proforma on which to record the patient's plan of care. Over time, different ones have evolved and are still in the process of development.

PROBLEM-ORIENTED RECORDING

The *problem-oriented medical record* is an approach first advocated by an American doctor, Lawrence Weed (1969). His central focus for organising care is what is happening to the patient, and he considers the patient's record to be the 'tool' which facilitates the accomplishment of goals set for and with the patient. Weed emphasises that *all* members of the health care team should contribute to the record, with the organisational basis being the patient. Despite being specifically patient-oriented, Weed uses the term

'problem-oriented *medical* record' rather than 'problem-oriented *patient* record'.

Weed advocates four basic phases of activity:

1 **The establishment of a data base:** what we have called assessment.

2 **The formation of a problem list:** which comes after the patient has been assessed.

3 **The preparation of an initial plan for each problem:** corresponding roughly to the planning stage discussed earlier in the module, i.e. goals and actions to achieve them. Weed, however, distinguishes between therapeutic, diagnostic and educational orders for care.

4 **The maintenance of progress notes on each problem:** written in a specific format, for which the acronym is SOAP. This format includes subjective data (S) related to the specific problem; objective data (O) related to the specific problem; an assessment (A) based on the subjective and objective data; the plans (P) to solve the problem. An example of patient notes structured around a single patient problem is illustrated in Figure 3.5.

COMPONENTS OF A CARE PLAN

A well-organised care plan should include the following four components:

1 **Present or potential nursing care problems:** their priority should be indicated and they should include all those which will be dealt with by nurses in this episode of care.

2 **Patient goals:** explicitly stated in terms of the patient's responses that will indicate that goals have been achieved.

3 **Nursing actions:** associated with each problem or goal, as a means of accomplishing the goal and relieving the problem. Nursing actions need to be stated in such a way that all nursing personnel, including auxiliary staff, will understand them.

4 **The signature** of the nurse or nurses responsible for writing the plan.

In addition to the plan, progress notes are necessary to record patient progress and responses so that nursing care may be evaluated and adjusted, where necessary.

BARRIERS TO WRITING CARE PLANS

Systematic approaches to nursing are dependent on how nurses conceptualise nursing. The written care plan is a synopsis of the thinking and knowledge which decide appropriate care. Yet nurses often resist writing care plans in the detail being advocated here. A number of reasons can be identified. Firstly, there are conceptual

Patient's name: Mr Glen		Problem no. 4: Nausea after stapedectomy	Date: 7.6.83	Time: 10am
Subjective	The problem from the patient's point of view, how he feels, changes he has noticed.	"My stomach feels upset. My head is dizzy."		
Objective	Information and observations, gathered from any other source: reports from lab, family, pertinent developments regarding the specific problem.	Had no breakfast, taking only sips of fluid; refuses to get out of bed because feels dizzy.		
Assessment	Impressions or conclusions about what is happening, as logically derived from the subjective and objective data collected.	Normal post-op dizziness and nausea.		
Plan	Immediate and future nursing actions to deal with specific problem. • diagnostic: likely to be medical tests to further investigate the problem or additional nursing investigations, by questioning patient further. • therapeutic: nursing interventions used to treat the specific problems. • education: what is taught to the patient and his family about the specific problem.	Re-assess every 2 hours. Offer anti-emetic as charted. Encourage fluids 100mls. every hour. Ascertain fluid preference. Start fluid balance chart. Explain nausea and dizziness are normal after an operation and that walking will help reduce dizziness. Encourage to keep own fluid balance chart.		

Progress notes on each problem are updated regularly. The goals for care could easily be added to these notes.
Part of a nursing care plan for this patient might then take the form:

Patient's name: Mr Glen			
Problem no.	Goals	Nursing actions	Signature
4 Nausea after stapedectomy	7.6.83/4.1 will report not feeling nauseated and will have begun to eat solid food by 6pm.	4.1 offer anti-emetic as charted until nausea disappears. Obtain food preferences for lunch and supper.	J. Crump
	7.6.83/4.2 will not show signs of dehydration by 10am on 8/6.	4.2 offer favourite drinks 100mls. every hour till 10pm. Ask patient to keep fluid balance chart and explain how to do so.	J. Crump
	7.6.83/4.3 report feeling less dizzy and be able to walk the length of the ward every half hour.	4.3 Explain that dizziness will gradually disappear if he walks more frequently. Walk with him twice from 10am then encourage him to walk alone. Observe that he does so.	J. Crump

This extract shows that it is useful to write the nursing action section adjacent to problems and goals, and care plans require sufficient space to do so.

Fig. 3.5 A problem-oriented record (adapted from Ulisse, 1978)

barriers associated with an unwillingness to commit oneself to paper and to identify clearly a plan of care, rather than only the desired outcomes or end results of care. Inherent in this is the uncertainty of what are the most appropriate goals for patients and ways of meeting them. However, such uncertainty is in itself an inherent feature of nursing because we deal with such complex physical, social and psychological problems. It is more difficult to decide how to encourage a disturbed new mother to accept her baby than it is to prescribe an antibiotic to combat an organism of known sensitivity. In nursing, there is sometimes no one right answer to a patient's problem, and it takes some courage to *write* a plan which may ultimately fail and which shows the uncertainty in which we often have to work.

However, unless we do write plans and make our proposed goals and actions clear, then it makes it more difficult to learn about the most successful ways of dealing with problems or to make the rationale for nursing actions explicit.

Secondly, there are organisational problems – the practical difficulties involved in introducing documentation into the current system of staff organisation. If no one nurse has major responsibility for a patient, then who is responsible for writing the care plan? Is it everyone's job or no-one's job? There is a need to allocate the responsibility for preparing each care plan to one individual. Nursing actions may be delegated but the planning should not.

Finding time to do the writing is not easy when staffing levels are poor, or when nurses seem to be in a state of perpetual motion. Initially acquainting oneself with, and acquiring the skills to complete new forms of documentation is time-consuming. It is important that a number of key staff should develop skills in writing care plans before they are used with all patients under their care. There remains a value judgment to be made on whether the time taken to produce good quality documentation is worth the effort, or whether the time spent doing this could be put to better use. It is a matter of deciding whether the methods of care planning advocated in this module and elsewhere do offer the potential for more individualised and co-ordinated care, as well as providing a valuable means of staff development.

A third kind of problem is the practical one of having appropriate forms of documentation on which to write care plans. In general, nurses themselves have had to evolve forms which are most appropriate for the settings in which they work. Problem statements may include a column to indicate whether problems are current or potential; an evaluation column may also be included. Because a variety of formats may be tested before a final decision is made on what is most appropriate, it is wise to use fairly crude forms for a small number of patients before going on to the stage of having them printed. If forms can be designed to be kept in a readily available form of storage, so much the better. It is all too easy to *begin* with a form and then to try to develop an approach which fits it. This is entirely the wrong way round. Documentation must incorporate what are regarded as the most appropriate and workable methods of recording for local purposes.

An adaptation and extension of the SOAP format for care planning, used by health visitors, is described by Clark (1982). Other examples of documentation are illustrated in some of the case notes included in the *Case Files* and in Module 6, as well as in some of the books on the nursing process included in the References.

REFINEMENTS OF CARE PLANS

DAILY CARE PLANS

All care plans must be updated at regular intervals. McFarlane and Castledine (1982) advocate the use of a daily care plan, shown in Figure 3.6, which is prepared for each patient as a means of specifying what it is hoped that the patient will be able to achieve at a specific time for that day. They find this to be particularly useful for patients who are confused or disoriented, and who need some form of daily routine. Such a plan specifying what patients, as well as nurses, will do at particular times seems a useful way of drawing attention to what is expected of *patients,* particularly those whose days may be very busy or very empty.

Wherever possible, patients should be involved in constructing their own daily plans, thereby increasing their responsibility for their own care and, at times, helping them to understand some of the constraints on flexibility imposed by the organisation and institution in which they are currently living.

STANDARD CARE PLANS

Another approach to formal care planning is the use of the standard care plan for patients with identical problems or common conditions, such as those requiring pre-operative preparation for a hysterectomy, a breast-feeding mother after a spontaneous vertex delivery, or those at risk of infection due to an indwelling urinary catheter. The case notes on Peter O. in the *Case Files* include standard care plans for children in hospital and other examples are included in Module 6. In each of these instances, patients will have some problems which are unique to them, while others are common. Mayers (1978) advocates distinguishing between common or usual patient problems, and unusual ones. Standard care plans are developed to deal with what are predictable interventions for common problems. They could be called 'core' plans; in other words, they have a consistent common basis, to which is added the unique plan for the individual patient.

University of Manchester – Department of Nursing. M5/Assessment Unit			
DAILY CARE PLAN FOR Mr. Dennis			
Times	Daily Activities/Sleep and Rest	Progress (Comments achieved or /X)
Awakening	Usually at 7am. likes to use commode at bedside and then have a cup of tea.	
8 a.m.	Sit out in chair by bedside for breakfast. Add extra bran to diet.	
9 a.m. to	EITHER – 1. Encourage to wash hands and face at bedside, plus shave with electric razor.	
10 a.m.	OR – 2. Encourage up, bath and shave in bathroom. Help with dressing.	
11 a.m.	Take B.P. and pulse. Encourage fluids min. of 180 mls. Likes coffee – no milk, no sugar.	
12 noon	Give medications prior to lunch at 12·15pm. Encourage patient to walk with special frame.	
1 p.m.	To dining-room, walk back to bedside and allow patient to either rest in chair or on his bed.	
2 p.m. to	For 1 hour– Take B.P. and pulse + temperature. Check pulmonary function with Wright's peak flow meter.	
3 p.m.	Record result in notes.	
4 p.m.	Exercises as per chart in day room. Encourage fluids min. of 180 mls. – likes tea, no sugar.	
5 p.m.	Walk to dining-room for evening meal	
6 p.m.	Usually likes sandwiches, fruit and tea	
7 p.m.	Encourage to walk to day room, likes to watch T.V. or read evening paper	
8 p.m.	Encourage to walk to day room, likes to watch T.V. or read evening paper	
9 p.m. to	Walk back to bedside, likes to be in bed by 9·30p.m.	
10 p.m.	Take to toilet prior to this – likes a drop of whisky (30mls.), no night sedation needed.	
NIGHT TIME		
1 a.m.	Usually wakes to use commode at bedside – may only need to pass urine. Therefore encourage use of urinal	
6 a.m.	Usually awake – but does not like to be disturbed until 7a.m.	

Fig. 3.6 Completed example of a daily care plan (McFarlane and Castledine, 1982)

By spending time in developing standard care plans – which, like all nursing interventions, need to be reviewed regularly – more time would become available in the long term to identify patients' unique problems and methods of alleviating them.

Patients have similarities as well as differences. There is now a greater emphasis on individualising care and major attention has been given to the unique nature of each patient. The individuality of a patient's problems can only be ascertained after a thorough assessment. However, Mayers says that "the critical element for effective care is *not* the dissimilarity of care from patient to patient, but rather the *relevance* of care based upon thorough, appropriately spaced nursing assessments". Therefore, good quality care is not a matter of the degree of individuality of care, but of the care given being matched to solving individual patient problems. Inevitably, some of that care will be identical for patients with identical problems, particularly in acute and short-term care settings where nurses have reported difficulty in using care planning.

A standard care plan is a protocol for nursing care. However, to be useful, it must be written in the same format as other patient documentation so that it can be easily integrated into it. That means that problems, goals and nursing actions should be set out in the same way as they are on the care plans used for individual patient problems. A standard care plan should evolve through the same problem-solving process of development as other care plans. It should be based on sound evidence agreed, written, tested and evaluated as the most appropriate care for the designated patient problem. Periodic revision is essential to take account of new research findings and changes in the environment, equipment or other resources. In effect, what is being written is an agreed standard and procedure for care for a patient with a particular problem or condition. Wherever possible, the research base of the plan should be made explicit in its background documentation.

In the United Kingdom, we do not yet have conclusive research evidence on the value of problem-oriented approaches to care. There is an intuitive and common-sense belief, as well as anecdotal evidence, about its effectiveness in improving the quality of patient care and the job satisfaction of nurses who are sufficiently interested to try it. However, because evidence is lacking, it is not possible to say whether standard care plans detract from individualised care or promote it. They do have value, however, in informing all grades of staff about some common aspects of patient care and this is useful when staff turnover is high. Their potential for in-service education, when they are being evaluated and reviewed, is enormous. More particularly, the use of standard care plans can help to avoid a great deal of unnecessary and repetitive writing, leaving more time to deal with unusual and specific patient problems.

More will be said about documenting the planning phase of problem solving when we deal with integrating the discrete steps of the nursing process in Module 6.

Activity 3.14   Allow 30 minutes

A care plan for Sharon Cox

You should now be able to write a good nursing care plan. This activity gives you some practice in doing so and enables you to check your response.

The final activity in this module involves listening to the audiotape of an interview between a sister and a newly admitted patient, Sharon, and writing a nursing care plan for her. Please turn to Activity 3.14 in Part II of the *Case Files*. You will require a tape recorder to complete this activity. It also relates to the next group session, so you are advised to complete it *before* you attend this session.

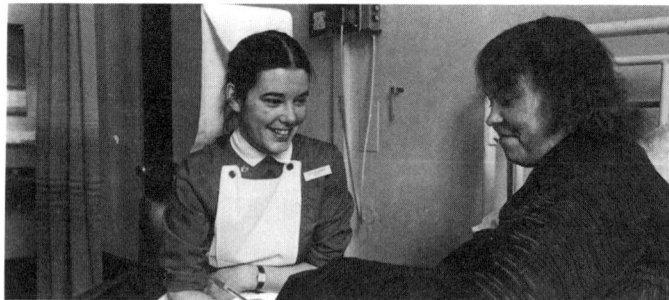

Sharon in hospital

In this module and in Module 2, you have covered a lot of ground relating to the preparatory work which goes on *before* nursing care actually takes place. In practice, these activities may occur very quickly – if a patient haemorrhages or has a cardiac arrest, we do not wait to ask whether he wishes us to intervene. On the other hand, an increasing number of our patients are with us for many years, suffering chronic conditions requiring care in hospital, at day centres or at home. Many are simply growing old. A goal-directed approach to care is as relevant for them as it is for the many who require nursing for very short periods in their lives.

In this module the importance of involving patients fully in their own care has been stressed. This is not merely a reflection of a belief that patients should have an increasing say in the recovery of their own health. It actually results in more effective care.

Effective nursing is not possible without also taking account of the plans other professionals have made with or for patients. These may be shared at wards rounds or staff conferences about patients. In some places, integrated *patient* plans are evolving, so that different professional groups share a comprehensive plan for a patient, of which nursing is one element. This removes the need for individual medical, nursing and therapy notes and promotes inter-professional co-operation.

The group session following this module deals with a doctor, social worker and nurse discussing Sharon's care.

COMMENTS ON ACTIVITIES

Activity 3.1 (p. 60)
Goal components
Your answers should read:

             5   1   2   4   3
After breakfast and before going to bed, / Joan / will carry out her knee exercises / for five minutes, / with the assistance of her mother.

 1   2   4   2   3   5
Mr Grey / will report / no more than two episodes of / giggling / in public, / when he comes to the clinic next week.

Activity 3.3 (p. 60)
Getting rid of "fuzzies"

Goal statement	Clear or fuzzy	Comments
1 Increase mobility	F	*This is quite unhelpful, except to tell us that the patient should increase some form of mobility. It gives no indication of what, how much or when, and so would be unhelpful without much greater specificity e.g. "walk 20 steps supported by tripod to affected side, 3 times each day".*
2 Drink at least 6 cups of fluid between 7 am and 8 pm	✓	*This is specifying a minimum fluid intake and it does not matter when or what the patient drinks. It is easily measured. Time is specified.*
3 Sleep 6 hours un-interrupted each night	✓	*Quite specific – although whether the patient requires any assistance to sleep may be ascertained in assessment.*
4 Accept her illness	F	*This is fuzzy. The goal statement does not specify which observations will tell us she has "accepted her illness". What "accepting an illness" means will be open to a number of interpretations. It would be better to write: "express her feelings about her illness".*
5 Make one or no self-deprecating remarks during follow-up interview	✓	*This specifies the number of a particular kind of verbalisation, indicating how the patient feels about himself. This would be a feature of a patient with depression and reducing this kind of behaviour would indicate improvement in his mental state. Other indicators would also be used.*
6 Communicate verbally and non-verbally		*The specificity of this goal would depend on the patient. For someone who is unconscious due to a head injury, a goal in the 'communicating' activity of living may be broad.* *However, for someone regaining speech, or someone expressing delusions the goal would have to be much more specific to be useful.*

The need to relate patients' goals to their assessed problems is obvious.

Activity 3.5 (p. 62)

Goal steps

Patient's name: Mr Wallace

	Goal	Target date	Achievement date
1st step	Will sit out of bed on chair, assisted by two nurses	1.3	
2nd step	Will rise from sitting to standing position, with the aid of two nurses	4.3	
3rd step	Will rise, with assistance of one nurse and a Zimmer frame	6.3	
4th step	Will rise from sitting to standing position, with no nursing assistance	8.3	
5th step	Will rise unaided and stand, using a Zimmer frame	9.3	
6th step	Will move unaffected leg forward and back, with the aid of a Zimmer frame	10.3	
7th step	Will move incapacitated leg forward and back, with the aid of a Zimmer frame	10.3	
8th step	Will take two steps, with aid of a Zimmer frame only.	12.3	

Steps 1-7 would all have to be successfully completed in sequence before the patient could move his legs in order to be able to walk. It is easy to identify whether the patient can achieve each step and, importantly, to note when he comes to something which he is unable to do, so that his plan of care can be adjusted accordingly. This sequence would, of course, be agreed with his physiotherapist and Mr Wallace would be involved in agreeing this plan. Both professions would be involved in assisting Mr Wallace to achieve mobility. The target dates would depend on the severity of hemiparesis.

Examine your own goal steps to see that they are sequential and contain all the elements of a well-stated goal, which were outlined on p. 59. If they are not, re-order them and amend them if they are "fuzzy".

Activity 3.8 (p. 67)

Stating goals positively

You have not been given much information to guide you about the particular patients in this activity, which should have permitted plenty of scope for your imagination. Possible answers given here illustrate the process of moving from problems to the identification of appropriate positive behaviours, which might be quite broad, and turning them into a specific goal or goals.

1 Mr Tate is constipated. His diet is without roughage and he takes no exercise.
(a) Mr Tate will increase the amount of roughage in his diet.
(b) Mr Tate will have bran or porridge for breakfast every day and fruit for his lunch.

2 Miss Miles has had two abortions and two unplanned pregnancies, and she cannot remember to take her contraceptive pills regularly.
(a) Miss Miles will use some other form of contraception to avoid further unwanted pregnancies.
(b) Miss Miles will attend the family planning clinic next week.

3 Fred gets his tablets mixed up.
(a) Fred will take the correct tablets at the correct time.
(b) Fred will count out and show his son which tablets he takes, at which times, tomorrow and every day, until he gets it right.

MODULE 4
THE THIRD STEP OF THE NURSING PROCESS
IMPLEMENTATION

Prepared for the Course Team by Alison Binnie and Ruth Roberts

CONTENTS

OBJECTIVES

After studying this module, you should be able to:

1 Describe three systems of organising nursing work outlined in the module.

2 Identify features of each of the three systems which either encourage or hinder holistic nursing practice.

3 Describe the way in which nursing work is allocated in your own field of practice.

4 Critically assess the suitability of this system for implementing individually planned care.

5 List the specific skills which nurses need to develop in order to implement individualised care.

6 Identify areas for further personal study which you feel would help you to extend your own managerial and interpersonal skills.

7 List the main elements of the kind of 'helping relationship' which will develop and sustain a genuine nurse-patient partnership.

8 Apply a planned, systematic approach to teaching patients and relatives, so that they can become actively involved in the implementation of care.

9 Critically assess the nurse-to-nurse communication system in your own work setting, identifying the extent to which it supports continuity of care.

INTRODUCTION

'Implementation' means putting the plan of nursing care into action. In the first four sections of this module, we shall examine the *practicalities* of providing a unique programme of care for each patient. We shall do this by discussing some recognised ways of organising nursing work and considering how much they may help or hinder nurses who wish to implement individually planned care. We shall also briefly look at how different styles of work organisation can influence the development of skills which nurses need in order to be able to implement individualised care plans.

We shall then consider how a genuine nurse-patient partnership can be developed and sustained during the actual provision of care. We shall examine the nature of the nurse-patient partnership in a little more depth and discuss ways in which nurses, patients and relatives can be helped to cope with, and benefit from, this close working relationship.

Finally, we shall look into the question of maintaining a consistent approach to dealing with a patient's problems when, as is usually the case, there are several people involved in putting the plan of care into effect. This means that we shall be touching on the subject of record-keeping and other ways in which nurses share information about their patients, but we shall limit our discussion to aspects of nurse-to-nurse communication which relate most directly to maintaining continuity in the implementation of nursing care. It could be argued that some of these issues have more to do with implementing the nursing process as a whole, than with implementing an individual care plan. However, we have included several broad organisational matters in this module because we have found, in our own experience, that failure to deal with them appropriately can make it impossible for nurses to put individual plans into action.

ORGANISING NURSING WORK

WORK ORGANISATION AND THE IMPLEMENTATION OF NURSING CARE

The authors of Module 1 claim that every person who becomes a patient has the right to be considered as a unique and complex being, with a variety of highly individual needs (p. 9). They see this *holistic* view of patients as fundamental to the practice of the nursing process. Modules 2 and 3 follow through this emphasis on acknowledging each patient's individuality and on recognising that each patient has his own unique pattern of daily living and his own way of responding to stress. In the first sections of Module 4, we want you to think critically about different ways of organising nursing work in fields of practice that are familiar to you and to consider the extent to which each of the various methods either hinders or fosters a holistic approach.

Taking a holistic approach to nursing means getting to know each patient as a person and as a member of a family unit. To find out whether a pattern of work organisation is compatible with the practice of the nursing process, we need to ask:

"Does this method provide nurses with opportunities to get to know their patients and are they encouraged and taught how to make the most of such opportunities?"

Getting to know people is never a one-way process. If the nurse is to get to know a patient, she must allow herself to be seen as a person. This means being open and honest and not hiding behind barriers such as a uniform or an air of being busy. Many nurses feel uncomfortable at the idea of getting close to patients in this way. Some may feel threatened because they lack confidence in their own professional ability; others may feel vulnerable because they fear the emotional impact of involvement with patients.

However, if we believe that a closer professional relationship between nurse and patient is necessary for holistic care, we need to find out whether nurses will be helped to cope with the new stress that this may entail and be guided towards finding the deeper satisfaction that should follow. We need to ask:

"Does the way in which nursing work is organised allow sufficient recognition of nurses as people? Does it allow them to be creative and to express their individuality? Does it teach them to gain insight into their own feelings and behaviour? Does it provide nurses with sufficient feedback to help them to mature and gain confidence?"

An appropriately established organisational system will not, in itself, ensure the provision of individualised care. Nurse practitioners must be able to make full use of the system. Putting an individualised plan of care into action demands organisational skill, and every new care plan presents a new organisational challenge. When caring for a group of patients, each with his own unique plan of care, the nurse will need to be extremely flexible for her pattern of work may need to be different every day. Nurses must have the ability and the authority to make decisions about how they use their time, and to select priorities when their workload is heavy. In a later section we shall therefore also consider how nurses can be helped to function effectively within a system that is flexible enough to allow individualised care.

NURSING AS TEAMWORK

In this country, it is very rare for a nurse to practise in isolation. In hospitals, the need for teamwork in order to provide a twenty-four hour service is obvious, but nurses working in the community also usually share their workload with others. Whatever the setting, the nursing team involved in implementing the care planned for a group of patients is likely to include nurses of a variety of grades and levels of training.

Nurses in charge of hospital wards or community caseloads cannot personally provide all the care for all their patients all the time. Although their employing authorities hold them responsible for their patients and they remain *accountable* for the nursing care which these patients receive, they have to *delegate* responsibility for some of their work to colleagues or subordinates.

Three systems of organising nursing work will be briefly outlined and then their relevance to the practice of the nursing process will be discussed.

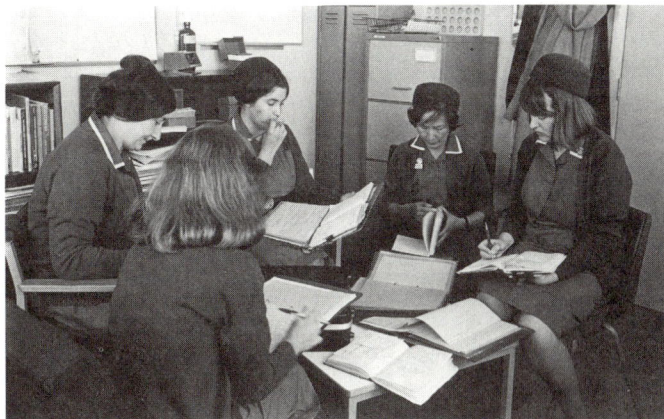
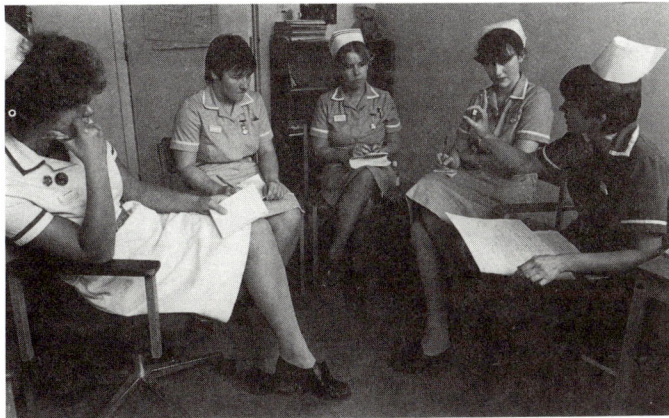

Hospital and community nursing teams

SYSTEMS OF WORK ORGANISATION

WHAT IS TASK ALLOCATION?

In this system, the care of patients is broken down into a series of tasks such as bed-making, blanket baths, washes, meals, 4-hourly observations, 'back rounds', drug rounds, care of intravenous infusions, collection of specimens and so on. Each nurse is made responsible for the completion of certain tasks for the duration of a shift. When next on duty, the same nurse may be allocated a different set of tasks. There is usually a preferred method for carrying out each task. This is established as local policy and is often written out in detail in a Nursing Procedures Book. The nurse is expected to adhere strictly to instructions laid down in this way. When task allocation is used in a hospital setting, a fairly rigid ward routine governs the sequence and timing of the various tasks which nurses have to perform. A nurse working within a task allocation system frequently has brief contact with a large number of patients and each patient encounters many different nurses. A nurse responsible for taking temperatures in a hospital ward, for example, may have to perform this task with perhaps thirty different patients.

There is often an unwritten hierarchy of tasks. Those of low status usually involve helping patients with daily living activities – such as washing, dressing, feeding and eliminating – and these tasks are allocated to untrained or junior members of the nursing team. Tasks accorded high status are usually technical, clerical or organisational and tend to involve less patient contact. Assisting doctors with diagnostic procedures, keeping nursing records, ordering supplies, talking with patients' relatives and liaising with paramedical staff are tasks which would fall into this category and they are generally allocated to senior learners or qualified nurses.

The tasks formally allocated to nurses in this system are usually those concerned with the physical care of patients. This does not mean that patients' emotional, social, and spiritual needs are always totally ignored. A sensitive, perceptive nurse may handle these less tangible aspects of care very effectively but, because they have no formal place in the task system, they are not the special responsibility of any particular nurse, will not be dealt with systematically and may easily be forgotten when nurses feel they are busy and have only enough time to complete the officially recognised tasks.

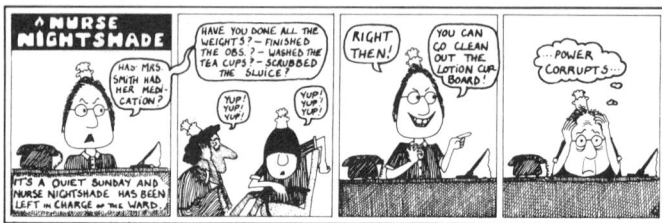

WHAT IS PATIENT ALLOCATION?

As the term implies, this is a system in which each nurse is delegated responsibility for the care of a specific group of patients, or just one patient, as in an intensive care or labour ward setting. This allocation may be for the duration of one shift only, or nurses may work with the same patients whenever they are on duty, over a period of days or weeks. However, when nurses go off duty their responsibility ceases and they hand over the care of their patients to other nurses. The nurse in charge of the ward or caseload remains ultimately accountable for the nursing care which the patients receive.

The way in which patient allocation is interpreted varies in practice. A nurse caring for a group of patients may only be expected to carry out the low status tasks described above, often referred to as 'basic nursing care'. She may be expected to organise her work strictly in accordance with established routine and recognised procedures, with the nurse in charge dealing with the less predictable and the 'more important' aspects of nursing care.

Alternatively, a nurse may be delegated responsibility for all the care of her patients and she may be given greater freedom to organise her work around their particular needs and wishes.

Having delegated responsibility for all aspects of nursing care, the nurse in charge has much more time to devote to the teaching

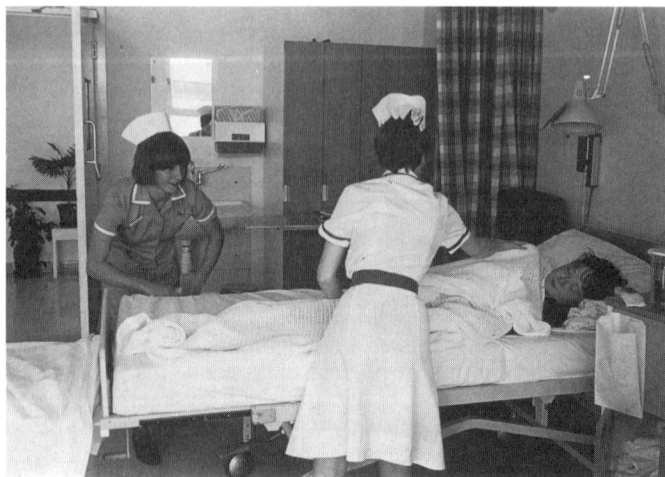

A patient allocation system does not leave nurses to work entirely alone

and supervisory parts of her role, giving particular attention to supporting, guiding and assisting unqualified or inexperienced staff, so that they can cope with and learn from their much heavier responsibility. Although, in this system, nurses are personally *responsible* and *accountable* (to the patient and to the sister/charge nurse) for the nursing care of their own patients, they need not necessarily carry out every aspect of care themselves and they do not need to work in isolation. Their responsibility is to ensure that appropriate care is provided in the right way, at the right time. Nurses continue to work as members of a team, and in planning their work they must consider what advice and physical assistance they may need from colleagues. They must also consider what help colleagues may need from them. Co-operation and genuine teamwork are essential for the success of patient allocation.

WHAT IS PRIMARY NURSING?

'Primary nursing' is a term which may be new to you for, as yet, it is not widely used in the United Kingdom. It is not to be confused with the term 'primary health care' which is used in this country to describe the first level care which patients receive from general practitioners, district nurses, health visitors, social workers etc. in the community.

Primary nursing is a system of work organisation that was first described by a group of American nurses (Manthey et al, 1970). These nurses were concerned by the fragmentation of patient care and by the vague, collective responsibility for care in hospital nursing. They felt that these two factors prevented hospital nurses from providing genuinely *professional* care to *individual* clients. They developed an organisational pattern which enabled each of their nurses to take responsibility for the total nursing care of between three and six patients, from admission to discharge. The authors described this as returning to the personalised concept of "my nurse" and "my patient".

Although the work of Manthey and her colleagues was carried out in an acute general hospital, their primary nursing system can be applied in a wide variety of health care settings. A **primary** nurse is responsible *and* accountable for the care of her own group of patients. This responsibility and accountability does not cease when the nurse goes off duty, but continues throughout each patient's stay in hospital, or for as long as nursing support is needed in the community. The primary nurse works closely with her patients and plans all aspects of their nursing care. When she goes off duty, she delegates responsibility to an **associate** nurse, who works according to the plan worked out by the primary nurse. Except in dire emergency, the plan of care is not altered without consultation with the primary nurse. As with patient allocation, teamwork is essential and primary nurses need to act as associate nurses and assistants for each other, as well as depending upon those specifically employed as associate nurses.

The primary nurse has overall responsibility for identifying her patient's needs, setting goals with him, helping him to make decisions about his care and evaluating outcomes. When she is on duty she also plays a major role in the implementation of his care. The primary nurse is responsible for liaison with doctors and paramedical staff and she will be the main nursing contact for relatives. Patient education, and the planning and preparation for discharge or transfer are initiated, and largely carried out, by the primary nurse. Whilst associate nurses make contributions to the patient's progress record when they participate in his care, the primary nurse is ultimately responsible for the patient's nursing record.

Because the primary nurse is fully accountable, both for the nursing decisions that concern her patients and for the nursing care which they receive, she should be an experienced registered nurse.

OTHER SYSTEMS OF WORK ORGANISATION

The three methods of organising nursing work described so far are probably the most widely recognised and they are the systems most commonly referred to in the nursing literature. However, in practice, these systems may be extensively modified or certain elements from the different systems may be combined. In team nursing, for example, a small group of nurses is allocated the care of a group of patients under the direction of a team leader. The leader may share out the group's work-load by allocating nursing tasks to each member of the team, so that it is essentially task allocation that is being practised, but with a smaller group of patients than when the system is applied to a whole ward. Alternatively, a team leader may subdivide the team's group of patients into smaller groups and apply the principles of patient allocation to the team's work.

In busy hospital wards, patient allocation is often interpreted in geographical terms. Individual nurses are allocated the care of patients in a particular area of the ward and they nurse them for as long as they remain in that area. If a patient is moved in the middle of a shift to another part of the ward, perhaps to be near an oxygen point, then his nurse hands over responsibility for his care to the nurse working in that area.

In long-stay hospital wards, patient allocation may be organised over a fixed time-span. Nurses work with the same group of patients whenever they are on duty for, say, four weeks. After this time, it might be felt that patients would benefit from the stimulus of forming new relationships and that a different nurse, taking a fresh look at patients' chronic nursing problems, may come up with some new ideas.

Sometimes nursing work is organised so that nurses simply follow an established daily routine. Where more than one nurse is involved in this routine pattern of work, individual responsibility for nursing care is extremely uncertain and implementing an individualised care plan is virtually impossible.

So far, it may seem as if we are talking more about nursing management than about implementing nursing care plans, but in reality the two go hand in hand. Nurses wishing to provide care specifically designed to meet individual patient's needs and wishing to provide it in the spirit of the nursing process as a whole, must organise their work in a way that makes these things possible. Inappropriate organisation can mean that an individualised plan of care simply cannot be implemented; it can mean that the nurse-patient partnership, which began to grow during the initial assessment and planning stages, is destroyed; and it can mean that lines of responsibility and accountability for nursing care become extremely blurred.

The activity which follows will ask you to think about the organisation of your own work and then, in the next section, we shall discuss what various systems of organisation have to offer to nurses who wish to implement individualised care plans. The central importance of work organisation in the implementation stage of the nursing process should then become clearer.

Activity 4.1	Allow 15 minutes

Your own system of work organisation

This activity is designed to help you to start analysing and critically appraising the way in which your own nursing work is organised.

1 Briefly describe the organisation of work in your own nursing setting. (It may be one of the systems described above, or a mixture, or something slightly different.)

2 List what you consider to be the advantages and disadvantages of your current method of work organisation.

Authors' comment
There will be no specific comments, but the next section is a critique of systems of organising nursing work and this should give you plenty of feedback and probably some more ideas.

A CRITICAL LOOK AT SYSTEMS OF ORGANISING NURSING WORK

TASK ALLOCATION

Well-organised task allocation has the advantage of being efficient in terms of completing practical tasks in the minimum time. It corresponds to the industrial production line model in which efficiency, in terms of maximum output with minimum labour costs, is increased by each worker repeatedly performing a standardised task, or series of tasks, to a strict time schedule.

Sociologists who have examined the effects of this kind of work pattern on workers in industry, have found that it produces boredom and frustration and that it provides minimal job satisfaction. A worker who has little control over the organisation of his work and who is distanced from the results of his labour, has been described as being *alienated* from his work and hence from his true self. Blauner (1964), for example, describes the alienated worker as experiencing a sense of powerlessness, meaninglessness, isolation and self-estrangement in his work.

The psychologist Isabel Menzies (1960) made a detailed study of a London teaching hospital which practised task allocation. She described this method of work organisation as part of a "social defence system", which had developed in the nursing service to protect individual nurses from the anxieties they would otherwise experience as a result of close contact with suffering and death, and with things which would normally be considered alarming or unpleasant. She saw task allocation as a means of splitting up the nurse-patient relationship. She suggested that it "prevents her [the nurse] from coming effectively into contact with the totality of any one patient and his illness and offers some protection from the anxiety this arouses".

The standardisation of procedures and the strict adherence to routine that accompany task allocation have the advantage of ensuring that a minimum standard of practice is maintained, regardless of which nurses carry out the work. Menzies, however, saw these features as yet another part of the nursing service's defence system. Making decisions which will affect the welfare of patients is another source of anxiety for nurses. Laying down precise instructions for

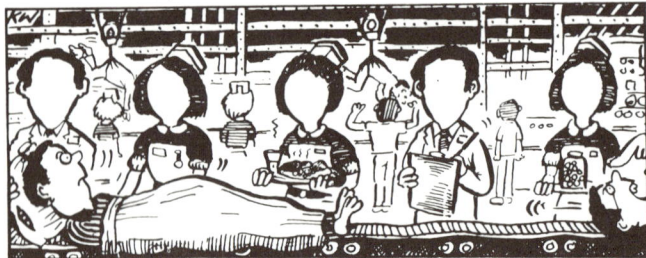

the performance of nursing tasks and following a rigid daily pattern of work minimises decision making, and transfers responsibility for nursing decisions from a personal to an institutional level.

In Menzies' analysis, nursing's defence system fails, because, whilst it enables nurses to avoid certain stresses in their work, it creates others which are damaging to individual nurses and which interfere with the main task of providing nursing care for patients. The system fails to provide personal satisfaction for individual nurses. In Menzies' words, "success and satisfaction are dissipated in much the same way as the anxiety. The nurse misses the reassurance of seeing a patient get better in a way she can easily connect with her own efforts".

The conformity imposed upon the nurse to protect her from decision making denies her the stimulus of challenge and the opportunity for creativity and self-expression. This kind of working environment actually hinders a nurse's personal development. Rarely able to act upon her own initiative or to exercise discretion, exploration of her own potential is thwarted. As Menzies states:

> The defences . . . inhibit the full development of the individual's understanding, knowledge and skills that enable reality to be handled effectively . . . The social defences prevent the individual from realising to the full her capacity for concern, compassion, and sympathy and for action based on these feelings which would strengthen her belief in the good aspects of herself and her capacity to use them.

Menzies' findings about nurses in a task allocation system have much in common with what is known from sociological studies about the alienated worker on an industrial production line.

You may be feeling that these are complex ideas to handle and may be wondering about their relevance to your own work, but there are important lessons here. Failure to analyse and modify the way in which your own work is organised may make it impossible to implement an individualised plan of care and reach the goals you have agreed upon with your patient. You may find, as Menzies did more than twenty years ago, that:

> The poignancy of the situation is increased by the expressed aims of nursing at the present time, i.e. to nurse the whole patient as a person. The nurse is instructed to do that, it is usually what she wants to do, but the functioning of the nursing service makes it impossible.

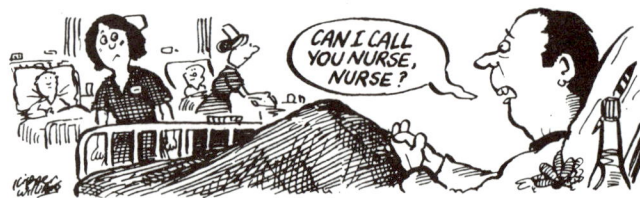

Activity 4.2

Allow 10 minutes

Analysis of task allocation

Even if you have never worked in a strict task allocation system it is worth thinking about for two reasons:

- *a great deal of traditional nursing practice still in use was developed within this system*
- *you are likely to work with other nurses who were trained in this system and it will help you to understand what their training experience was like and to understand how they may feel about changing to a less structured system.*

Using the material which you have just read and, if you have worked in a system of task allocation, using your own experience, try to answer the following questions about this system of work organisation.

1. What opportunities does task allocation provide for a nurse to get to know her patients as whole people?

2. What opportunities does task allocation provide for junior nurses to use their initiative and be creative in their work?

Authors' comment

You may have answers based on your own experience that you would like to discuss; if so, take your ideas to the next group session.

Our comments relate to what has been discussed so far in this section.

The evidence which we have mentioned suggests that task allocation interferes with the process of getting to know patients as people and may have been adopted specifically to discourage this kind of involvement.

On the question of allowing the nurse to express her individuality through initiative and creativity, our evidence suggests that task allocation has little to contribute. It follows from this that experience of task allocation during training is unlikely to prepare a nurse for the decision making and the organisational flexibility which must be very much part of her work, if she is to put highly individualised plans of patient care into action.

One final word about task allocation. It is not our intention to condemn this system out of hand. We recognise that much good nursing work has been carried out within this system in the past. It does have advantages and there are difficulties associated with abandoning the system at a time when resources are scarce. However, attitudes and expectations, both within nursing and amongst the general public, change with time and circumstances, and research produces new knowledge and insights which rightly make us question established practices.

If nurses become committed to a holistic view of nursing care, and if public demand for recognition of the patient as a responsible individual continues to grow, then we are likely to find that task allocation has outlived its usefulness.

PATIENT ALLOCATION

Where patient allocation is applied within a highly structured routine, with nurses providing standardised 'basic nursing care' for a group of patients, much of what has been said about task allocation also applies. The major difference is that with this system nurses have more contact with fewer patients; therefore, the opportunity to get to know them is greater and it is possible for the nurse to have a broader, but still not complete, view of her patients' problems.

Where the nurse is delegated responsibility for all the nursing care of her patients and is given a free hand in organising her work, the situation is quite different.

Using one aspect of the care of four patients, we shall try to make a detailed comparison between routine, standardised care and a more flexible organisational approach.

Nurse Edwards is given responsibility for the care of a group of patients in hospital. For different reasons, four of her patients spend most of their day in bed and early nursing assessments showed that they were all at varying degrees of risk of developing pressure sores. An individual plan of nursing care has been drawn up for each of these patients.

Mrs Adams is frail and her skin reddens easily if she remains in one position for more than two hours. She sleeps very soundly and says she hardly notices when nurses change her position at night. A plan of 2-hourly change of position, which includes helping her into a sitting-up position at meal-times and when her daughter visits at 8 pm, is agreed upon.

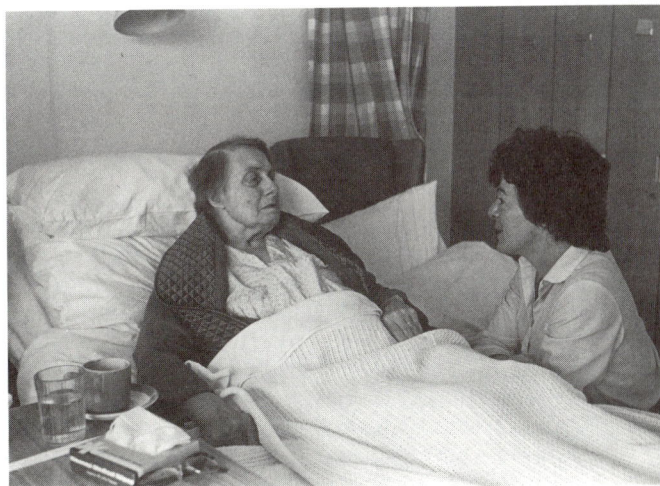

Mrs Adams

Mr Burrows is deeply unconscious. He is a very large gentleman and it takes three nurses to lift him clear of his bed. Turning him from side to side every three hours is currently keeping his pressure areas intact.

Mrs Clark had been bedridden at home for several weeks before her admission. Her husband had helped her to get out of bed at meal-times and whenever she needed to use the commode, day or night, and she had liked sitting in her chair for half-an-hour between 10.30 and 11.00 in the evening before she settled for the night. She found that this activity had been sufficient to keep her skin in good condition. Mrs Clark is very ill and knows that she is going to die, but she wants her nurses to help her to continue this pattern for as long as she can.

Mr Davis is able to move himself in bed, but has tended not to do so and the skin over his sacrum is reddening. He understood the problem when it was explained to him. He is a meticulous man and likes to do things for himself. He has worked out his own schedule of position change which should relieve the present problem. His nurse is simply to inspect his pressure areas once a day, at 5 pm, when his wife comes to help him to have a bath.

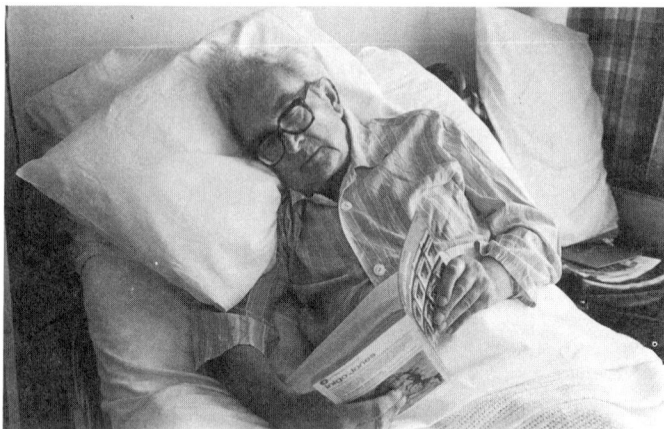

Mr Davis

Under a system of task allocation, or any system which followed a fixed routine and standardised procedures, it is likely that these four patients would have received '2-hourly pressure area care' as Nurse Edwards and a colleague went to each bedridden patient in the course of their 2-hourly 'back round'. It is very probable that this routine care would have been highly successful in terms of preventing pressure sores in these four patients. The routine might, however, be criticised on two levels:

Firstly, it is wasteful of resources. Turning Mr Burrows takes three nurses ten minutes. On a 2-hourly schedule, that is a total of *six hours* nursing time in twenty-four hours. On the 3-hourly schedule, which his individual assessment showed is quite adequate, a total of only *four hours* nursing time is required. Two whole hours of precious nursing time is saved. Mrs Adams can move quite easily with the help of one nurse, and once things have been carefully explained to him, Mr Davis doesn't need the nurses to 'bother' him at all over this aspect of his care, so more time is saved.

Secondly, the rigid system denies patients the right to participate in their care and to make choices. Many patients expect nurses to tell them what to do and they expect to have to fit in with the nurses' routine. Mrs Clark probably would not have complained about the nurses' 2-hourly regime, but it would have meant totally disrupting an established and highly satisfactory pattern of activity at a time in her life when security, familiarity and physical comfort are particularly important to her. Mr Davis would probably also have submitted to the standard care, but he would have resented the loss of independence. He would have suffered a loss of self-esteem and he would probably have begun to see himself as an old man and an invalid. It is very likely that his behaviour would have mirrored this change in self-concept and that he would have gradually become increasingly dependent, both physically and emotionally, upon his wife and his nurses.

Following a strict routine and standardised procedures is rather like trying to fit patients into nice neat boxes, forgetting that patients are people who come in all sorts of shapes and sizes.

Using a more flexible approach, leaving the nurse to organise her work in relation to patients' needs, means that there is much greater scope for making nurses' work fit more comfortably around each individual patient. Starting with her patients' care plans, Nurse Edwards can begin to plan her day's work. She will need to consider fixed points in the hospital day so that, for example, she can work out Mrs Clark's schedule around meal-times. Nurse Edwards will have to liaise with other nurses in the ward, so that they know at what times they will be needed to help turn Mr Burrows and so that they take this into consideration in planning their own work. It may also be useful for Nurse Edwards to talk to the physiotherapist when she first arrives on the ward to find out what plans she has for treating Mr Burrows' chest that day, so that this can also be considered in the planning of his turning schedule.

Considering the work of other hospital departments is also important. Mrs Adams, for example, is booked for a barium X-ray at 10.30 am, so it would be wise for Nurse Edwards to help her to change her position at 10 o'clock in case she has to wait in the department for a long time. Checking with Mr Davis that his wife is

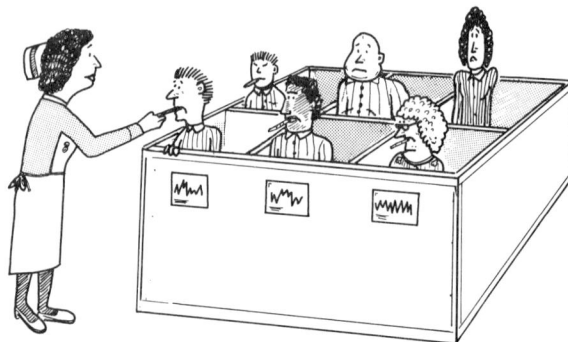

Patients don't fit into nice neat boxes

coming in as usual would be sensible, so that alternative arrangements for his bath can be planned well in advance if she is not expected.

These are factors which concern only one aspect of the care of four patients. Similar thinking and planning is necessary for the whole range of care required by Nurse Edwards' group of patients.

Activity 4.3   Allow 10 minutes

Constraints on the organisation of nursing work

The purpose of this activity is to help you to relate our discussion on work organisation to your own field of practice.

Write down:

- fixed points in your own working day
- activities of other people which you would have to consider if you were planning how to implement individualised care for your own group of patients.

Authors' comment

If you work in a hospital setting, you may try to plan your day much as Nurse Edwards did. The functioning of a large institution would put certain constraints on your plan and you would have to liaise carefully with nursing colleagues, with other members of the health care team and with other hospital departments.

If you work in a community setting you will have quite different things to consider, but the principles of careful planning, setting work priorities and retaining organisational flexibility are just the same. You may have to work around fixed points such as regular clinic sessions or meetings of the primary health care team, there may be geographical constraints, and you may have to plan home visits to coincide with a G.P.'s visit or the times when relatives are at home.

This flexible approach to planning your day's work is much more complicated than simply following a set routine and it clearly demands considerable organisational skill, but it is absolutely essential if individually planned care is going to be put into practice.

PRIMARY NURSING

As a system of work organisation, primary nursing clearly has a great deal to offer to nurses who wish to base their practice on the principles of the nursing process. It provides opportunities for nurses to get to know patients and their families well and, through working with them over a period of time and being involved in all aspects of the nursing care, nurses are well placed to establish genuine partnerships with individual patients. The closeness and continuity of the working relationship make the implementation of individually planned care feasible.

The question, then, is can this concept be applied to the British nursing service? Though not given any particular title, nursing work in many community nursing settings is already organised on broadly similar lines. Community nursing services have a high proportion of qualified staff, so caseload allocation to health visitors, community

midwives, community psychiatric nurses and district nurses attached to general practices is quite practicable. These nurses can attend the same patients for as long as they require community nursing support and, when they are off duty, colleagues or relief nurses usually take on the role of associate nurse. The problem-oriented approach to nursing may not yet be thoroughly established amongst community practitioners, but from an organisational point of view they are certainly well placed to implement highly personalised care.

Many acute psychiatric hospital units are developing a system of **key workers.** One nurse acts as the key figure for a patient throughout his stay in the unit, planning and co-ordinating all his care and establishing a close therapeutic relationship with him. The charge nurse allocates each patient to the nurse whose talents, abilities and special training or experience are most appropriate for his particular needs. This system is again very similar to primary nursing.

After a lot of hard work and a supportive educational programme specifically aimed at changing staff attitudes and developing interpersonal skills, primary nursing has been successfully introduced at Burford, a small, Oxfordshire cottage hospital caring for elderly patients. This scheme has been well documented in the British nursing press (Alderman, 1983; Punton, 1983; Swaffield, 1983).

In acute general hospitals, where there is a rapid turnover of patients and staff and where, unlike the American system, there is often heavy dependence upon learners for the provision of care, the introduction of primary nursing would present a considerable organisational challenge. However, some British hospital nurses have succeeded in using many elements of Manthey's concept to apply a modified form of primary nursing in their own acute nursing settings.

Two sisters in a Leeds hospital gradually introduced a form of primary nursing to a busy, acute medical ward with all the usual problems of rapid turnover and staff shortages (Cavill and Johnson, 1981). They were pleased with their results: "We feel strongly that learners are now able to see the patient as a whole being and that staff nurses and enrolled nurses are allowed to develop their *nursing* skills to high degree". They also report a reduced length of in-patient stay for the chronically ill and a greatly improved after-care service, and they say that their team spirit is stronger because of better communications.

McFarlane and Castledine (1982) found that they developed a modified system of primary nursing in their acute hospital ward "more by accident than design". As the nursing process approach was gradually introduced to the ward, the need to change the pattern of work organisation became obvious; practice similar to primary nursing evolved naturally as a method which provided continuity and the close personal contact necessary to implement individually planned care.

So from an organisational point of view it seems that, with effort and determination, primary nursing – at least in a modified form – could become a realistic proposition in British hospitals.

Activity 4.4   Allow 10 minutes

Wider implications of changes in organisation of nursing work

This activity aims to help you to look beyond your own work role and to consider the implications of changing systems of work allocation for your nursing organisation as a whole.

Consider your own work environment. Then, make a note of any organisational constraints or potential areas of conflict which might make adopting a system of primary nursing difficult in your work setting.

Authors' comment

Wherever you work, you have probably identified problem areas in at least some of the categories shown in Figure 4.1 and you may well have thought of others.
The text which follows this activity looks back to the early American work on primary nursing and discusses some of the problems associated with introducing it to practice.

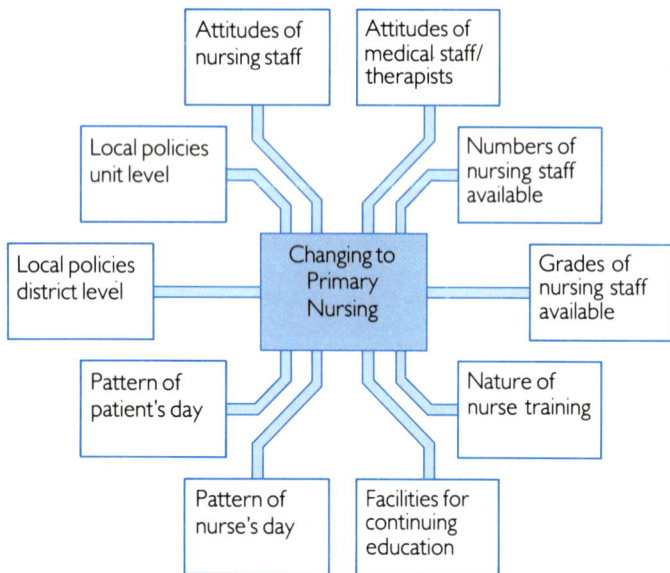

Fig. 4.1 *Some potential constraints to the introduction of primary nursing*

The original paper by Manthey and her colleagues gives clues as to why primary nursing, with all its obvious advantages for those wishing to implement individually planned nursing care, has so far not been more enthusiastically welcomed in Britain. Firstly, primary nursing demands that the staff nurse takes on an entirely new role. Instead of working as part of a large system where major responsibility lies at a higher administrative level, the staff nurse becomes a much more independent practitioner, responsible for her own decisions and actions. Manthey and her co-authors suggest that this requires an organisational climate "in which individuals feel free to learn, to risk, to make mistakes and to grow". They say that nurse leaders must trust and support individual nurses "whose attempts at comprehensive patient care lead to unorthodox activities". This is a totally different philosophy from the prevailing view in British nursing management, which tends to try and protect both staff and patients by creating firm rules and policies.

According to the American authors, the second prerequisite for the successful use of primary nursing is adequate preparation of staff nurses to accept the personal responsibility which their new role implies. The traditional training of nurses in the United States and in Britain has not fulfilled this function. Primary nursing therefore presents a major challenge to nursing education, which must seek to provide each nurse with a sound knowledge base, an ability to relate sensitively to others, and an ability to determine priorities confidently and to make valid judgments.

Primary nursing could then be used in Britain, if nurse managers and educationalists commit themselves to supporting the concept of a truly professional nurse practitioner.

NEW IDEAS IN WORK ORGANISATION

Perhaps we should emphasise that the three systems discussed above are not the only ones available to nurses. Other work organisation patterns exist and there is nothing wrong with inventing new ones to meet the particular needs of your client group and your nursing colleagues.

An example of an exciting organisational innovation is the work of Caroline Flint and her midwifery colleagues at the St George's Hospital Maternity Unit in London (Flint, 1981 and 1982). They were disturbed by the impersonal 'conveyor belt' system of maternity care, in which a mother may receive care from as many as twenty or thirty different midwives in the course of her pregnancy and be greeted by a total stranger at the labour ward door. An excellent initial assessment may be carried out and an individual care plan devised, but implementation of really personalised care in the spirit of a mother-midwife partnership is virtually impossible in such a system. Flint has described several schemes which aim to overcome these problems. One of these involves a team of four midwives who share responsibility for all aspects of hospital maternity care for a caseload of 200 women, from the time of ante-natal booking right through to transfer to the care of the community midwife on post-natal discharge from hospital (Flint, 1981). Mid-wives are trained as independent practitioners and the opportunity to practise their full range of professional skills afforded by this new system increases their job satisfaction enormously. Having maternity care, including delivery, supervised by only four midwives whom a mother really gets to know and trust, can transform the whole process of childbirth for her.

Implementing individually planned care involves taking a hard, critical look at the way in which your own nursing work is organised and being prepared to make ambitious changes in your system, if that is what is really needed. Imagination and determination are often more necessary than more staff or more money (Flint's scheme requires no extra staff and in the long run may actually be more economical than the old system). Handling organisational change, however, is not easy and that is why, in Module 7, you will be looking at the whole question of implementing change in much more detail.

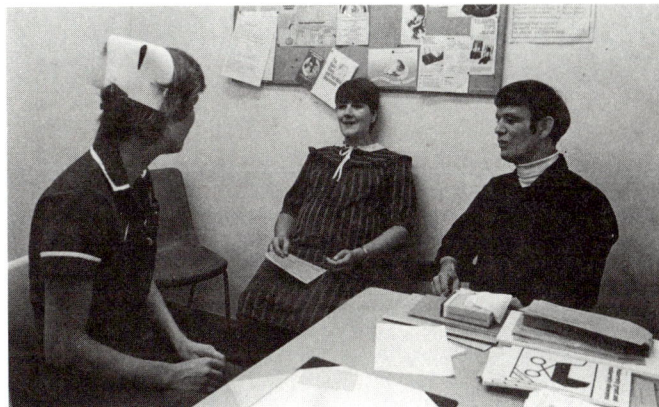

Mother and father-to-be in the ante-natal clinic, with a midwife they are both getting to know well

DEVELOPING SKILLS TO IMPLEMENT INDIVIDUALISED CARE

We have explained that, to implement nursing care planned to meet patients' individual needs, nurses have to be:

- flexible in the way in which they organise their work
- able to make decisions, on a day-to-day basis, about how individualised care can be implemented
- able to work in a way that provides opportunities for them to get to know their own patients.

Working in this way demands special skills which fall into three main categories:

- organisational skills
- decision-making skills
- interpersonal skills.

In this section, we shall discuss these skills in relation to implementing individualised care and we shall place particular emphasis on considering how more experienced nurse practitioners can help others to develop these skills.

ORGANISATIONAL SKILLS

For a nurse providing truly individualised care, every working day may need to be organised differently. In order to be efficient and effective, but also sufficiently flexible, a nurse needs to be able to apply the *systematic problem-solving process* to the organisation of her work.

First, she must be able to **assess** her workload for the day. This will involve:

- examining patients' care plans
- finding out what resources are available
- establishing the needs of other nurses in the team
- considering the activities of other health workers.

Secondly, she must be able to make a **plan** for her day's work. This will involve:

- deciding what can realistically be achieved in the time available
- setting priorities so that the most important aspects of her work are sure to be completed
- outlining the order and timing of her work
- communicating her plan to those whom it involves, i.e. patients, relatives, other nurses, other health workers.

Next, she must be able to **implement** her work plan. This will involve:

- using her time carefully
- not being too easily distracted by trivia, but
- being sensitive to new circumstances or new patient needs which may necessitate modification of the original plan.

Finally, she must be able to **evaluate** the way in which she works. This will involve:

- checking her own progress through the day, so that if she finds she has set herself unrealistic goals she can modify her plan accordingly
- examining the results of her work at the end of the day, so that she can communicate what she has achieved or failed to achieve to the nurse taking over from her
- questioning whether the way in which she assessed, planned and implemented her work could have been improved, thereby learning from her day's experience
- checking that unnecessary nursing work is not being perpetuated.

Asking nurses to work in this way creates a major organisational challenge for those who lead a nursing team. How can they create a learning environment which allows juniors to experiment with planning and decision making, without causing chaos and endangering patients? It can be done, but it means that the team leader (for example, the ward sister or the community nursing sister) may need to change her role.

Let us consider two styles of leadership which may be used in nursing and see what they offer.

An **authoritarian** leader does all the thinking and decision making for her team and issues precise instructions which team members are expected to follow to the letter. This kind of leadership may produce a very obedient and efficient team, but individuals may be quite unaware of how their leader reaches her decisions and they may not understand why they are performing the tasks which they have been given. Opportunities for juniors to learn and develop are minimal.

With little stimulus to think for themselves, team members are unlikely to generate new ideas; the leader is rarely challenged and the whole team can easily become rather narrow, fixed in its ways and resistant to change, and it can have difficulty in maintaining the flexibility required to implement individually planned care.

Alternatively, a **democratic** leader can ask nurses, from their earliest days in training, to think about how their own work should be organised, to try making suggestions about work priorities and ways in which they can make best use of their resources. If reasonable ideas are put forward, juniors can be given permission to try them out and see what they can learn from the experience. If there are obvious serious pitfalls the leader can point them out and suggest

Supervision is

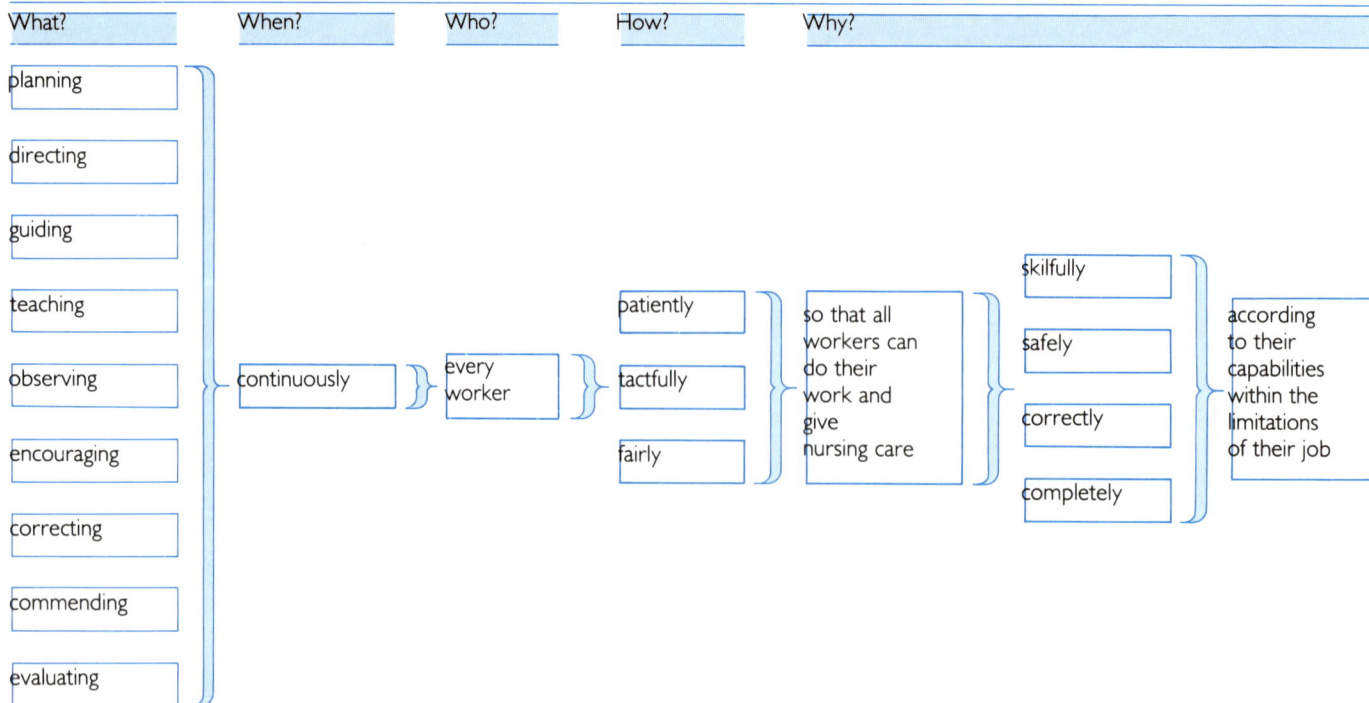

What?	When?	Who?	How?		Why?		
planning							
directing							
guiding							
teaching			patiently	so that all workers can do their work and give nursing care	skilfully		according to their capabilities within the limitations of their job
observing	continuously	every worker	tactfully		safely		
encouraging			fairly		correctly		
correcting					completely		
commending							
evaluating							

Fig. 4.2   Kron's summary of supervision (Kron, 1981)

alternatives, so no harm is done. Learner nurses in a new setting can often come up with original ideas, which those more habituated to the work had never thought of, so this can be an exciting way for everyone to work. Healthy questioning, innovation and change can become part of everyday life.

The democratic leader retains control and has the final say in decision making. Nurses' abilities are stretched: they have to be imaginative and creative, they discover their own strengths and weaknesses, they have the satisfaction of seeing the results of their own efforts and they are constantly learning and developing.

The key element of a democratic leader's role is **supervision**. The leader delegates the task of organising nursing work to individual team members and then makes herself available to guide and advise them, so that they can develop their skills in an atmosphere of security, support and encouragement. The leader is also available to make sure that patient care is implemented safely and effectively. Kron (1981) gives a succinct diagrammatic summary of the senior nurse's supervisory role, shown in Figure 4.2.

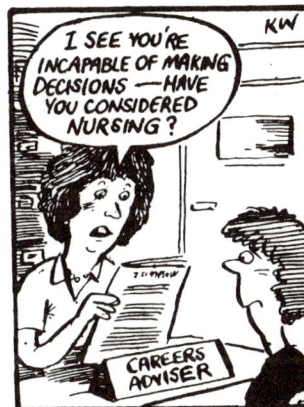

DECISION-MAKING SKILLS

As you work through this course, you will appreciate that nurses have to make decisions at all stages of the nursing process.

At the implementation stage, they need to make decisions about how to organise their work and about priorities within their workload.

It seems appropriate to consider decision making in a little more detail at this point, because the way nursing work is organised and the way in which the team leader functions can greatly influence the development of decision-making skills in more junior nurses.

It has already been said that making decisions can be stressful for nurses, especially when a wrong decision may adversely affect a patient (p. 88). On the other hand, making decisions can be challenging and satisfying. There is always an element of risk in decision making: a judgment has to be made about possible choices. If the choice were obvious there would be no need for a decision. Coping with the stressful risk element depends upon whether nurses feel that they can confidently justify the decisions which they make. This confidence will only come from knowing that decisions have been based on accurate information, sound knowledge and a thorough assessment of the choices available.

Helping nurses to develop confidence and competence in decision making is another vital part of the leader's role when individually planned care is being implemented.

Practice that is governed by tradition, ritual, routine or strict rules leads to *illogical* decision making which can only be justified by statements such as:

"That's the way it's always been done here."
"That's the way I was taught."
"That's what sister always uses."

Nurses who are eventually to be accountable for their own actions will need to give better answers than these. So here are just a few ideas on how a senior nurse may lead others towards making sound, *logical* decisions.

Take every opportunity to help less experienced nurses to extend their knowledge base by:

- showing a willingness to impart information

- relating relevant theory to practical situations

- promoting discussion of research literature that relates to specific clinical problems

- making relevant reading material available in the clinical setting

- emphasising the importance of responsible nurses being able to explain the reasons for their actions

- learning not to feel threatened by difficult questions and being able to say "I don't know".

Help less experienced nurses to apply logical thinking to their everyday work by:

- formally applying systematic problem solving to the care of each individual patient

- taking nurses through the steps of systematic problem solving as they organise their work (as described earlier on p. 93).

- explaining the rationale behind her own decisions.

Feeling confident about decision making not only helps nurses to feel comfortable with professional responsibility, it also enables them to take an active and assertive role when group decisions concerning their patients need to be made by the whole health care team.

INTERPERSONAL SKILLS

Interpersonal skills are important at all stages of the nursing process. In Module 2, you have seen that one of the purposes of an initial assessment is to lay the foundations of a good nurse-patient relationship. Module 3 stresses the importance of working in a partnership with patients when setting goals and planning nursing care.

During the *implementation* stage, it is vital that nursing care is carried out in a way which makes the patient feel that he is recognised and respected as a person. Failure to act in this way can undermine the trust and confidence that was beginning to grow. Nursing can often involve performing activities which, for the patient, are potentially embarrassing and humiliating. Being catheterised, having an unsightly wound exposed, discussing sexual difficulties, or acknowledging irrational fears and behaviour can be traumatic – even devastating – experiences for a patient if the nurse concerned, however well-meaning, behaves insensitively and inappropriately.

Consider two patients:

An attractive 40 year-old woman has had a mastectomy. She now believes that she is grotesque, unfeminine and repulsive to her husband. She is unable to focus on any of the good features of her body or her personality. Her distorted body-image is seriously hindering her rehabilitation.

A 50 year-old company director has had a stroke. He has no speech deficit, but he has become withdrawn and uncommunicative, especially at meal-times, and he refuses to eat. He cannot control the left side of his mouth. He dribbles saliva, and food and drink spill down his chin. He feels like a baby. He feels disgusting, helpless and worthless. His self-concept is so negative, his self-esteem so low, that he would rather be dead than disabled. He will not even discuss a rehabilitation programme.

Nurses' behaviour can either confirm or negate what these two people feel about themselves, so the way in which nurses relate to them, as they carry out even the simplest of nursing tasks, can profoundly affect their recovery. For example, tactfully encouraging the woman to use her make-up and do her hair would be useful practical steps which, if accompanied by sensitive, gentle signs of approval of her appearance, could begin to mend the shattered self-image. Simply spending time sitting with the man, conveying a liking for him and an interest in what he has to say, could be the nurse's first step towards helping him to value himself more highly.

It needs to be remembered that, whilst assessment and care planning may be closely supervised by experienced nurses, it is often a very junior member of the team who actually helps the woman who has had the mastectomy to undress and get into the bath, or who takes the disabled man his lunch; the junior's manner of relating to these patients can be as significant as anyone else's.

As the interpersonal skills of *all* nurses are so very significant when care is being implemented, it seems appropriate at this stage to mention just what these skills are and to consider how nurses may be helped to develop them. However, we must state that this is a vast and complex field and detailed discussion is beyond the scope of this course. Some further reading will be recommended at the end of this module.

We have suggested that nursing work should be organised in a way that provides nurses with *opportunities* to get to know their patients and to establish close relationships with them – but opportunities alone are not enough. Indeed, the close contact may trigger stronger defences, as nurses struggle to protect themselves in relationships which they feel unable to handle. So how can they be helped?

Experience and research in the field of psychology is particularly valuable here. For example, it is helpful for nurses to know that when a person finds himself in a relationship in which he feels he is accepted uncritically for what he is, valued in his own right and genuinely understood, then psychologically he is likely to grow, gaining insight, emotional independence, self-respect and confidence in handling reality. Carl Rogers (1967) describes this kind of relationship as a "helping relationship", that is, "a relationship in which at least one of the parties has the intent of promoting the growth, development, maturity, improved functioning, improved coping with life of the other". This is the kind of relationship which nurses can beneficially try to provide, not only for their patients as they work with them, *but also for each other.*

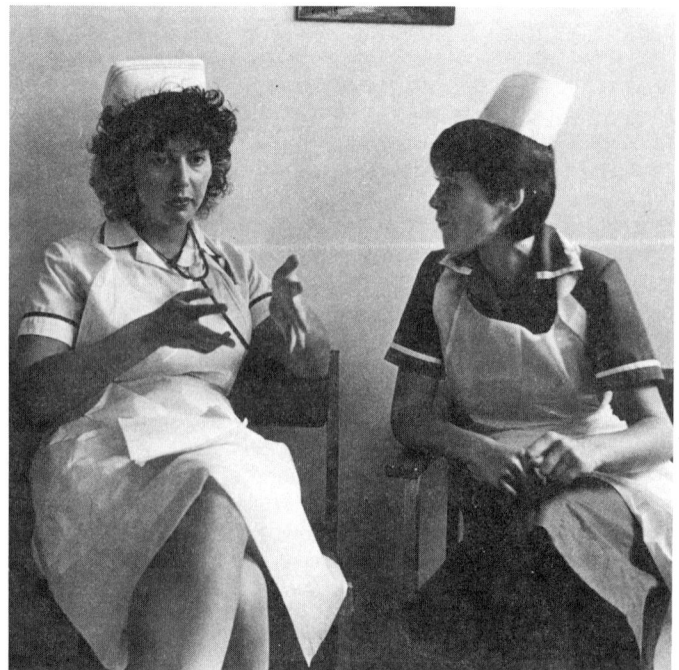

Sister discussing a problem with a staff nurse

How can this be achieved? Rogers makes some suggestions based on his work as a psychotherapist and on his own experience of life:

> The relationship which I have found helpful is characterised by a sort of transparency on my part, in which my real feelings are evident; by an acceptance of this other person as a separate person with value in his own right; and by a deep empathetic understanding which enables me to see his private world through his eyes. When these conditions are achieved, I become a companion to my client . . .

The work of another psychologist, Sidney Jourard (1971), helps us to see what this kind of relationship can mean in nursing. Jourard, who taught and worked with nurses, is not very complimentary about their traditional professional behaviour, describing it as "the contrived, tense, even frantic, and sometimes silly specimen of behaviour that we have called the bedside manner". However, he is sympathetic and looks at ways in which nurses might be helped so that "they will not have chronic need to hide their real self behind a professional mask". He emphasises the importance of senior nurses and nurse teachers allowing, indeed encouraging, juniors to express fear, embarrassment, disgust, sadness and all the other emotions that they will naturally feel when they first encounter sick and distressed people. Accepting these emotions as normal, the senior perhaps acknowledging that she once felt the same, allows the junior to come to terms with her experiences and to mature without feeling any sense of shame at her initial reactions. On the other hand, if the junior is made to feel that her reactions are inappropriate, that "nurses shouldn't behave like that", she will feel obliged to deny and repress her true feelings, and mimic the 'more acceptable' behaviour of her superiors. Having been made to feel ashamed of her real self, she no longer trusts or respects her own feelings and she hides behind the professional mask, unable to grow and unable to get close to others.

Jourard suggests that nurse teachers (i.e. any nurse who influences other nurses) can prevent this unhappy process, simply by showing more interest in getting to know their students as individual people. This is likely to prompt a response from the students which acknowledges the real self of the teacher. Jourard says that openness and genuine interest in others is contagious, "just as contagious as impersonality and indifference to inner experience". Jourard and Rogers are saying quite simply that if people, including nurses, feel valued and cared for themselves, then they will be free to care for and get close to others.

This thinking has important implications for the whole nursing service. Menzies (1960) discovered a widespread "depersonalization" in the hospital nursing world which she studied and she found that "support for the individual is notably lacking throughout the whole nursing service within working relationships". Considering effects of this "depersonalization" on the individual nurse she says "The implied disregard of her own needs and capacities is distressing for the nurse, she feels she does not matter and no one cares what happens to her".

If nurse managers, teachers and senior practitioners want nurses who work with them to implement personalised nursing care, it is important that they examine their own nursing organisation and try to weed out any remnants of "depersonalization". They need also to examine the kind of relationships which they provide for their subordinates.

Once again, dipping into the world of psychology, we have touched upon some quite complicated ideas. It might be helpful if we try to summarise what has been said and point out areas which you might usefully explore further at a later date, if this material is new to you.

Implementing nursing care planned specifically to meet the needs of a unique, complex human being demands mature, sensitive behaviour. If nurses experience relationships with senior colleagues in which they feel trusted and valued, they can develop the insight and self-confidence which they need in order to relate appropriately to their patients. *The experience of feeling cared for in a supportive relationship enables nurses to care.*

The key elements of a helping relationship are:

Self-awareness: this means being in touch with your own feelings and emotions, being honest about your strengths and weaknesses, and understanding your motives and actions.

Authenticity: this means genuinely being yourself and not hiding behind a facade, not trying to be what you think a staff nurse/sister/midwife etc. *ought* to be like.

Acceptance of others: this means showing a genuine interest in others, acknowledging and valuing what they are in a non-judgmental way.

Empathy: this is a sensitivity to and understanding of the other person's feelings and experience.

Of course, effective communication is vital for building up this relationship. Self-awareness includes being sensitive to what your appearance, manner, expression and gestures communicate to others. Authenticity requires you to put into words and gestures what you really think and feel. Showing an interest in others requires active listening, a very important skill in nursing. Empathy may be conveyed in facial expression, by the use of touch and by the use of silence, as well as by words.

The teaching of communication theory and the use of experiential learning techniques to develop self-awareness and communication skills are relatively new in nursing education programmes, but they are proving extremely valuable. In an adventurous scheme at the Burford Nursing Development Unit (Swaffield, 1982) a group of actors participated with trained nurses in role play activities. Results, in terms of nurses' personal development and ability to relate effectively to patients, have been impressive. Dowd (1983) has described the use of experiential learning with student nurses at The London Hospital and reports that "one of the most noticeable results . . . is the rapidity of development in the students' interpersonal skills".

Showing empathy

You should find this activity quite easy. It is intended simply to emphasise how nurses and patients can convey clear messages to each other without the use of words. Without knowing what is being said between nurse and patient, you should be able to identify signs of the presence or absence of empathetic understanding by noting in the photographs factors such as body posture, facial expression and gestures.

Look carefully at the photographs. For each, write down whether you think the nurse is conveying empathy towards the patient.

State, in each case, what it is about the nurse and the patient that has brought you to your conclusion.

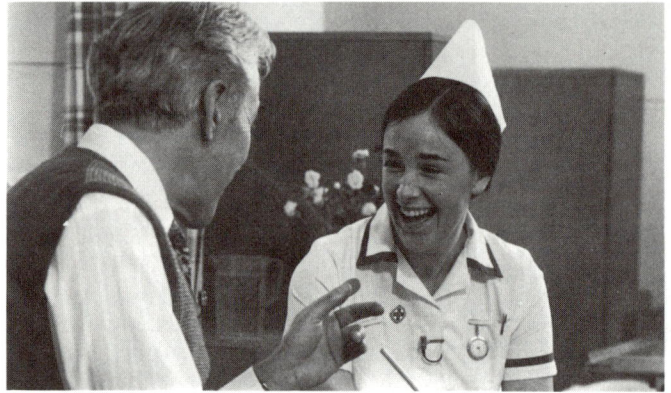

PHOTO 2

Authors' comment

PHOTO 1: this nurse is talking to her patient but is busy studying her chart at the same time, and so is missing the messages she is giving out. The patient's expression is anxious and questioning and she is sitting up tensely as if she is about to say something important. She is getting no encouragement from the nurse, who has not noticed her agitation and so is unable to empathise with her.

PHOTO 2: this nurse is conveying empathy towards her patient. She is sitting close to the man, giving him her time and attention and she is reflecting his relaxed posture. She shows she appreciates his jovial mood by laughing warmly as he talks.

We shall look at empathy in more depth further on in the module.

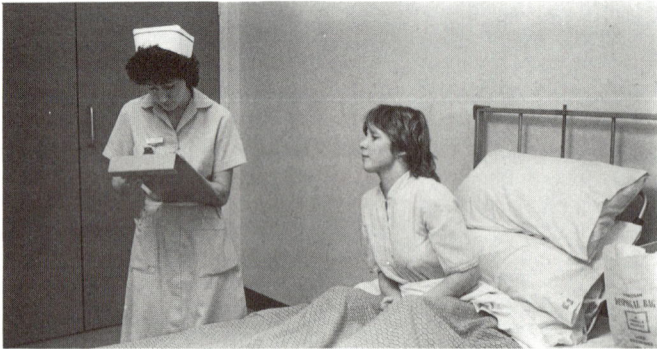

PHOTO 1

MAINTAINING THE NURSE-PATIENT PARTNERSHIP

The idea of the nurse working in partnership with her patient runs very clearly throughout this course. The initial patient assessment was described in Module 2 as forming the basis for a close working relationship between nurse and patient. Module 3 describes the nurse as a professional, offering specialist advice to a responsible client who is free to make choices about the aims of his care and the actions needed to achieve them. At the beginning of this module, we looked at ways of organising nursing work which would create opportunities for this nurse-patient partnership to grow and develop during the actual implementation of care; we also explained why and how education and management in nursing should focus on helping nurses to cope with this new kind of relationship.

A PERSONAL APPROACH

Inherent in the word 'partnership' is the idea of sharing – not only sharing knowledge and information at the assessment and planning stages, but also sharing in carrying out the work planned. If a patient is to take an active part in his care, he must be treated as the responsible human being which he is. Partners are equal and nurses' behaviour should reflect recognition of this fact.

It is still not uncommon to hear well-meaning nurses using inappropriate pet names for patients, using baby-talk and uttering patronising platitudes. Treating mature people like children is likely to provoke either resentment and hostility, or else regression to a dependent child-like role. This is no basis for co-operation and partnership. All members of the nursing team, including auxiliaries, need to be made aware of the importance of addressing and talking to patients respectfully. It doesn't mean that relationships have to become starchy and formal and that Christian names can't be used, if that is what the patient likes. There is plenty of scope for friendliness, warmth and laughter between equal partners.

Over the last decade or so, many nurses have been making strenuous efforts to provide a more personal service for their patients. The need to counteract the dehumanising effects of institutional life is being recognised, particularly in areas where long-stay or

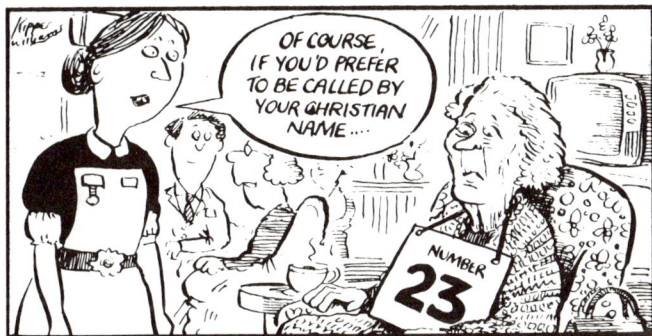

OF COURSE, IF YOU'D PREFER TO BE CALLED BY YOUR CHRISTIAN NAME....

NUMBER 23

elderly patients are nursed (Royal College of Nursing and British Geriatric Society, 1975). For example, nurses are being taught the importance of remembering the formalities of normal social interaction as they provide care for their patients. Introducing themselves by name, sitting at eye-level when talking to patients and being careful not to exclude them when speaking to colleagues in their presence, are simple examples of ways in which nurses can show respect and help patients to retain dignity. These changes in attitude and practice must continue if individually planned care is to be successfully implemented.

THE HELPING RELATIONSHIP

During the implementation stage of the nursing process, nurses have an opportunity to build a strong element of trust into the partnership. A nurse's behaviour as she carries out nursing activities can confirm to her patient that the partnership is genuine. If the patient can still relate to his nurse as a person while care is actually being given, if he feels that he can comfortably participate, question and criticise, and if he sees that his nurse is still interested in him and responsive to him, then he will feel that the self-disclosure involved in assessment was worthwhile. The promises of the planning stage will be realised and his personal needs met. The way in which care is implemented proves to the patient whether or not his nurses mean what they say, whether or not they can be trusted. You need to remember that, like any good relationship, the nurse-patient partnership doesn't just happen; it needs to be worked at. With this in mind, you can consciously make constructive use of the time you have with a patient, while care is being implemented.

So what do you actually need to do? Let us now look in a little more detail at what is involved in building up this partnership while you are there doing things with and for your patient.

So far, we have talked about telling your patient who you are, letting him see you as a person, and showing respect for him as an individual. These really quite simple things form the basis of "the helping relationship" described by Rogers, which we discussed in the last section. This relationship is very much a partnership and it is one in which an individual can mature, learn to cope and become more emotionally independent. This kind of relationship is particularly appropriate in nursing. If you look back to the three models of nursing discussed in Module 1 you will see that, within different frameworks, the role of the nurse is consistently shown as being to help her patient along a health continuum, away from dependence towards independence. Even for the dying patient, the nurse can facilitate an emotional and spiritual strengthening, a coming to terms with the reality of death.

Having established, in the way you approach your patient, that there is mutual respect, your "helping relationship" can be sustained and developed through empathy. This again is something which you can convey in your manner as you work with and for your patient. Kalisch (1973) defines empathy as: "the ability to enter into the life of another person, to accurately perceive his current feelings and their meanings". Empathy is different from sympathy. Sympathy means actually feeling the other person's emotions so that you get upset/angry/scared with him. Empathy means that you understand the other person's emotions and what they mean for him, but you don't actually experience them for yourself (Sundeen et al, 1981).

In order to empathise with your patient you need to be receptive to what he is conveying to you about his own experience. As you perform nursing duties, such as helping a patient bath, changing a surgical dressing, or supervising breast-feeding, you will have many opportunities to listen to your patient and to watch for non-verbal cues, which may either confirm or contradict what your patient actually says.

Listening involves:

- showing that you are interested in what your patient has to say
- allowing him time to put his ideas and feelings into words
- allowing silence to let him develop his thoughts
- helping him to continue with what he is saying by using encouraging gestures and noises: for example, nodding, "I see", "Mmmm", "Yes, carry on"
- summarising what he has said in your own words, so that he can see you have understood and can then build on what he has said.

Non-verbal cues are messages which a person gives out without using words. You can consciously watch:

- his facial expression
- the way in which he positions his body
- his gestures
- the way in which he looks at you, or away from you.

Conveying receptivity to what another person really wants to communicate is an active, skilful process which can be studied and learnt. It is invaluable in nursing.

Activity 4.6　　　　　　　　　　　　　　　　Allow 5 minutes

Active listening

This activity, like the last one, uses photographs and is quick and easy to do. These photographs are intended to make you more consciously aware of the non-verbal messages associated with listening.

As you look at the following two photographs, imagine that *you are the patient*. State, in each case, whether you think that the nurse is listening to you in a way that really makes you feel she is concerned to hear what you have to say. Write down what it is about the nurse that tells you whether or not she is listening.

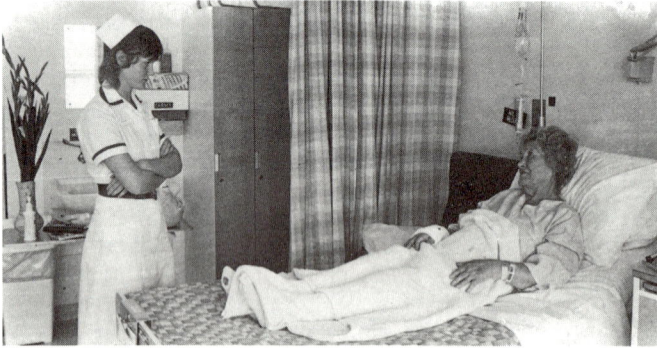

PHOTO 1

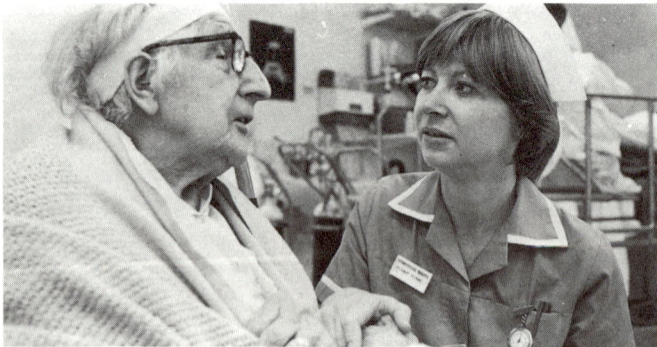

PHOTO 2

Authors' comment

PHOTO 1: this nurse appears to be paying attention to what the patient is saying, for she is looking directly at her. However, the nurse is standing up and has placed herself further away from the patient than is usual for someone who is genuinely interested in developing a conversation. The nurse also has her arms folded so that she is unconsciously creating a physical barrier between herself and the patient. The message which the patient receives from the nurse is to keep her conversation brief and superficial.

PHOTO 2: this patient is being listened to. The nurse has positioned herself close to the woman and at her eye level. She shows no sign of hurrying away. She is looking directly at her patient and her face shows that she is concentrating on what is being said. The way the nurse is leaning slightly towards the woman suggests genuine interest, and her touch shows warm concern. The patient should be aware that the nurse wishes to hear what she has to say and indeed, she appears to be quite relaxed and comfortable in the conversation.

Communication is a two-way process. Once you have *perceived* what your patient is telling you, you need to *respond* in a way that shows you understand.

You can convey empathy in your words and your actions. For example, you can use words which simply reflect an understanding of what is being said:

"I can see that is very painful for you to talk about."
"You are really very worried about going home."

You can avoid words that imply an opinion or judgment and thereby focus attention away from the patient and onto yourself.

"That's good", "That's wrong", "I think you should . . ."

Touch can convey a great deal of warmth and understanding, but needs to be used sensitively. Inappropriate invasion of personal space can be discomfiting and irritating and will not be received as an empathetic gesture. However, holding the hand of a woman in labour or a patient undergoing a painful procedure, cuddling an unhappy child or literally providing a shoulder for a distressed patient or relative to cry on are examples of ways in which touch can be used to give comfort. Touch can also be invaluable in conveying empathy when there are major communication barriers, as with a blind person, a patient being artificially ventilated, or a patient who cannot understand English.

Allowing the patient to cry, or to express anger or any other emotion is important. "There, there don't cry", or "try to calm down" imply that you don't think that the emotions being expressed are appropriate, or at least that the person shouldn't be sharing them with you.

Of course, empathy isn't something which you deliberately set out to create – it evolves within a relationship; but a deeper understanding of the elements of communication involved and a heightened self-awareness can make you a much more effective partner to your patient. If this material is new to you, further study in the field is strongly recommended (see *Further Reading* at the end of the module).

Activity 4.7　　　　　　　　　　　　　　　Allow 10 minutes

Getting involved with your patients

This activity aims to help you think about the practicalities of forming close relationships with your own patients and their families.

List any practical difficulties or personal anxieties which you think may occur if you get more closely involved with your patients and their families.

LIMITING AND TERMINATING THE PARTNERSHIP

A helping relationship is obviously a very close one. In the nurse-patient partnership, a degree of emotional involvement is inevitable for both parties. If the relationship is a long one, or if the patient's experience is intense, strong emotional bonds may form. However, there will be limitations to the relationship, both in terms of how much time the nurse and the patient can spend together and how long the relationship will last. It is very important that both nurse and patient know, at an early stage, what the boundaries of their relationship will be, so that they are both emotionally prepared.

Establishing the boundaries and preparing for the end of the relationship should begin soon after the nurse and patient first meet.

For example, the student nurse coming to work on a long-stay geriatric ward as one allocation in her training programme, should make it clear to her patients, soon after she arrives, that she will only be working in the ward for eight weeks. It may also be helpful, as the weeks pass, to remind them how much time is left.

The community nurse visiting an elderly lady recently discharged from hospital after having had a fractured neck of femur repaired, needs to explain how often she will call and for how long her visits will continue. If a time limit cannot be stated, the achievement of certain goals may be the limiting factor – she will continue to call once a week, until the lady can get in and out of the bath without help.

Many psychiatric nurses have found that they and their patients are able to handle very close therapeutic relationships by actually making a formal contract. For example, the nurse and patient may agree to spend exactly one hour together each Monday and Thursday for six weeks and then review their progress. Both partners know exactly what to expect and they can both prepare for these occasions in order to make the best use of the limited time available.

The boundaries of the partnership are often implied at the care planning stage. Goals stating the expected outcome for the patient often indicate the degree of independence which he is expected to achieve, but gradual withdrawal of nursing support may need to be discussed and reinforced as care is being implemented.

Usually, if both parties have known what to expect, the relationship can be ended comfortably with the nurse and patient feeling satisfaction at having achieved the goals which they planned together. When a patient dies at the end of a long illness his nurse may well feel loss and sadness, but she should also feel satisfaction at having provided a close, supportive relationship which enabled her patient to die peacefully.

If the nurse – or the patient – is finding difficulty in ending a close bond, the nurse should discuss the matter with a senior colleague. It may be helpful for the nurse simply to share her emotions, or she may need to examine critically the kind of relationship which she is providing for her patient. Preparation must be made for terminating the partnership. An emotional response to the termination should be acknowledged, shared and discussed.

PATIENT AND FAMILY PARTICIPATION IN CARE

Partnership means working together towards some common goal. It implies a positive, active role for each participant in the partnership. Clearly, there are times in nurse-patient relationships when the patient cannot participate in his own nursing care and when the nurse has to act on his behalf; the anaesthetised patient on an operating table and the premature baby in an incubator are obvious examples. However, there are occasions when a patient, highly dependent upon nurses in some ways, may be able to function independently in others. Nurses' recognition of healthy functioning, as well as of weaknesses, and their utilisation of any remaining independence, can greatly enhance a patient's sense of identity and sense of having some degree of control over what is happening to him. An artificially ventilated patient may be able to do little for himself, but he may be conscious and still perfectly able to perform cerebral activities. Nurses who provide this patient with intelligible and appropriate information will help him to form a rational interpretation of what is happening to him, to adopt healthy attitudes to his situation and to exert a degree of control over his own responses. Ashworth (1980) discusses this problem in her work on communication with patients in intensive care units. She gives an example of a man who found tracheal suction very distressing until he learned that the procedure cleared his chest and that it hurt less if he did not resist the passage of the catheter down his trachea. Once he understood what was happening and why, he was able to control his response to the procedure and thereby make a helpful contribution to his nursing care. He then found that 'suction' was no longer as unpleasant. A ventilated patient receiving tracheal suction may initially appear to be a passive recipient of care, but this example illustrates very well how nurses could actively involve even highly dependent patients in the implementation of their care, to the benefit of all concerned.

The patient's participation in his nursing care can often be anticipated at the planning stage. In discussing components of nursing prescriptions (Module 3, p. 72), it was suggested that:

A clear definition of what the patient will do not only makes for a more useful prescription of care, but also promotes awareness that patients have an important – and often the major – role to play in achieving goals.

It is important that the roles of the nurse and of the relatives are also made explicit. Orem's self-care model of nursing is particularly helpful here, for it focuses on Man's ability to care for himself and it lays particular emphasis on the agent of care – whether it is the patient himself, the nurse or some other person.

As you will remember from Module 1, Orem describes the patient as progressing from having his needs met for him, through being helped to meet his needs, to finally meeting them independently.

Figure 4.3 is a diagrammatic representation of Orem's model. Part (a) indicates the nursing contribution necessary when a patient cannot care for himself unaided, or to use Orem's term, when there is a self-care deficit. Part (b) illustrates the nurse's aim to help the patient in a progression away from dependence and towards independence.

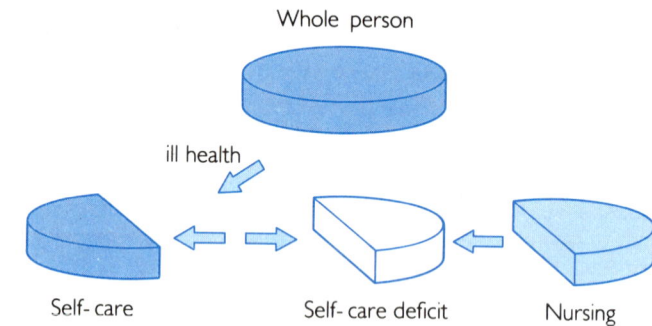

Part (a)

The wholeness of the person is disrupted by ill health leaving the person unable to care fully for himself, i.e. with a self-care deficit. Nursing compensates for this deficit, maintaining the integrity of the whole.

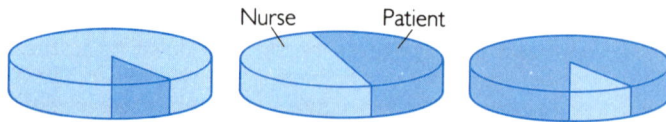

Part (b)

Progressive reduction in the compensatory role of the nurse as the patient moves away from dependence towards independence.

Fig. 4.3 Diagrammatic representation of Orem's self-care model of nursing (after Ewing, 1983)

The nurse's helping role may involve:

- acting or doing for the patient
- guiding
- supporting (physically or psychologically)
- providing an environment which promotes personal development
- teaching.

The work of Gail Ewing in Edinburgh (Ewing, 1983a) provides a practical example of how Orem's model can be used to clarify the role of each participant in a particular aspect of nursing care. Ewing uses elements of Orem's model alongside guidelines devised to help patients with the management of stoma appliances. She has developed a self-care preparation plan in order to co-ordinate more effectively the nursing care of patients with stomas (Figure 4.4). A patient may learn to handle some aspects of his own care faster than others. For example, with the removal of the old appliance, the patient may progress quite rapidly from the initial point where the nurse acts for him, through teaching and guidance, to being finally independent. However, he may be slow to learn about skin protection and so have to spend longer at the teaching stage, before he progresses towards independence in this aspect of his care.

Ewing provides working definitions of the "helping methods" which she has specifically designed for use in stoma appliance management (other definitions could be devised for other fields of nursing). Her definitions are:

Acting: this refers to the nurse undertaking the care for the patient.

Teaching: this is done in conjunction with acting, and refers to the nurse teaching about a guideline (one aspect of care, as shown in Figure 4.4); this involves more than just explaining what is about to be done, but teaches how it is done.

Guiding: this refers to the patient taking over the care, with the nurse instructing how to do it.

Supporting: this refers to the patient taking over the care without any instruction from the nurse, but with moral support.

Home/self-care: this refers to the patient becoming self-caring for one guideline; the home situation in relation to the guideline is discussed where appropriate.

Provision of a developmental environment: this refers to providing a positive atmosphere during the appliance change by:

- the provision of privacy
- the use of professional terminology
- a positive facial expression
- the avoidance of the use of gloves.

The aim of using the plan is to enable a nurse to decide upon the care which she is going to give, on the basis of knowing what has been done before. By looking at the progress which the patient has made

Guideline	Acting	Teaching	Guiding	Supporting	Home/self-care	Developmental environment	Date of change
Preparation of equipment						Privacy	1
						Uninterrupted care	2
Preparation of patient						Exposure of stoma only	3
Removal of old appliance						Screening of patient	4
Skin care						Terminology	5
							6
Skin protection							7
Selection of new appliance						Facial expression	8
							9
Preparation of new appliance							10
Application						No gloves	11
							12
Disposal							13

Fig. 4.4 Part of Ewing's self-care preparation plan for patients learning to change a stoma appliance (Ewing, 1983a)

in relation to each guideline, the nurse should be better able to take the patient another step forward in his care.

The nursing staff involved in the trial at the Edinburgh Royal Infirmary were "very positive that it enabled them to co-ordinate the self-care preparation of their stoma patients" (Ewing, 1983b).

If the patient cannot be self-caring for a particular need, a friend or relative may be willing to be the self-care agent. When we were beginning to introduce the nursing process and were looking at our own practice, a situation occurred which made us realise that we had to reconsider the family's role in implementing care.

Mrs Jones, a widow in her early sixties, was in the last stages of a terminal illness. Her only daughter, Mrs White, lived nearby with her husband and two young children. Mrs White worked part-time. The family, the G.P. and the community nurse had discussed various ways of providing care. Mrs Jones decided that she would prefer to be in hospital on the ward where she had previously received treatment.

On her mother's admission, Mrs White explained that she had regularly helped her to have a bath and wash and set her hair and that she wanted to continue doing this. Mrs Jones said that she always felt relaxed afterwards. Mrs White continued to carry out these elements of care, always indicating any days when she would be unable to bath her mother.

When Mrs Jones died, Mrs White was with her and she asked the nurse if she could help with 'laying out'. This request momentarily threw us; our initial reaction was "yes, but what did the hospital system say?" Then we realised that for nurses the last offices represent the last act of care for a patient, and we frequently gained 'satisfaction' from this. Why should the daughter feel any differently and what right had we to deny Mrs White her wishes?

During a discussion later on, we wondered how many other relatives might have wanted to become involved with the care but were afraid to ask, or didn't ask because they felt that the hospital would not allow it or that the nurses might think that their care was being criticised. Nurses automatically tend to take over many simple 'non-technical' activities, such as cutting nails, shaving, setting ladies' hair and so on, when a person becomes 'a patient'.

The family may want to be involved, but need to be told that they can be. Some relatives may not want to be physically involved with care but may not want to be excluded – when the screens are drawn it does not always imply that the relative has got to leave the bedside.

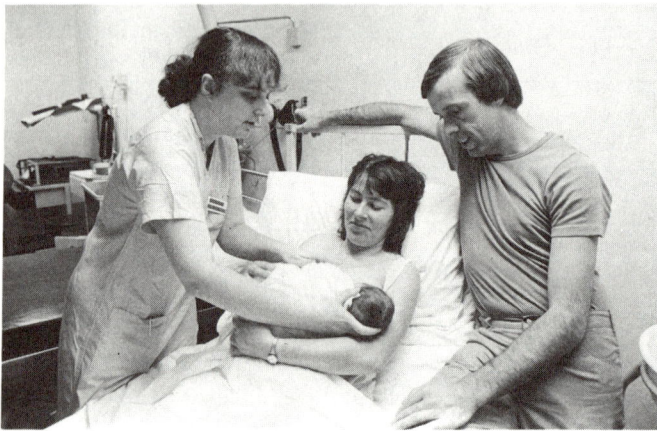

A proud father looks on as his newborn son learns to breast-feed

Many patients appreciate the involvement of relatives or close friends in their care, but it is also worth remembering that some people do not feel comfortable seeing their relatives in the role of carer. In the article *Every day is a bonus for us* (Dopson, 1983), Sue Coffey, a nurse herself, welcomed the opportunity to 'special' her husband, Paul, while he was in the intensive care unit, but he found it confusing: "The nurse role is not a role in which I see Sue . . . so far as I am concerned, she is a wife and a friend".

Activity 4.8   Allow 5 minutes

What is it like to be a patient's relative?

The purpose of this activity is to try and help you to get 'inside a relative's shoes' and to help you think about the role of patients' relatives in your own work setting.

Imagine yourself as the close relative of a patient for whom you have recently cared.

1 What was your relationship like with the nurses?
2 In what ways, if any, would you have liked this relationship to have been different?
3 What did you do to help the patient?

Authors' comment
It is difficult to give specific feedback on this activity because every situation will be so different.

If, as 'the relative', you felt that your relationship with the nurses could have been better and if you would have liked to do more for the sick member of your family, the section you have just read should give some ideas on how nurses may improve the situation.

So far, we have talked of the nurse as the initiator of care, but in order for the patient and/or the family to participate fully in care they may need special knowledge.

Research has shown that adults do not retain a great deal of what they are taught unless they have opportunities to practise new skills under supervision. Adults learn better by 'doing'. Patient and family therefore need to be actively involved in care with the nurse.

THE NURSE AS A TEACHER

The role of the nurse as a teacher is not new. For instance, the scene of a nurse teaching a person with diabetes how to inject insulin, which sites to use and how to draw up the required dose, is familiar.

At present, teaching may be done when there is time and on an ad hoc basis, but for it to be effective, like other aspects of care, teaching needs to be planned.

Just as the nursing care of an individual patient can be managed in a problem-oriented fashion, and just as nursing work can be organised using the steps of the problem-solving cycle, so the same systematic process can provide a framework for patient teaching. An assessment of the patient's abilities, goals for his learning and a plan of teaching activities can all be incorporated into his nursing care plan.

In any rehabilitation process, nurses can use much of the time which they spend carrying out practical activities with patients to implement a planned programme of teaching. We shall consider one common example. Cerebrovascular accident is a major cause of disability in this country and the recovery period can extend for a period of eighteen months to two years, with slow sustained improvement. Not all patients with strokes are admitted to hospital; many remain at home receiving the care of the community nursing services.

An integral part of the multi-disciplinary care of patients with strokes is teaching them how to recover function and to overcome disabilities. The nurse plays a major role in this rehabilitation and in preventing complications such as pressure sores and contractures. As the nurse spends more time with the patient and family than any other person, she can also act as a co-ordinator of care.

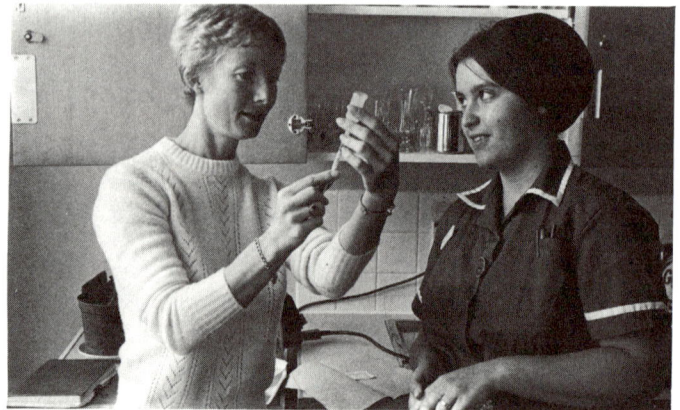

The community nurse in a teaching role

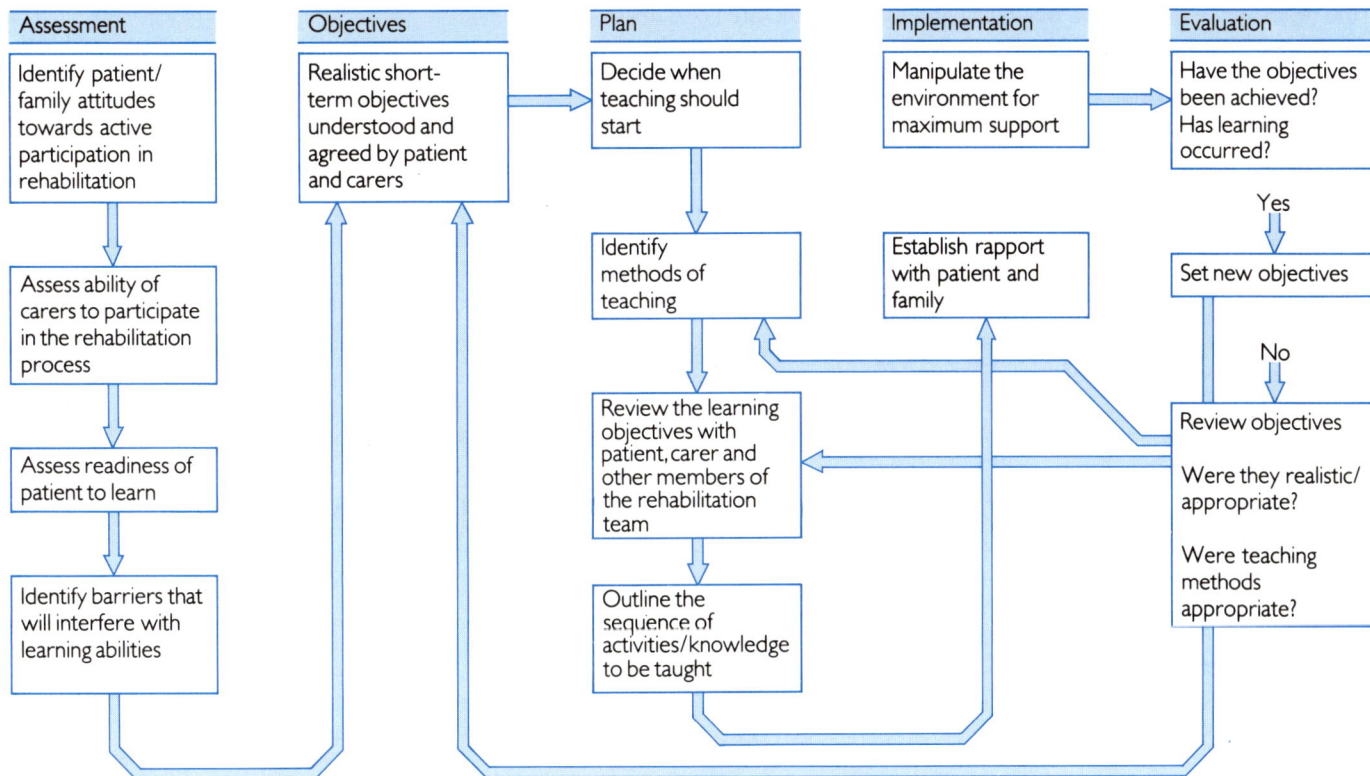

Assessment	Objectives	Plan	Implementation	Evaluation
Identify patient/ family attitudes towards active participation in rehabilitation	Realistic short-term objectives understood and agreed by patient and carers	Decide when teaching should start	Manipulate the environment for maximum support	Have the objectives been achieved? Has learning occurred?
Assess ability of carers to participate in the rehabilitation process		Identify methods of teaching	Establish rapport with patient and family	Set new objectives
Assess readiness of patient to learn		Review the learning objectives with patient, carer and other members of the rehabilitation team		Review objectives

Were they realistic/ appropriate?

Were teaching methods appropriate? |
| Identify barriers that will interfere with learning abilities | | Outline the sequence of activities/knowledge to be taught | | |

Fig. 4.5 Framework for stroke patient/family teaching (Batehup, 1983)

The Manchester Stroke Study (1978) found that the majority of patients with strokes have someone to care for them following discharge – out of 135 patients, 97 had a chief carer and only 9 of those relatives were unable, because of ill health, to have the patient return home. Garraway et al (1980) and Hamrin (1981) found that once discharged home, patients often lost the abilities they had achieved during hospital rehabilitation. This deterioration was attributed to carers at home not being aware of the patient's full potential and, anxious to 'care', tending to do more for the patient than was necessary. This highlights the need for patient and carer to be involved together in teaching and rehabilitation programmes.

Lynn Batehup (1983) has used the problem-oriented approach to develop a framework for stroke patient/family teaching (Figure 4.5). She states that "taking the time to write a teaching plan will ensure an individual approach to each patient".

An area in which a nurse may wish to share her nursing knowledge, with both the patient who has had a stroke and his carer, is the prevention of contractures. The topics she may wish to include in a teaching plan might be:

- an explanation of the importance of prevention
- ideas on practical management

- a demonstration of care
- the involvement of the patient and carer in care
- observation of the carer when confident
- further tuition, if required.

What better time to teach all of this than when the nurse is actually carrying out the care?

In health visiting, the implementation of care is often almost entirely concerned with teaching, for the major emphasis of a health visitor's work is on health education and prevention. A health visiting study (Luker, 1982) confirmed that planned, rather than unplanned, intervention is more effective in terms of improving health problems. Investigating a group of elderly women living alone, the common health problems identified included:

- weight maintenance
- mobility
- dentition
- sensory function.

The findings indicate that focused health visitor intervention has the potential to improve up to 43% of health problems. Also highlighted in the report is the fact that the well-being of clients was generated through another person taking an interest in their welfare, or what Luker termed "therapeutic anticipation", so it needs to be remembered that implementation covers psychosocial as well as physical care.

Activity 4.9　　　　　　　　　　　　Allow 15 minutes

Planning patient teaching

This activity will give you practice in developing teaching plans.

Using the ideas we have presented in this module, draw up a simple teaching plan which could have been used for a patient whom you have nursed recently. You need only concentrate on one aspect of this patient's care.

Authors' comment

We have no specific comments for this activity because you all work in different environments and will have selected different aspects of nursing care. However, it is likely that your teaching plan will reflect the following main points:

- *identifying the patient's present knowledge and ability*
- *identifying the patient's learning needs*
- *assessing the patient's level of motivation and identifying motivating forces*
- *identifying and obtaining the resources needed*
- *selecting suitable teaching methods*
- *demonstrating and supervising practical skills*
- *evaluating the effectiveness of teaching.*

MAINTAINING CONTINUITY OF NURSING CARE

THE NEED FOR CONTINUITY OF CARE

In this section of the module, we shall consider the issue of maintaining a consistent approach to dealing with a patient's problems, when, as is usually the case, there are several people involved in implementing the plan of care. We shall discuss nursing notes relating to care given and the handling of information about patient care at nursing report sessions.

Activity 4.10　　　　　　　　　　Allow 10 minutes

The need for continuity

This activity should help you to appreciate the need for maintaining continuity of nursing care in your own setting.

Think about one particular patient whom you have nursed during the last month.

1　Make a note of the number of nurses involved in that particular patient's care during any twenty-four hour period.

2　Calculate or estimate the number of different nurses involved in that patient's care over a period of seventy-two hours.

Authors' comment

The number of nurses involved in a patient's care will vary according to many factors and will depend upon whether you work in a hospital or a community setting. In the community, the number will be quite low and you may have been the only nurse involved, but in a hospital the number can be quite high, especially if the ward or department has several part-time or agency staff.

In a situation where several nurses are involved in implementing nursing care, there is a danger that each nurse's approach to the patient's problems will be entirely different. A written record helps to provide accuracy and continuity of care.

Even when a nurse works alone on a one-to-one basis with patients, she will have numerous patients 'on her books'. She will be unable to remember what each patient needs, and she will require the written record as a guide.

The written care plan is part of the nursing record which is there for everyone working with the patient to use. It needs to be easily *accessible* to the nurses who are caring for the patient. If it is inaccessible, there is a danger that the nurse will not refer to it nor up-date the plan as required.

A variety of locations may be used for storing records. In the community, the care plan may stay with the patient or the nurse or health visitor may keep a locked box containing the records in the car. In hospitals, some wards keep the care plan at the patient's bedside; some have one central holder at the nurses' station; others may have several holders, each containing plans for a group of patients, which can be taken to the patient's bedside when care is implemented. Each unit will need to consider the most appropriate location in the light of local circumstances.

Activity 4.11　　　　　　　　　　　　Allow 5 minutes

Communicating with other nurses

This activity may help you to stop and look critically at how you approach communication in your own work area.

How do *you* communicate information about patients to other nursing staff?

You have probably mentioned several of the following:

- *written records*
- *spoken handover – either face-to-face or by telephone*
- *discussion with one nurse, or group of nurses, about patient care*
- *transfer forms/letters to nursing colleagues in other departments*
- *day/night reports on patients for nurse managers.*

NURSING NOTES

"Where do I record that I have given the care?"
"Is there a need for me to record that I'm giving the care, if there is a detailed care plan and date set for evaluation?"

These are questions that nurses often ask.

In practice, many nurses find that a care plan and an evaluation record are insufficient. They may feel that in order to ensure continuity, some of the elements shown in Figure 4.6 need to be included in the record.

In addition, district or unit policies may specify certain types and frequency of recording; for example, a daily statement on patient care.

There are also statutory requirements about the frequency of record keeping. The United Kingdom Central Council for Nursing, Midwifery and Health Visiting recommends that midwives should maintain records on a mother and baby for the first ten days after delivery. Some midwives use a progress record for this, others have developed mother and baby observation records on the reverse side of care plans or in addition to care plans.

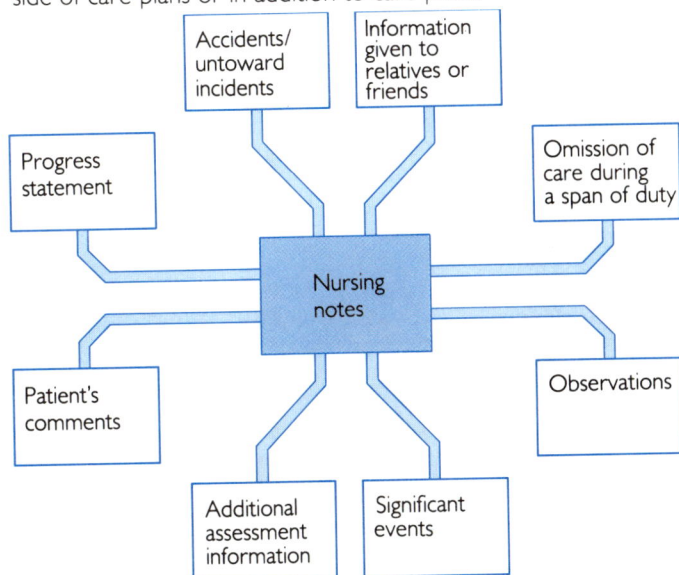

Date	Time	Progress notes	Signature

Or

Date	Problem no.	Progress record	Signature

Fig. 4.7   Examples of formats for nursing notes

Hence, most nursing records now contain a section called 'nursing notes' or 'progress records'; an example of one hospital's nursing notes is included in Module 6 (pp. 134–141).

Other examples of formats for nursing notes are shown in Figure 4.7.

The advantage of including a column headed 'problem number' is that statements which relate specifically to a problem stated on the care plan can be recorded without having to write out the problem every time it is mentioned.

With the use of a care plan system, the quality of information included in the nursing progress record tends to improve. Nurses are encouraged to emphasise a patient's response to nursing care, as well as to state what has been done, and they are taught to use language that conveys an exact meaning. Vague, ambiguous statements, such as "position changed frequently", "up for short periods" tend to appear less often.

Written records help to ensure that a comprehensive picture of a patient's progress is available at all times and is not simply held in the mind of the person allocated to care for the patient.

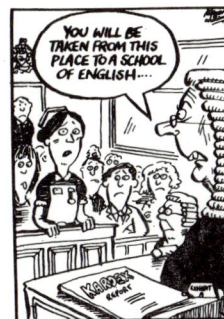

Fig. 4.6   Some important components of nursing records

TRANSFER OF NURSING INFORMATION ABOUT PATIENTS

Surveys have highlighted the problems of maintaining continuity of care between hospital and home (Skeet, 1970; Hockey, 1968) and nurses are still looking at ways of improving communication when a patient is transferred from one health care setting to another.

Nurses involved in shared care, for example community, day hospital and holiday relief care, need to know exactly what care is being implemented in each location in order to co-ordinate help and support for the patient and family. The ideal is to have only one set of patient's nursing records, which travels with the patient. This system is easier to maintain in an urban area, especially if the community nurse is based at the hospital.

Midwives also find that the care plan can be transferred more easily with the mother during the post-natal period, if the community midwife has her base at the hospital. In Portsmouth Health District the expectant mother holds her own records so that care can be continuous.

Some districts have re-designed the 'transfer form' to include details of patients' problems, the aims of care and the intervention planned, so that the 'new' nurse can maintain continuity of care.

An example of a completed transfer summary is shown in Figures 4.8(a) and (b).

SPOKEN NURSE-TO-NURSE COMMUNICATION

In this section, we shall consider information related to the implementation of the nursing care plan, which passes between nurses by the spoken word.

NURSING TRANSFER SUMMARY

Name of patient Alec Banarby

Transfer date 24th August

Date of birth (age) 6th April 1921 (60 yrs)

Method of transport Ambulance

Patient's address following transfer 14, The Dell Cottage, Ambleside

Home address (if different from opposite) 17, Sort Street, West Gorton, Manchester

Next of kin or significant person to contact in emergency Daughter Mrs Gee at above address

Length of stay in hospital 3 weeks

Clinic visits scheduled Anticoagulant clinic 28th August Out-patient follow-up 24th September

Patient's family/friends involved in post-transfer care Daughter and son-in-law taking father for a few days convalescence to their home

Referrals/community resources (including dates contacted and by whom) District Nurse (18th August) Meals on wheels (20th August) Social Worker - Mrs Plant - 20th August

Medications Sinthrone - see patient's drug chart Digoxin 0.0625 mgs daily

G.P. (name & address) Dr Sinner, 14, Septic Street, West Gorton

Profile/summary of patient Admitted on an emergency call with acute breathlessness and chest pain for investigation and assessment of physical needs. Lives alone and has received no help from outside sources except the odd visit from a social worker. Lost his job last year due to ill-health. Wife died 2 years ago. Two children - one away in America - one daughter in Ambleside. Several friends - well known in community.

Fig. 4.8(a)   Completed example of a nursing transfer summary: sheet 1 (McFarlane and Castledine, 1982)

A *Handbook for Nurse to Nurse Reporting* (King's Fund, 1983) describes two kinds of communication by the spoken word, distinguishing between 'oral' and 'verbal' communication:

- oral communication: refers to the spoken word only
- verbal communication: refers to the spoken word that will eventually be written down as part of the formal record.

Traditionally, nursing information has been passed on by the spoken word at a change of shift, or when one nurse hands over responsibility for her group of patients to another; this usually includes both 'oral' and 'verbal' communication. The spoken handover is still used when a nursing process approach is adopted, but the quality of the information communicated and the style of conducting reports may well be different.

Activity 4.12   **Allow 30 minutes**

A nursing report session

This activity gives you an opportunity to compare different approaches to spoken communication between nurses.

For this activity, you will need to listen to the middle section on side 2 of the audiotape and to read the audio notes in the *Case Files*.

On the tape you will hear two spoken handover reports on the same patient, Mrs Hall, the first made in a traditional style and the second following a nursing process approach.

You will then hear a brief report on another patient, Mr Barker. You will see a more detailed nursing report about him on the videotape, which will be shown during Group Session 4.

Comments about these different nursing reports will be made on the tape, as you work through the activity.

PATIENT'S PROBLEMS ON TRANSFER AND ON-GOING NURSING HELP

Patient's Problems	Help being Given	Expected Outcome
① Potential problem of bleeding due to anticoagulant therapy	① Teaching regarding signs and symptoms of bleeding and who to report to	① Patient able to verbalise the signs and symptoms of bleeding and knowledge of physical condition
② Limited mobility due to poor heart condition. Difficulty walking long distances of 50-100 yards and getting up and down stairs	② Physiotherapy advice regarding climbing stairs and importance of rest when taking long walks	② Able to get out to shops and pub. Climb stairs 2 times daily
③ Small 1"x1½" pressure sore on sacrum dry and healing - no signs of infection.	③ Dry dressing daily	③ Healed area of skin and tissue by two weeks

Potential Risks

① "Blackouts"? cerebral ischaemia? hypotension

② Depression due to state of health and loneliness

③ Maintenance of an adequate diet

Contact nurse responsible .....*T Small*.....
(Signature)
Address..*The General Hospital*...
.........*Ward A*.........

Date *24/8/81*

Fig. 4.8(b)   Completed example of a nursing transfer summary: sheet 2 (McFarlane and Castledine, 1982)

PREPARING FOR GROUP SESSION 4

The videotape which you will see in Group Session 4 shows a handover report at a patient's bedside. The patient is Mr Barker, whom you have heard about on the audiotape. You will need to read his case notes in the *Case Files* and to take them and the notes which you made for Activity 4.12 to the group session.

There may be some time at the end of the group session for you to raise any points about this module with your group leader and your colleagues, including any ideas that you would like to discuss relating to Activities 4.2 and 4.4.

PREPARING FOR MODULE 5

Before beginning Module 5, you are again asked to collect some material from your own work area.

If you are working in an area where the nursing process is already practised and where documentation includes specific goals for specific patient problems on the care plan, then you will be able to bring your own data for use with this module.

If possible, choose a patient/client in whose care you have been involved. Remember that you must omit any information by which the patient might be identified. Select one patient problem which is due to be evaluated and then collect the information required for evaluation, as directed by the goal (the goal should indicate what you will be able to see, hear, smell or measure when it has been achieved).

Copy into your notebook the assessment data relevant to the chosen problem and the appropriate section(s) of the nursing care plan for that problem, and then record what you did in order to decide whether the goal had been reached. Keep all these notes with you when you work through Module 5, as you will be asked to refer to this information.

Don't worry if you are not in a position to carry out the above exercise. If necessary, you can use the care plan for Mrs Harris in Part I of the *Case Files*, which provides the necessary information for the relevant activities in Module 5.

FURTHER READING

Bridge, W. and Clark, J. M. (eds.) (1981) *Communication in Nursing Care*, London, HM & M Publishers.

Fielding, J. (1983) 'Teaching is part of nursing', *Journal of District Nursing*, February.

French, P. (1982) *Social Skills for Nursing Practice*, Beckenham, Croom Helm.

Hewitt, F. S. (1981/2) 'The nurse and the patient – communication skills', *Nursing Times, monthly series* Jan. 1981–Jan. 1982.

Jourard, S. M. (1971) *The Transparent Self*, New York, Van Nostrand Rheinhold Co. Especially chapters 20–22.

Mayerhoff, M. (1971) *On Caring*, New York, Harper & Row Publishers Inc.

McFarlane of Llandaff and Castledine, G. (1982) *A Guide to the Practice of Nursing Using the Nursing Process*, London, C.V. Mosby Co. Especially chapter 8.

McIntosh, J. B. (1977) 'The nurse-patient relationship', *Nursing Mirror*, (Supplement) 152, Jan. 25.

Rogers, C. R. (1967) *On Becoming a Person*, London, Constable & Co. Ltd.

Sundeen, S. J., Stuart, G. W., Rankin, E. D. and Cohen, S. A. (eds.) (1981) *Nurse-client Interaction – implementing the nursing process*, St Louis, C.V. Mosby Co.. Especially chapters 3–6.

MODULE 5
THE FOURTH STEP OF THE NURSING PROCESS
EVALUATION

Prepared for the Course Team by Karen Lowe

CONTENTS

OBJECTIVES

After studying this module, you should be able to:

1 Describe your current method of evaluation.

2 Discuss the importance of evaluation in relation to the other steps of the nursing process.

3 Outline the different approaches of structure, process and outcome evaluation.

4 Describe the application of outcome evaluation.

5 Recognise that the patient is the focus of evaluation.

6 Specify and use sources of information for the purpose of evaluation.

7 Use appropriate information from evaluation in the modification of care plans.

8 Outline some of the ways in which evaluation can be organised.

9 Identify methods of determining the quality of nursing care.

10 Appreciate that evaluation is not an end in itself, but may generate further activity.

11 Discuss the constraints upon evaluation in nursing today.

THE PURPOSE OF EVALUATION

This module is devoted to the evaluation step of the nursing process. This is the fourth and final step in the systematic approach to nursing, but it is not an end in itself. As you will see, evaluation often leads to further activity: it generates questions and can lead back to other steps in the process of nursing. So don't think you've reached the end as you approach evaluation – you might be only just beginning.

The major part of this module is concerned with the kind of evaluation which you, as a practising nurse, are most likely to carry out; that is, deciding whether goals for specific patient problems have been achieved. Towards the end of the module, some consideration is given to evaluation from a broader perspective – for example, evaluation of the quality or standard of nursing care in a ward as a whole.

Evaluation has been the last step of the nursing process to be developed in practice. It cannot occur unless the other stages – assessment, planning and some implementation – have taken place and because it is a relatively new concept within clinical nursing, little has been written about exactly how it can be done in practice. Therefore, although various suggestions are made throughout the text as to how evaluation might be carried out, no one method is seen as the 'ideal' way. Nurses working in varying clinical settings may find certain ways of organising the practice of evaluation more suitable than others, because of the varying needs of different client groups.

Many functions of evaluation in nursing are suggested in the literature:

- to determine whether patient goals/expected outcomes have been achieved
- to measure standards of nursing care
- to measure the quality of nursing care
- to discover which nursing actions are most consistently effective in solving a particular patient problem
- to measure staff performance.

This module will concentrate on the first function: determining whether patient goals/expected outcomes have been achieved.

APPROACHES TO EVALUATION

Whatever is being evaluated, be it nursing actions, the quality of care or nurses' performance, there are three elements which can be studied. These are:

- **structure**   - **process**   - **outcome**

STRUCTURE EVALUATION

This approach involves examining the setting in which care is given and looks at such factors as patient dependency, numbers and grades of staff, styles of management, patterns of organisation and nursing education. One of the assumptions of this method is that if such factors reach satisfactory levels and are well co-ordinated, the care will be of a satisfactory standard.

PROCESS EVALUATION

This method focuses on nurses and what they do. Two approaches can be taken: concurrent process evaluation (while the patient is still receiving nursing care) and retrospective process evaluation (after the patient's discharge from care).

Concurrent process evaluation can be carried out in two ways:

- observation of a patient while he receives care
- observation of a nurse as she gives care.

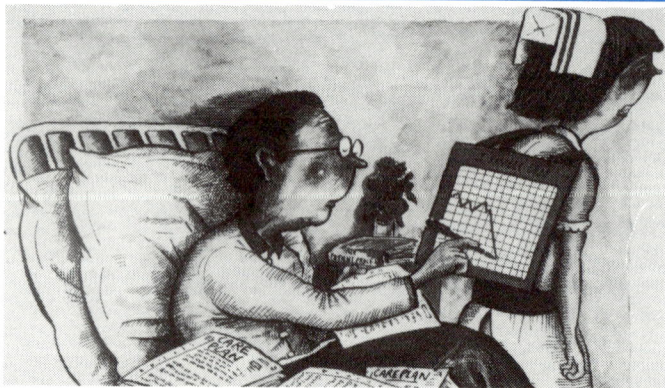

Retrospective process evaluation involves examining the records and charts of patients after discharge, searching for evidence that nursing care has been given to a required standard.

Process evaluation is based on the assumption that, if evidence suggests that the care given was of a satisfactory standard, then the nursing actions will have resulted in certain outcomes which benefit the patient. With concurrent process evaluation, there may also be some opportunity to observe outcomes of care as well as its delivery. Some examples of ways in which these approaches can be used are given later in this module.

Process evaluation is not widely practised in this country, mainly because the ways in which nursing care and records are assessed are complex and time-consuming and are not yet well developed.

OUTCOME EVALUATION

The patient is the prime consideration of this method. In particular, attention is paid to *patient outcomes* – the end result of care, as demonstrated by the patient's behaviour, physiological status or verbal expression. The actual outcome of care is compared with the expected outcome to assess the patient's progress towards or away from the goal.

Outcome evaluation, like process evaluation, can be carried out concurrently or retrospectively.

Concurrent outcome evaluation takes place while the patient is receiving care and concentrates on the patient's progress towards the desired goals.

Retrospective outcome evaluation takes place after discharge and uses the patient's records to determine whether goals were achieved.

The major assumption of outcome evaluation is that the observed patient outcome can be attributed to the prescribed nursing action. Obviously not all patient outcomes can be attributed to nursing care. For instance, a headache will often resolve itself without any nursing action being attributed to its resolution. If evaluation of nursing care is to follow this method, the contribution of other health workers and other factors (such as patients' own defence mechanisms) must be recognised.

Activity 5.1	Allow 5 minutes

The multi-disciplinary team

The purpose of this activity is to help you to appreciate the contribution of other team members to patient outcomes.

The calf measurements of a patient with leg swelling have reduced by 5 cm. over three days.

The prescribed nursing actions were to elevate his legs when he was sitting or lying down, and to walk with him a minimum distance of ten metres at least three times a day. Who and what else might have contributed to this outcome, i.e. reduction in calf swelling?

Author's comment
You might have included:
- *the prescription of diuretics by the physician*
- *leg exercises recommended by the physiotherapist*
- *a low sodium diet suggested by the dietitian*
- *spontaneous resolution without further intervention.*

This example illustrates that other members of the health team and other factors can contribute to patient outcomes. It is important that you bear this in mind when carrying out evaluation and do not see the nursing input in isolation from that of the rest of the multi-disciplinary team. This topic is discussed further in Module 6.

THE FOCUS OF THE MODULE

So far, you have been introduced to the functions of evaluation in nursing and the three different ways in which it can be studied i.e. structure, process and outcome. The focus of this module is on evaluation within the context of the nursing process and the aim of this kind of evaluation is to determine whether patient goals have been achieved. This is done by comparing the *expected outcome* for a specific patient problem with the *actual outcome*, and then modifying the care plan as appropriate. For example:

Patient's problem	Expected outcome
11/4 Difficulty in administering 'Indocid' suppository at night.	By 17/4, Meg will be able to insert her own suppository at night, correctly and unaided.

Determining whether the expected outcome for this problem had been reached would have involved the nurse watching the patient insert her own suppository on the evening of 17/4 and deciding whether she was able to carry out this action correctly and unaided.

This kind of evaluation concentrates on both the expected and the actual outcomes of nursing intervention.

In an ideal world, with no financial constraints, shortages of resources or staff, a combination of process and outcome methods of evaluation would be adopted. Not only could it then be determined whether goals had been reached, but the contribution of specific nursing actions in bringing about specific patient outcomes could also be analysed. One study which has linked process and outcome is that carried out by Jenny Boore (1978), which showed that giving patients relevant information pre-operatively affected their progress favourably post-operatively.

Researchers are trying to develop ways of measuring the relationship between nursing actions and patient outcomes, but until significant developments are made it is difficult to adopt a process-outcome approach to evaluating the care of individual patients.

This module is concerned with the evaluation of the results of planned nursing interventions, carried out in response to specific, identified problems. It concentrates on concurrent outcome evaluation, for the following reasons:

1 Whilst the study of structure provides data about the adequacy of facilities and equipment, it does not produce information about the direct effect that nursing has on the patient.
2 The process approach involves the time-consuming use of complex forms, which require the development of special skills and involve an 'observer' watching nursing care as it is being given and received. Resources and staff are currently scarce within our health system and this method is not practical for 'everyday' evaluation as part of the nursing process.
3 Outcome evaluation involves only those resources or staff which are readily available. Nurses planning and giving care can, for instance, measure outcomes of nursing interventions.
4 Outcome evaluation is suggested by several writers as the most suitable approach to adopt (see *Further Reading*).

THE DIFFERENCE BETWEEN ASSESSMENT AND EVALUATION

These two steps of the nursing process share some common components, such as data collection (information has to be sought as part of both assessment and evaluation) and the sources of data used (patients, patients' relatives, nursing colleagues, other members of the health care team and records). There are also some differences between the two:

1 Evaluation takes place only *after* goals have been set and some goal-directed activity has been performed, whereas assessment is concerned with the collection of information in order to identify the patient's problems.

2 The end result of assessment is a statement of the patient's problems. The end result of evaluation is feedback to, and possible modification of, the care plan.

3 In assessment, the data to be collected is determined by the model of nursing chosen; in evaluation, the goal statement determines what data is to be collected.

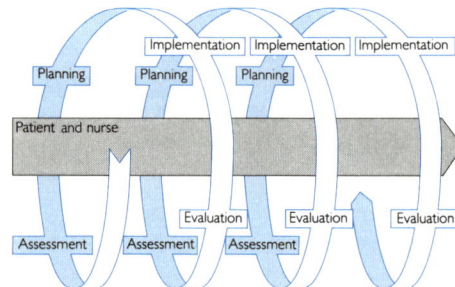

Fig. 5.1 The problem-solving process

Although evaluation is presented as the final step in this systematic approach to nursing, it can be intimately linked with assessment, because the information gained from evaluation can provide cues for further assessment. Figure 5.1 reminds you of the spiral nature of the nursing process.

SOURCES OF INFORMATION AND SKILLS INVOLVED IN EVALUATION

The sources used for data collection in evaluation are, as might be expected, similar to those used in assessment. Whenever possible, the patient is the focus for data collection in evaluation, as in assessment. Additional sources of information for use in evaluation are the same as for assessment. These are:

- members of the patient's family and/or significant others
- nursing colleagues
- other members of the health care team
- records: medical and nursing.

Activity 5.2   Allow 5 minutes

Collecting data for evaluation

This activity is designed to help you appreciate the various sources of information which can be used for evaluation purposes.

For this activity, you will need to use the data on a patient problem, which you collected in preparation for this module. Alternatively, you can use problem 1 on the care plan for Mrs Harris which you will find in Part 1 of the *Case Files*.

Suggest possible sources of information which you might use in the evaluation of this problem.

Author's comment

If you used your own data on a patient problem, you might have included any of the sources of information listed above. If you used the care plan for Mrs Harris and looked at problem 1, which concerned her anxiety, you might have suggested:

- *the patient herself*
- *Mr Harris, her husband*
- *other members of the nursing team caring for Mrs Harris*
- *other members of the multi-disciplinary team, for example, doctors.*

So you can see that there are many people who can provide data for evaluation.

There are a number of charts currently in use in nursing which can provide information for both assessment and evaluation. For example, a sleep chart or an incontinence chart might be used during the initial stages of a patient's care as a method of assessing a pattern of sleep or incontinence. Once the pattern has been established and a plan of care developed, then the same chart might be used to evaluate the success of the plan of care implemented for this particular problem.

Activity 5.3   Allow 5 minutes

Using charts for evaluation data

Nurses always seem to be filling in charts. This activity is designed to stimulate your thoughts on how some charts can be used in evaluation.

List some more examples of charts or scales which can be used as tools for both assessment and evaluation.

Author's comment

Some of the charts or scales which you might have listed have already been referred to in Module 2, such as the Glasgow Coma Scale and the pain thermometer. You might like to remind yourself of these by looking back at the section on Use of special data collection instruments. Figure 5.2 shows an example of a chart used in psychiatric nursing to record patient behaviour, for both assessment and evaluation.

Such measurements can be very useful in evaluation. For instance, a pain thermometer could be used both before analgesia is given and again, after a suitable time has elapsed for the drug to take effect. Thus the effect of the analgesia could be evaluated.

The skills involved in the data collection component of evaluation are again similar to those used in assessment, namely:

- observing
- measuring
- interviewing

For example, you might:

- *observe* a patient's interaction with other patients during a group therapy meeting
- weigh a baby at the clinic (*measuring*)
- spend time talking with a patient to elicit her feelings about her recent spontaneous abortion (*interviewing*).

The particular skills you will need to draw on when carrying out evaluation will vary according to the goal.

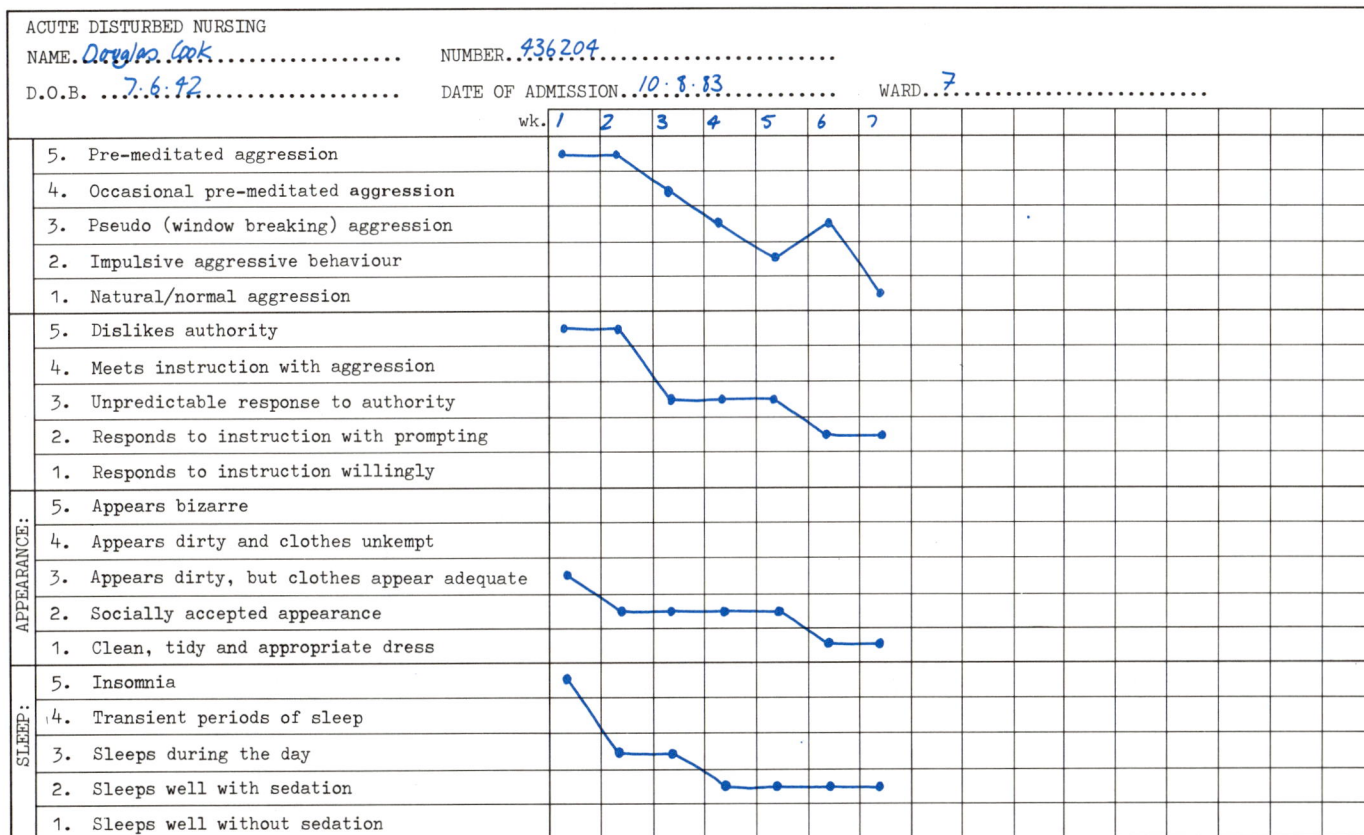

ACUTE DISTURBED NURSING
NAME. Douglas Cook   NUMBER. 436204
D.O.B. 7.6.42   DATE OF ADMISSION 10.8.83   WARD 7

		wk. 1	2	3	4	5	6	7
	5. Pre-meditated aggression	●	●					
	4. Occasional pre-meditated aggression			●				
	3. Pseudo (window breaking) aggression				●		●	
	2. Impulsive aggressive behaviour					●		
	1. Natural/normal aggression							●
	5. Dislikes authority	●	●					
	4. Meets instruction with aggression							
	3. Unpredictable response to authority			●	●	●		
	2. Responds to instruction with prompting						●	●
	1. Responds to instruction willingly							
APPEARANCE:	5. Appears bizarre							
	4. Appears dirty and clothes unkempt							
	3. Appears dirty, but clothes appear adequate	●						
	2. Socially accepted appearance		●	●	●	●		
	1. Clean, tidy and appropriate dress						●	●
SLEEP:	5. Insomnia	●						
	4. Transient periods of sleep							
	3. Sleeps during the day		●	●				
	2. Sleeps well with sedation				●	●	●	●
	1. Sleeps well without sedation							

Fig. 5.2 Nursing process assessment and evaluation chart

MODELS OF NURSING AND EVALUATION

In the previous modules you have seen how the different nursing models may influence data gathering in assessment, problem identification and goal planning. Their influence on the evaluation stage of the nursing process is less direct. However, the values inherent in each model of nursing will be reflected in the goals of nursing, and therefore will guide the selection of criteria for measurement in evaluation.

In Orem's model of care, for example, self-care is highly valued and goals are developed which aim at the patient achieving self-care. In evaluation, therefore, the nurse will be measuring the patient's ability to carry out self-care. The type of sub-goals illustrated on p. 117 might be useful in the context of this model, as they could be used to show how the patient is progressing towards self-care.

Similarly, Roper, Logan and Tierney's model emphasises activities of living, and evaluation will involve the assessment and/or measurement of the patient's ability to achieve objectives related to these activities of living.

In Saxton and Hyland's model, objectives are concerned with the interruption of stress-adaptation cycles, and nursing interventions aim to contain or prevent maladaptive responses and to promote adaptive responses. However, Saxton and Hyland do not identify how, when using their model, evaluation of nursing care takes place. They say that "If the patient's symptoms have been reduced, the nurse can conclude that the measures have assisted the adaptive mechanism". Evaluation, using this model, centres on determining if the patient's symptoms have subsided.

Models of nursing do not affect the *way* in which evaluation is carried out in practice, but they may influence the *kind* of information you are directed to seek.

Let us take the example of a patient with a problem of constipation, caused by inadequate fluid intake. Using Orem's model, goals would be directed towards the patient achieving optimum self-management of this problem and might involve evaluating the patient's ability to monitor his own fluid intake, to walk to the toilet and to manage his own clothing.

Using the Roper, Logan and Tierney model, goals would be aimed at the achievement of an activity of living – in this case, elimination. The goal would direct the collection of data for evaluation towards measuring the frequency of bowel movements and monitoring the patient's ability to manage his own elimination.

Using the Saxton and Hyland model, evaluation would consist of ongoing assessment of the patient's adaptation levels. On admission, the nurse might have assessed the adaptation level of the patient to be level four (where the patient's usual mode of functioning is interrupted: see p. 21), because the patient was experiencing nausea and vomiting as a result of constipation. Evaluation would involve assessing the patient's level of adaptation, with the expectation that, if there had been some resolution of the constipation, the level of adaptation would have been reduced to a lower level. This might mean that the patient was at the second level of adaptation (limitation) where he was eating normally, without nausea or vomiting, but still needed suppositories to facilitate bowel movements.

THE FIVE STEPS OF EVALUATION

In this part of the module, evaluation will be broken down into its five component parts and discussed in detail.

The five steps (after Luker, 1979) are:

1 Selection of criteria which will guide observation.

2 Collection of data.

3 Comparison of actual patient outcomes with expected patient outcomes.

4 Making a judgment about the patient's response and the extent to which expected outcomes have been achieved.

5 Feedback to, and modification of, the care plan.

Although these five steps are discussed separately, they sometimes take place in very rapid succession as, for instance, in giving artificial respiration when you would evaluate the effectiveness of your intervention (breathing into mouth) by observing the chest wall for

movements. This evaluation has taken only a few seconds to complete and may not be documented until much later. The five steps have taken place implicitly rather than explicitly.

1 SELECTION OF CRITERIA

In evaluation, you determine whether goals have been met; therefore information relating to the goal in question will be collected.

Activity 5.4   Allow 7 minutes

Collecting information for evaluation

How do you decide what information to collect for evaluation? Have a go at this exercise and you will realise how important the goal statement is.

Consider the following two goals:

[A]	[B]
Normal development for a one year-old.	Reduction in anxiety by 18/5 as shown by facial expression, reduced fidgeting and verbal expression of feeling less anxious.

What information would you collect if you had to decide whether these goals had been reached?

Author's comment

It is likely that you found it easier to determine which information to collect for goal B than for goal A. This is because goal B tells you how you will know that a reduction in anxiety has taken place – by facial expression and reduced fidgeting, and by the patient expressing that she is feeling less anxious. In contrast, goal A does not tell you what to do nor precisely when to do it. You may think that it is unlikely that goals like A would be written in a care plan but they frequently are, and you can see how difficult it is to measure whether goal A has been achieved when the goal is non-specific. One of the prerequisites for evaluation is specific goal statements.

As already suggested in Module 3, in order to be effective goals must indicate:

- who will perform the desired behaviour
- the actual behaviour to be performed
- the relevant conditions under which the behaviour will take place
- the standard used to evaluate the behaviour
- the expected time frame within which the behaviour will have been achieved.

The importance of the specificity of goal statements in relation to evaluation cannot be overemphasised. If you don't know where you're going, how will you know when you get there? If the goal statements are nebulous, vague and unmeasurable you will not know what to measure or when, in order to determine the effectiveness of your actions. In such circumstances, evaluation will not take place.

In Module 3, it was suggested that, when the desired goal might take a long time to reach, identifying goal steps can be helpful. This can help to direct data collection for evaluation. Inzer and Aspinall (1981) suggest that desired patient outcomes should be broken down into steps, which act as intermediate goals progressing to the final patient outcome.

An example of a goal could be: "the patient will care for his colostomy without assistance by 13/8". This goal breaks down into the following components:

- remove the soiled bag
- irrigate the stoma
- clean the stoma
- apply a new bag.

The steps, building up towards achieving the final goal, are:

Step 1: Can do none of the above, without assistance
Step 2: Can do one of the above, without assistance
Step 3: Can do two of the above, without assistance
Step 4: Can do three of the above, without assistance
Step 5: Can do all of the above, without assistance
(Step 5 indicates the criterion for goal attainment).

No particular order or time for achieving the goal components is suggested because individuals differ in the order and speed in which they are able to learn a task. The achievement of all four components of this goal may take a few weeks for some patients. Awareness of achieving a goal, a step at a time, increases the sense of achievement for both patient and nurse, and may mean the difference between reaching the ultimate goal and giving up half-way because the patient or the nurse feel the overall goal is too difficult to accomplish. The use of intermediate goals has been compared with staging posts on a long journey, which indicate how far you've come and how much further you have to go until you reach your destination.

2 COLLECTING THE DATA

Since the patient is the focus of evaluation, an interaction between patient and nurse will take place in most stages of data collection. This may involve trying to elicit the patient's feelings about his progress or actively listening to what he is saying and what he is not saying (trying to perceive non-verbal cues). Both subjective and objective data should be collected, where possible.

If a patient verbally expresses that he feels less anxious (*subjective*), this should be substantiated by *objective* data such as facial expression of calm and the absence or reduction of any previously demonstrated nervous mannerisms.

Interviewing may sometimes involve relatives or significant others in addition to – or instead of – the patient/client, for instance

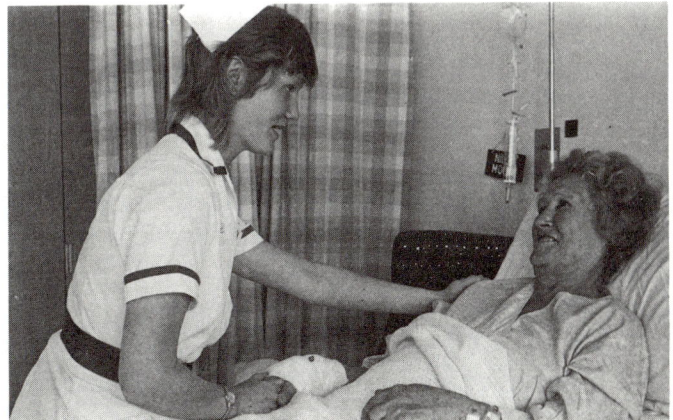

The patient is the focus of evaluation

for patients who are unable to communicate fully with nurses due to language difficulties or speech problems.

Interviewing patients and relatives to obtain data for evaluation involves more than simply asking "any problems?" It can mean spending time finding out what a patient really feels about something, especially when the problems are of a psychological nature. Measuring feelings and emotions can be difficult. The use of scales, such as the Hospital Anxiety and Depression Scale, can be useful in such instances.

Activity 5.5   Allow 30 minutes
A bedside evaluation

Involving the patient is an essential component of evaluation. This activity gives you the opportunity to listen to a bedside evaluation and to comment on the nurse's approach to patient involvement.

Read the audio notes on May Bradley in Part II of the *Case Files*. Now listen to the last section of side 2 of the audiotape, paying particular attention to the extent to which the nurse involves May as a partner in the evaluation process.

Measuring and counting are perhaps the simplest skills used in evaluation and, although there are plenty of opportunities to use them, nurses have been slow to do so. Instead of measuring the size of a pressure sore when a patient is admitted to hospital or seen at home and then repeating the measurement a week later, nurses tend to say "I think the sore is smaller". There are numerous simple measurements which could be made to provide data both for assessment and for evaluation, such as weighing, taking temperature and measuring calf diameter. Examples of counting are:

- how much analgesia is required
- how many interactions take place
- the number of heartbeats per minute.

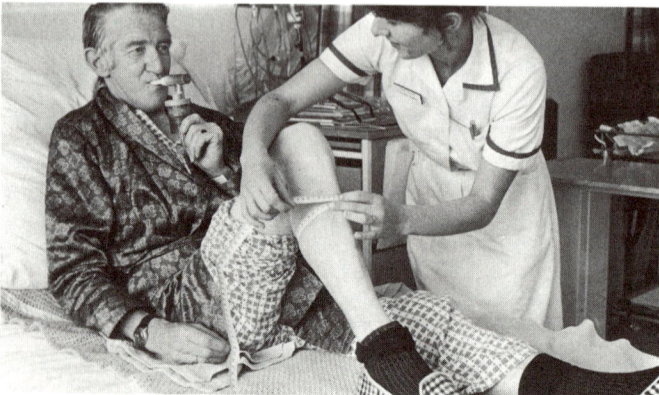

Measuring – one of the simplest skills used in evaluation, but one of the most valuable

Activity 5.6   Allow 7 minutes
Measuring and counting

These two ways of collecting information are simple, yet they can provide a great deal of data for evaluation, as you will see when you have completed the activity.

Write down a list of at least five activities which might provide data for evaluation under each category below:

1 Measuring
2 Counting.

Author's comment
You will probably have thought of many examples. This will help you to realise that these simple skills could be used much more to provide data for evaluation. Here are a few more examples:

Measuring:
- *fundal height in centimetres*
- *pain, anxiety, depression (using scales)*
- *the risk of developing pressure sores (Norton scale)*
- *the apgar score of a baby*
- *the amount of drainage from a wound*

Counting:
- *the number of cigarettes smoked in 24 hours*
- *the number of times a patient is incontinent in 24 hours*
- *the number of bowel movements over 24 hours*
- *the number of days without an alcoholic drink*
- *the number of beats per minute of the foetal heart.*

Observation to collect information is the third skill involved in both assessment and evaluation. This may involve watching a patient perform an activity or skill, such as walking or breast-feeding, or interacting with relations, or it may mean inspecting a wound or a particular part of the body. Where observation of a patient performing an activity is involved, you should try not to let your presence affect the patient's performance. If the nurse who is most familiar with the patient is carrying out the evaluation, this is likely to increase their feeling of comfort and ease with each other, and this should promote the collection of information which accurately reflects the patient's abilities at that time.

Observation and measurement are often combined; for example, when evaluating the progress of a pressure sore by measuring its size, observations can be made for inflammation, infection or granulation. Another example of combining observation and measurement is post-operative care, which involves measuring blood pressure, pulse and wound drainage as well as observation of the patient's colour and the dressing over the wound.

If patients have been involved in their care plans right from the beginning, they are more likely to demonstrate a keen interest in the outcomes of care, and be willing to participate in data collection for evaluation. *Creating a partnership with patients* is therefore beneficial to both the recipients and the providers of nursing care. 'Informed'

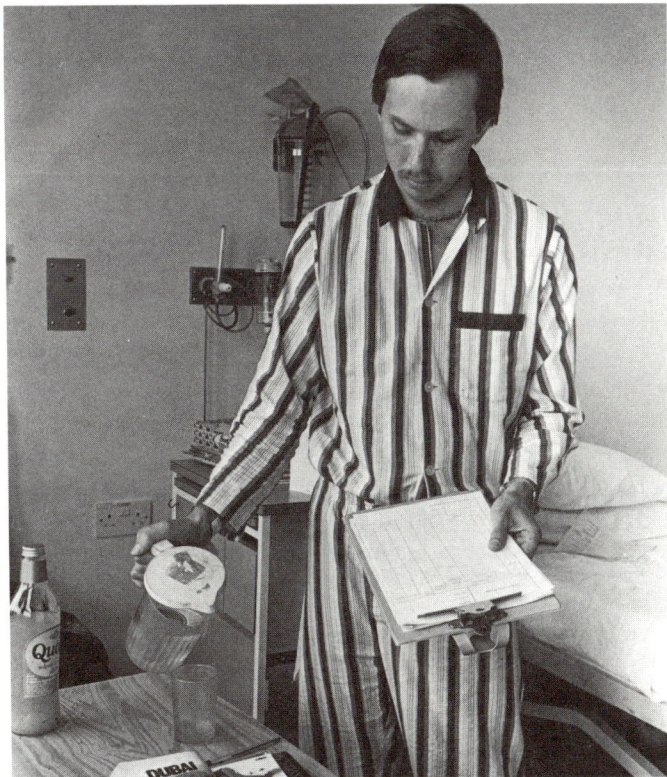

Patients can record their own data for evaluation

patients who know what their goals of care are will probably want to tell nurses when they feel they have achieved a goal.

Where practical, patients can be encouraged to record their own evaluation data, for instance filling in their own stool charts or rating their levels of pain, anxiety or depression. The keeping of a diary may help patients undergoing psychiatric care to record their thoughts and feelings. If you believe that nurses and patients should be partners, then you will feel happy to facilitate self-monitoring for evaluation.

Activity 5.7	Allow 5 minutes

Self-evaluation

This activity is designed to help you to consider possible ways in which patients can themselves record information for evaluation.

What further suggestions do you have on how patients might carry out self-evaluation?

Author's comment

You will have an opportunity to share these ideas at Group Session 5. No further examples will be provided here.

To summarise, the second step of evaluation is the collection of pertinent information from various sources using skills of interviewing, measuring, counting and observing on the pre-determined evaluation date/time.

3 COMPARISON OF DATA WITH EXPECTED PATIENT OUTCOMES

Having obtained information about the *actual* outcome of care, the next step is to compare this with the *expected* outcome.

For example:

Actual outcome	**Expected outcome**
18/7 Weight: 58 kg.	Target weight: 55 kg. by 18/7. Minimum loss of 1 kg. per week.

Here you can see that the actual outcome does not match the expected outcome but, from the data presented above, it cannot be seen whether the patient is moving towards or away from the goal. For this particular example, and also for similar types of problems where size, weights, frequency or intensity are involved, information from assessment needs to be inspected before a judgment can be made.

Examining the above example, we could say that if on 28/6 the patient had weighed 60 kg., then the evaluation would show a movement towards the goal. If, however, the patient weighed 56.6 kg. on 28/6 then the evaluation would suggest that she is moving away from the goal.

This is a simple example to illustrate the necessity, with this type of goal, of having more than two measurements from which to make a judgment. Of course not all goals can be quantified in this way but, where possible, measurements should be used.

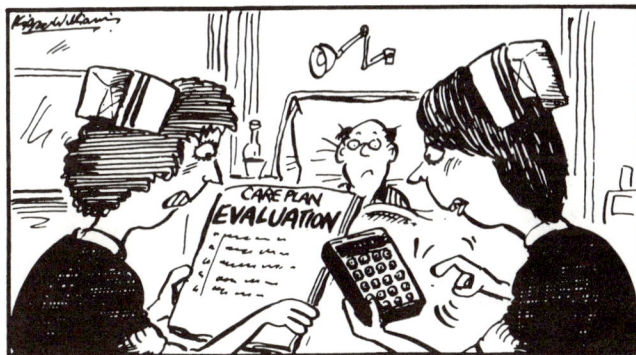

4 MAKING A JUDGMENT

Having collected all the necessary data, a judgment is then made about the patient's response to care and the extent to which the desired outcomes have been achieved is determined.

The possible outcomes are:

1 Attainment of the goal.
2 Progress is being made towards the goal.
3 No movement, position is static.
4 Movement is away from the goal.

Activity 5.8   Allow 3 minutes

Making a judgment

The outcome of evaluation will affect what further action takes place. Try this activity to see if you can categorise what the outcome of your evaluation was.

Consider the information which you collected for the evaluation of a patient problem, or the information on one of the problems included in the care plan for Mrs Harris in Part I of the *Case Files*. Compare this information with the expected outcome (and, where appropriate, pertinent information from the assessment). Decide which of the four outcomes listed above relates to the chosen problem.

Author's comment

This activity should give you a little practice in determining outcomes of evaluation. Further discussion on such outcomes of evaluation can be found after this activity.

Attainment of the goal: this is demonstrated when the actual outcome matches the expected outcome. For example:

Expected outcome	Actual outcome
By 16/5 defaecation will be painless, no blood loss.	16/5 Patient says he has had no pain on defaecation. No blood loss since 12/5.

Here the actual outcome matches the expected outcome and so it can be concluded that the goal has been attained.

Progress is being made towards the goal: at evaluation, the data may indicate that progress is being made towards the goal, but has not been fully achieved. For example:

Expected outcome	Actual outcome
Will eat at least half of each meal given to her by 19/12.	19/12 Eats half of first course and no pudding.

Assessment data shows that the patient ate no solid food on 12/12, so progress has been made towards the goal, but it has not been fully attained.

No movement, position is static: this can be interpreted either positively or negatively.

If the goal relates to a potential problem, it may be that no change since assessment is a *positive* outcome. For example:

Potential problem of pressure sores due to enforced bed rest (Norton Score:12).

On admission: skin intact, no redness.

Goal: skin remains intact. No signs of redness at pressure areas.

Actual outcome: skin intact, no redness over pressure areas. Therefore the goal has been attained.

When there is no change in a problem which was expected to improve, a static position can be interpreted as meaning movement away from the goal. This could be interpreted as a *negative* outcome.

Movement is away from the goal: this is demonstrated when the actual outcome for a problem which is expected to improve shows a deterioration since the last review date or since assessment. Figure 5.3 illustrates an example of increasing incontinence, a movement away from the goal.

Having determined the outcome of evaluation, it is then necessary to decide what to do with this information. This is step five.

5 FEEDBACK TO AND MODIFICATION OF THE CARE PLAN

This section will consider the actions to take arising from the four possible outcomes, which are:

1 Attainment of the goal.
2 Progress is being made towards the goal.
3 No movement, position is static.
4 Movement is away from the goal.

Attainment of the goal: the goal has been achieved, but it needs to be considered whether a higher level of goal could have been set.

The goal for a patient having difficulty walking because of the poor condition of her feet could be "able to walk 5 metres unaided in two weeks' time". However, after two weeks she is walking around the ward unaided. The goal has indeed been reached, but would it have been possible to have aimed higher, either in terms of a more difficult or strenuous behaviour for the patient and nurse to achieve, or by setting a shorter time-span?

Although it is at the moment very difficult in nursing to predict goals and target dates with accuracy, it is only by persevering that knowledge can be built up about which nursing actions are most consistently effective in solving a particular nursing problem and the span of time required to do so. Having checked that the goal is not

TIME \ DAY	ASSESSMENT 1 Sept 10	2 Sept 11	3 Sept 12	4 Sept 13	5 Sept 14	6	7	8	9	10
00.00										
01.00										
02.00			○	○ □	○ □					
03.00										
04.00					● ■					
05.00		● ▲	● ■	● ■						
06.00					○ □					
07.00	● ■									
08.00		● ■			● ■					
09.00			○							
10.00	● □	● ▲		○ □						
11.00	○				○ □					
12 Midday		○								
13.00	● ▲	● ▲	● ■		● □					
14.00					○					
15.00			○							
16.00	● ▲	● ▲		○ □	○ □					
17.00										
18.00										
19.00	● ■	● ■	● ■							
20.00				○ □	○ □					
21.00	● □	● □								
22.00	○ □	○ □	○ □							
23.00										

KEY:

Incontinent ○	Aid offered – urine not passed □	Asked for aid, did not use △	Absent ✖
Continent ●	Aid offered – urine passed ■	Asked for aid, urine passed ▲	

Fig. 5.3 An example of movement away from the goal

set too low, the reaching of a goal means that one of the problems has been alleviated and can be crossed off the care plan. It does *not* mean that the problem is erased from the care plan, since it can provide valuable information for research, teaching and monitoring of standards of nursing. There needs to be some indication on the care plan that the problem has been resolved. There are at least two ways of doing this. Figure 5.4 (p. 122) shows the use of a column on the care plan to indicate that an intervention has been discontinued. Another way of indicating the discontinuation of a nursing action is by drawing a vertical line through the appropriate parts of the care plan, as shown in Figure 5.5 (p. 122).

Whatever method is used to 'cross off' a problem from a care plan, the nurse doing this must sign and date the record, so demonstrating *accountability* for that action. The signature should only be that of the nurse who is accepting responsibility for that evaluation.

Crossing off a problem from the care plan is not necessarily the end of the story. Figure 5.6 shows the possible steps which can then be taken (p. 122).

Date commenced	Patient's nursing problem	Nursing care plan	Expected outcome	Date discontinued
10/11	POTENTIAL PROBLEM OF WOUND INFECTION.	DRESSING CHANGED ON ALTERNATE DAYS: CLEAN WITH SAVLODIL, APPLY MELOLIN AND TAPE WITH MICROPORE. REMOVE SUTURES ON 15/11.	BY 20/11 SUTURE LINE WILL BE HEALED, NO SWELLING OR REDNESS.	20/11 Y.Cole

Fig. 5.4 Using a 'discontinued' column to show that a problem has been resolved

Date	Problems	Actual (a) Potential (p)	Expected outcome	Evaluation date	Nursing actions	Date discontinued
2/5	Feeling that she never finishes anything properly. "I start doing something and never complete it".		Will set the tables for a meal time, for all the other patients.	7/5 ✓Completed	3/5 Direct Anne to set tables and do task with her. 4/5 Allow her to start task, help with last few tables. 5/5 – 7/5 Gradually decrease assistance.	7/5 C. Emmett

Fig. 5.5 Crossing off a problem in the care plan

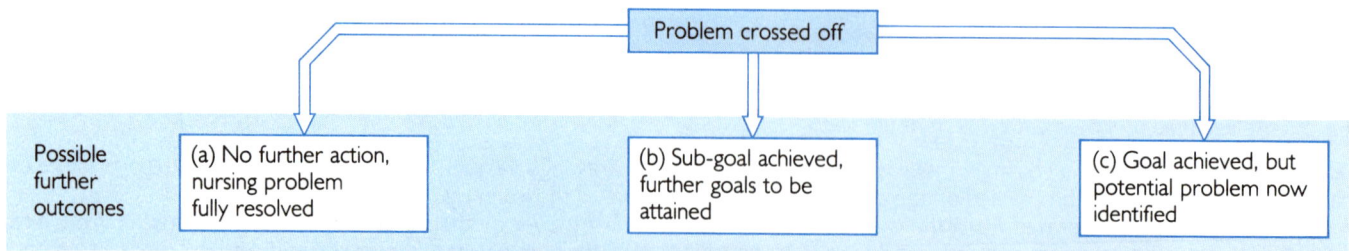

Fig. 5.6 What happens after a problem has been crossed off in the care plan?

(a) Problem has been completely resolved, all short and long-term goals reached, no potential problems identified.
(b) Goal step attained, but still further steps to be taken; next goal step added to care plan and further nursing actions as appropriate.
(c) Problem resolved but potential problem remains, which is added to care plan.

An example of further steps would be as follows:

Problem	Goal
12/8 Mouth infected with candida albicans (thrush).	By 17/8 buccal mucosa will be moist, pink and clean.

On 17/8 the goal has been achieved, but a potential problem of recurrence is identified because the patient is apt to forget to carry out oral hygiene, so this would be added to the care plan.

Progress is being made towards the goal: if the decision, after evaluation, is that movement is towards the goal, this does not always mean that the care plan will remain the same. Look at the following example:

Date	Problem	Goal	Action	Evaluation data
10/4	Not yet gained bladder control (wets × 8/day).	Bladder control will be gained by 25/4.	Toilet after meals.	17/4 Passes urine in toilet after meals. Very wet after diuretic.

In this example, there has been some resolution of the problem. The question has then to be asked – is this satisfactory? Should anything be changed? Could the evaluation date be brought forward? Should the frequency or timing of toileting be increased? The nurse responsible for planning, implementing and evaluating care will make the decision about whether a change in the care plan is needed, based on her knowledge of the individual patient, combined with experience in caring for other patients with similar nursing problems.

If the progress is thought to be satisfactory, another review/evaluation date may be added to the care plan.

No movement, position is static: if it is considered that a static position can be interpreted positively (as for a potential problem), then it is likely that no alteration will be made to the care plan.

If it is interpreted negatively (as for a problem which was expected to improve), then this indicates a need to review the care plan.

Movement is away from the goal: this indicates the need to review the care plan. There are numerous reasons why the goal may not have been attained, some of which are amenable to nursing intervention whilst others are outside the sphere of control of nursing.

If the medical condition of the patient alters significantly this will call for a reassessment of the patient, since it is likely that most of the goals will require review. Sometimes a care plan may be drawn up for a patient whose prognosis is unknown. This can make the prediction of realistic, attainable goals very difficult. In such circumstances, regular review dates may help in setting realistic goals.

When goals are not reached or when it is felt that progress towards the goal is unsatisfactory, and the medical condition of the patient is such that it is expected that problems should be resolved, then a review of the care plan is called for.

> The need to modify a care plan does not connote failure of nursing care. Failure takes place if the plan of care is not relevant to the client's needs and is not revised as the needs change or are clarified. (Sundeen, Stuart, Rankin and Cohen, 1981).

Reviewing the care plan

Luker (1979) suggests that the actions which may be taken when a goal has not been reached are:

- alteration of goals
- alteration of nursing actions
- alteration of evaluation dates.

This assumes that the problem has been accurately identified and that the assessment was complete and valid.

A review of the care plan can include each part of the care plan: the goals, the nursing actions and the statement of problems, as well as assessment data. Figure 5.7 (p. 124) suggests *one way* in which this review might take place. The aim of the flow chart is to help you to go through each part of the care plan and to check that it meets the criteria outlined.

Activity 5.9	Allow 10 minutes

Reviewing the care plan

Nobody ever writes a perfect care plan, but there are ways of ensuring that it meets certain criteria. This exercise will help you to appreciate how valuable reviewing the care plan can be.

Spend a few minutes studying the flow chart shown in Figure 5.7. Now turn to the care plan for Mrs Jane Harris in Part I of the *Case Files* and read the care plan for problem 4. You will see from the evaluation data that the goal has not fully been achieved.

Assuming that there is no physiological cause for the increase in oedema, use the flow chart to suggest possible reasons for the goal not having been achieved.

Author's comment

Here are some suggestions on what you might have included in your answer:

The nursing actions do not specify which leg exercises to teach the patient. No timing was indicated for calf measurement, which may vary according to the time of day.

The goal might have included a positive goal statement relating to the calf measurements. For example, by 29/6 calf measurements will be 32 cm. on both legs.

The problem: without further data, it must be assumed that the anaemia is the cause of the oedema. There are, of course, other possibilities such as congestive cardiac failure.

Fig. 5.7 flowchart

Goal not achieved →

Nursing action
1 Does it tell the nurse:
   what to do?
   when to do it?
   how to do it?
2 Is the action the most appropriate?
3 Is the frequency of action appropriate?
4 Has the prescribed care been implemented?

Yes →

Goal
1 Is it realistic?
2 Does it specify who will do what, by when?
3 Is evaluation date appropriate?

Yes →

Problem statement
1 Has problem been stated specifically?
2 Has problem been correctly identified?
3 Has cause of problem been correctly identified?

Yes →

Assessment
Is assessment complete/accurate?

Yes →

If all these criteria have been met and there is no apparent physiological or psychological reason why the goal cannot be achieved, then identify further questions to ask and possible actions to take.

No ↓
1 Reword nursing action so it is clear and specific
2 Select alternative action
3 Increase or decrease frequency
4 Ensure implementation of care

No ↓
1 Change goal
2 Reword goal to specify who will do what and when
3 Change evaluation date

No ↓
1 Rewrite the problem
2 Identify correct problem
3 Identify correct cause of problem

No ↓
Carry out re-assessment

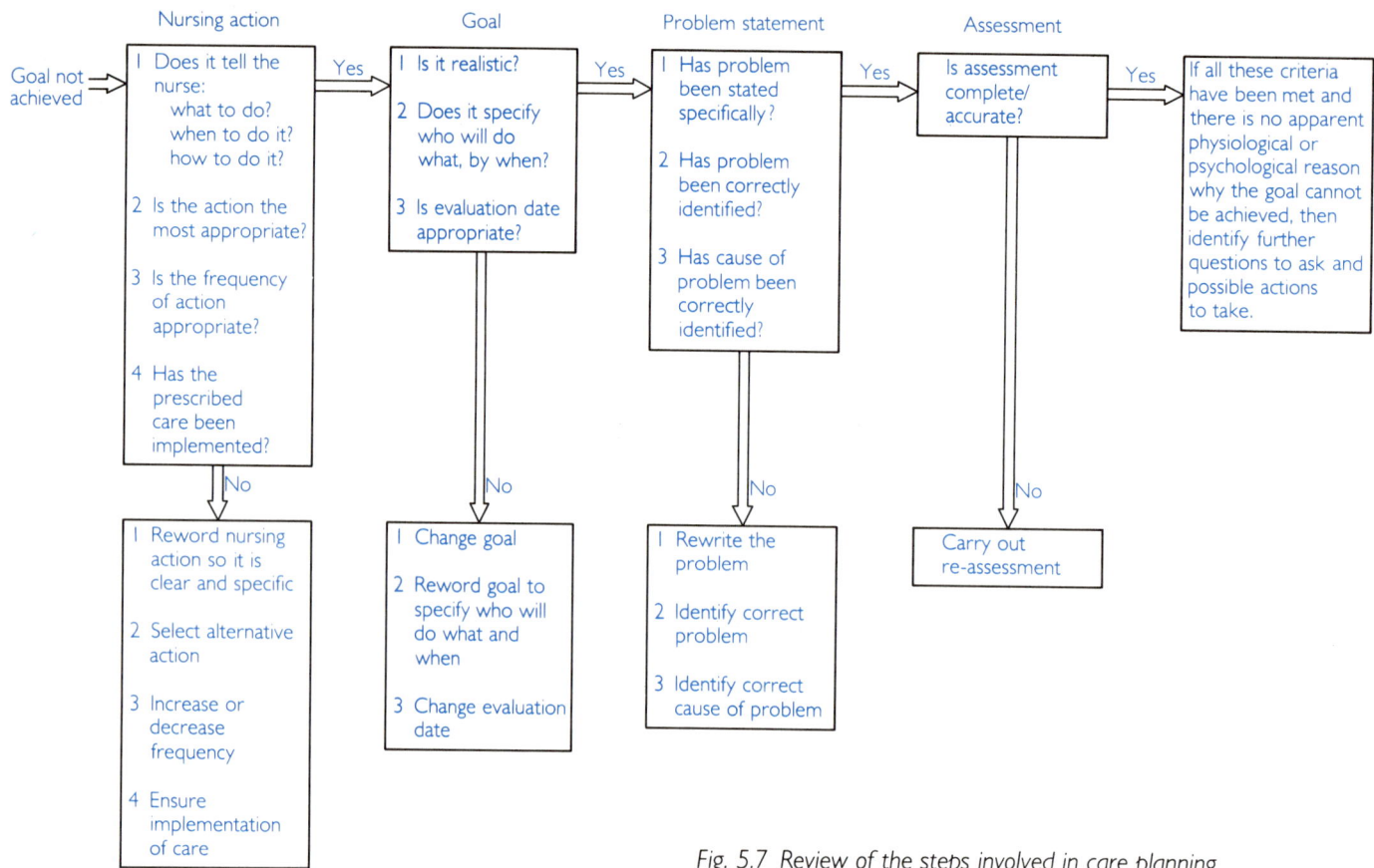

Fig. 5.7 Review of the steps involved in care planning

EVALUATION – WHEN AND HOW?

Every written goal statement should indicate a date by which it is expected that the goal will be achieved. For example: "By 19/4, Susan will weigh 50 kg." To evaluate this goal, Susan would be weighed once on 19/4.

With some goals, evaluation may take place over a span of time. With a goal such as "By 11/7, Mrs Brown will void urine in the toilet more times than she is incontinent of urine over 24 hours", information would have to be collected over 24 hours to determine if this had been achieved. Thus a record (incontinence chart) would have to be kept and more than one person would be involved in data collection.

When the resolution of a problem is expected to take a long time, there are likely to be both long and short-term goals, all of which, where possible, should indicate an appropriate time for evaluation. So for this kind of problem, evaluation will take place three or four times before the final goal is reached.

Occasionally it may not be possible to predict evaluation dates for all sub-goals within a long-term goal. In the case of an unsupported mother, suffering from post-natal depression, who is in a psychiatric hospital, one of the identified problems is her inability to cope with all household tasks. Her mother is currently caring for the baby. The long-term goal for this problem is that she will be able to perform the necessary tasks, without anxiety, by 12/10. Intermediate goals might be as follows:

1 The patient will be able to go home with a nurse and decide which tasks need to be done and when, by 11/9.

2 She will draw up a weekly timetable for necessary tasks.

3 She will go home with the nurse, spend two hours at home and perform one household task.

4 She will go home with the nurse for a whole day and be able to carry out necessary tasks.

5 She will go home alone for the day and carry out necessary tasks.

Obviously, the resolution of this problem will be influenced by the degree of depression experienced by the patient and so it may not be possible, when planning care, to decide on appropriate dates for the achievement of each intermediate goal. When the first evaluation takes place on 11/9, a further date for evaluation can be made.

If you find it difficult when writing a goal to predict when it might be achieved, don't be put off and leave out a date. Decide on a date for evaluation and write underneath the problem "Evaluate on . . .". The purpose of stating such a date is not only to predict the achievement of the goal, but also to predetermine the date for evaluation. I have seen far too many goals written without *dates*, and the end result is that nobody bothers to evaluate the care plan until a significant event takes place or the patient is discharged from care.

What can you do if you are uncertain as to when a goal is likely to be reached and don't know when to evaluate the outcome? Look at the problem statement: if it concerns something which is likely to change frequently, you may need to carry out evaluation frequently. With a pyrexial patient, evaluation may take place every hour to determine the effect of nursing interactions such as tepid sponging or the administration of soluble aspirin.

If, on the other hand, the problem is likely to begin to be resolved over several days then it may be pertinent to evaluate several days after the problem was identified. A patient attending a psychiatric day hospital may have a problem of being unable to perform simple word exercises, because of a lack of concentration and a lack of confidence in his own abilities. In this case, evaluation could first take place at the end of the week in which he starts attending and then further dates for evaluation could be set, maybe at weekly intervals.

The frequency of evaluation, then, depends on the nature of the problem in question. The nurse planning care is accountable for determining evaluation dates.

Griffith and Christensen (1982) describe two forms of evaluation – formative and summative – and their recording.

FORMATIVE EVALUATION

This is seen as an ongoing process where each intervention is judged as it is carried out, or just afterwards. This kind of evaluation can be practised by all nurses giving care. If two glycerol suppositories are the nursing prescription for a patient with constipation, the nurse who is caring for the patient on that day will record the outcome of this intervention in the progress notes.

Sometimes the recording of formative evaluation data is useful in demonstrating movement towards the goal. The goal for a mentally handicapped child who has difficulty in self-feeding might be: "Will be able to use spoon independently by 2/6". Formative evaluation recording might include such statements as: "25/5 Can scoop food onto her spoon, but needs maximum assistance in directing the spoon to her mouth". This kind of information might be recorded in the 'Kardex' or in progress/evaluation notes, as referred to by McFarlane and Castledine (1982).

SUMMATIVE EVALUATION

Summative evaluation data is that information obtained on the dates predetermined for evaluation. It incorporates the five steps discussed earlier, from data collection through to feedback to the care plan. The type of nursing records used vary enormously from area to area and so, accordingly, will the space available for recording evaluation data vary. Two examples are shown in Figure 5.8.

Fig. 5.8 Recording summative evaluation

A separate sheet from the care plan can be used to record evaluation data. For example:

Date	Signature	Problem no.	Evaluation

or the care plan and evaluation sheet can be combined. This would require two pages in order to accommodate the relevant information.

Date	Problems	Goals	Nursing plan	Date for review	Evaluation	Signature

RESPONSIBILITY FOR EVALUATION

This section will consider whose role it is to carry out evaluation.

Responsibility for evaluation

Use this activity to assist you in working out where responsibility for evaluation lies within different systems of nursing.

In Module 4, the practice of the nursing process was discussed with reference to several systems of work organisation and, in particular, patient allocation and primary nursing. For each of these systems identify who you think should be responsible for evaluation.

1 Patient allocation

2 Primary nursing.

Author's comment
You will probably have found that it was easy to identify the primary nurse as the person who should have responsibility for evaluation in primary nursing, whereas the term 'patient allocation' is open to so many different interpretations that it may have proved difficult to cite any one person with responsibility for evaluation.

In Module 4, it was suggested that evaluation is part of the role of the primary nurse. In theory this is fine: in practice it may need careful organisation and planning. Because of the shortened working week for nurses it may not always be practical for evaluation times/dates to coincide with the period on duty of the primary nurse; on occasions, therefore, this function might be delegated to an associate nurse, which again requires careful planning of off-duty periods. The other possible way of ensuring that the primary nurse carries out evaluation is to time the evaluation dates to coincide with those when the primary nurse is on duty.

Patient allocation is practised in many different ways. Sometimes when nurses say that they "do patient allocation" they mean that two teams of nurses work in the two halves of the ward, whilst at other times patient allocation may mean that one nurse is allocated to a group of patients for one span of duty. Yet another interpretation is the allocation of a group of nurses to a group of patients for as long as they remain on that ward. You can see that, within these three examples, differences will occur in relation to who does evaluation and how it is documented. There are no strict guidelines except that, if at all possible, a *qualified* nurse should accept responsibility and accountability for evaluation.

The degree of responsibility for evaluation within this range is proportional to the amount of nurse-patient contact. The more a nurse is involved in the preceding steps of assessment, planning and implementation, the more she is able to accept responsibility for the fourth step, evaluation. If a nurse has interviewed a patient on admission, identified problems, planned appropriate interventions, set goals and participated in giving care, then it is logical that she should also take responsibility for evaluation.

Accountability and evaluation are intimately linked:

> Evaluation is a way to demonstrate accountability ... Accountability implies responsibility for one's behaviour; it requires the ability to define, explain and measure the results of nursing actions. (Griffith and Christensen, 1982)

It is unlikely that the responsibility for evaluation will fall upon one nurse alone; it is more likely to be a collective responsibility. The practice of this collective responsibility will now be discussed.

EVALUATION IN PRACTICE

In community care settings, nurses, midwives and health visitors work alone for a great proportion of their time. This means that they might actively have to seek out their colleagues and/or superiors to confer about evaluation. Thus, in the community, individual nurses may accept total responsibility for evaluation.

In hospital, usually more than one nurse is significantly involved in assessment, planning, implementation and therefore evaluation. There are several different ways in which evaluation can be organised within the ward setting.

1 When one nurse is primarily responsible for the patient, she carries out evaluation, modifies the care plan and then communicates it to other team members, perhaps at a handover report.

2 A team of nurses together carry out the process of evaluation.

3 One nurse collects the necessary data, and then a group of nurses together decide on the appropriate feedback to the care plan.

When more than one nurse is involved, *nursing care conferences* are one way of conducting joint decision making. An example of this will be seen on video during Group Session 5. The nurse who has been primarily responsible for the care of the patient, or the team leader, presents the relevant information. Assessment data, the care plan and evaluation data are presented, discussion takes place and a decision is reached as to the most appropriate actions to take. This kind of conference is particularly useful in those care settings where learners are encouraged to carry out the steps of the nursing process. Such a meeting can also serve several other functions as suggested by McFarlane and Castledine (1982):

1 It provides time for reviewing assessment, problem identification and the nursing care which has been given.

2 Plans for the transfer of the patient to his home or to another hospital can be made.

3 Nurses can develop a new and wider understanding of patients.

4 Any relevant research findings and their possible application can be discussed.

5 It provides an opportunity for nurses to develop skills of leadership and interpersonal communication.

If the 'membership' of such conferences is extended to include teachers or managers, nursing care conferences can also:

1 Provide opportunities for teachers and managers to get to know members of staff more personally.

2 Enable teachers to keep in touch with current clinical practice.

3 Provide opportunities for teachers and managers to share their knowledge with clinical nurses.

4 Provide opportunities for appraisal of student nurses and trained nurses by teachers and managers respectively.

The exact way in which you can carry out evaluation and communicate the outcomes will depend on several factors:

- how much time is available
- how many nurses are available to meet together
- who carries out evaluation
- the system of nursing practised in your work area.

OTHER TYPES OF EVALUATION

This section will briefly consider methods of evaluation other than concurrent outcome evaluation, which has been the focus of this module. These other methods are:

- concurrent process evaluation
- retrospective process evaluation
- retrospective outcome evaluation.

These methods are *not* used to determine whether patients have achieved expected outcomes for specific nursing problems: they are used in a wider context, as you will see.

CONCURRENT PROCESS EVALUATION

An example of this type of evaluation, in which patients are observed as they receive care, is the Quality Patient Care Scale Nursing Audit (Wandelt and Ager, 1974). The use of this scale in Britain is described by Wainwright and Burnip (1983 a and b).

This particular tool of evaluation has sixty-eight items for consideration, which are divided into six categories: psychosocial (two sections), physical, general, communication and professional implications. An individual patient is studied by one observer for a set period of time, every interaction between nurses and patient being categorised and scored. Scores can be obtained for individual patients and nurses. This instrument can be used for several purposes:

- to determine whether care has reached an acceptable standard
- to identify any patients not receiving adequate nursing care
- to appraise individual nurses.

Wainwright and Burnip feel that, although the instrument was American in origin, it still has some use in this country.

RETROSPECTIVE PROCESS EVALUATION

The nursing audit, pioneered by Phaneuf (1972), is one example of a tool used to determine the extent to which care and records meet established standards.

Phaneuf describes the use of a nursing audit in an American hospital in her book *The Nursing Audit: profile for excellence*. The sole source of information for the nursing audit is the patient's records. The audit is divided into seven categories, reflecting the seven functions of nursing as seen by Lesnik and Anderson (1955).

1 Application and execution of physician's legal orders.

2 Observation of symptoms and reactions.

3 Supervision of the patient.

4 Supervision of those participating in care, except physicians.

5 Reporting and recording.

6 Application and execution of nursing procedures and techniques.

7 Promotion of physical and emotional health by direction and teaching.

In total there are fifty components, for which various systems of scoring are used. The outcome of the audit is a judgment (based on the score obtained) about the quality of nursing care as reflected in the nursing records. The care can be rated as unsafe, poor, incomplete, good or excellent. An auditing committee which directs and implements auditing is advocated by Phaneuf.

Two basic assumptions are made in this method of evaluation:

- if nursing actions are documented, they have been carried out
- if there is no record of a nursing action, it has not taken place.

The audit is really a tool for use by nurse managers to assess the standard of care in the area for which they have responsibility.

RETROSPECTIVE OUTCOME EVALUATION

This is the least developed of all methods of evaluation. There are several ways in which it can be approached:

- by the use of specially designed instruments which examine the records for evidence of achieved patient goals
- by interviewing patients, after they have been discharged from care, to ascertain if goals were reached
- by sending questionnaires for patients to complete after their discharge from care.

We have considered in this section some of the ways in which standards of nursing care and nurse performance can be evaluated. It seems likely that these types of evaluation could have only limited application within the health care system currently operating in this country, the main constraints being paucity of finance, resources and expertise.

Nurses can, of course, get together within their own units, or in the community, to carry out *peer review*. In a similar setting to that of the care conference, a sample of care plans is examined to look at standards of care planning. A predetermined set of criteria – such as

the questions listed in Figure 5.7 – could be applied to the plans to see if they meet these criteria. This type of peer review can have several functions:

- colleagues can receive and give support to each other
- good practices can be identified and reinforced
- information can be collated on problems commonly experienced by patients in the unit or area
- learning needs can be identified.

USES OF INFORMATION COLLECTED IN EVALUATION

All of the methods discussed in this module generate information which can be used to determine which nursing actions are most consistently effective in solving particular problems for individual patients. In time, as information is built up, it may be possible to determine the most effective nursing actions for common patient problems. This would help to facilitate accurate prediction of the time factor in goal planning.

CONCLUSION

Throughout the module, reference has been made to other stages of the nursing process – assessment, planning and implementation. The evaluation step demonstrates the intimate links between the four stages. Evaluation cannot take place unless goals have been set and some of the planned nursing actions have been implemented. Goals can only be set in response to the identification of a problem amenable to nursing intervention, and problems are only identified after an assessment has been made. After evaluation, there may be ramifications for each of the other stages, when goals may be rewritten, actions changed or a need for further assessment identified.

Thus evaluation can be seen as the axle upon which the process turns, which can start or end a revolution!

Fig. 5.9 Evaluation in relation to the other steps of the nursing process

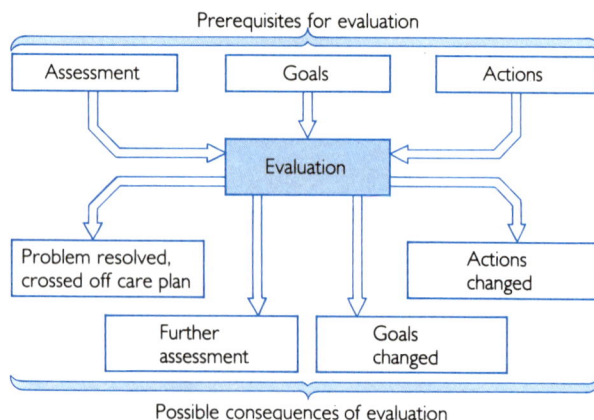

FURTHER READING

Hunt, J. M. and Marks-Maran, D. J. (1980) *Nursing Care Plans: The Nursing Process at Work* , London, HM & M Publishers. Ch. 9.

Griffith, J. W. and Christensen, P. J. (1982) *Nursing Process: Application of Theories, Frameworks and Models,* St Louis, C.V. Mosby Co. Ch. X.

Luker, K. A. (1979) Evaluating nursing care *in* Kratz, C. (ed.) *The Nursing Process,* London, Baillière Tindall, pp. 124–146.

McFarlane of Llandaff, and Castledine, G. (1982) *A Guide to the Practice of Nursing Using the Nursing Process,* London, C.V. Mosby Co. Ch. 9.

MODULE 6
REVIEWING THE NURSING PROCESS

Prepared for the Course Team by Gladys M. Law

CONTENTS

OBJECTIVES

After studying this module, you should be able to:

1 Demonstrate an understanding that the four steps of the nursing process – assessment, planning, implementation and evaluation – form an interrelated and continuous activity, when actually used in practice.

2 Recognise that putting the theory of a systematic approach to nursing into practice requires flexibility in approach.

3 Identify areas where you will use the nursing process flexibly in your own practice.

INTRODUCTION

In the previous modules the four steps of the nursing process have been discussed separately and in depth. This separation has been necessary for teaching purposes but in practice the steps are inter-related, frequently overlapping, and may need to be used on repeated occasions for various aspects of a patient's care. The nursing process has been described in Module I as 'a systematic problem-oriented approach' to nursing, but there are no rigid rules about its application. For example, decisions on the style and content of assessment or on the storage of nursing records will need to be made locally in the light of the needs of particular patients, available resources, constraints and local circumstances.

It is this cohesiveness yet flexibility of the nursing process in action which allows it to be used as an aid to the nursing of all patients in a variety of settings.

The nursing process is not a magic formula. Conscious and deliberate effort must be exerted by the users.

> "There is no expedient to which man will not resort to avoid the real labour of thinking" *Sir Joshua Reynolds.*

Successful use of the nursing process is dependent on nurses having the knowledge, insight, and confidence to use it to assist their practice and to enable efficient and effective nursing to take place. Nurses of all grades have to be aware of their responsibility for, and be involved in, making appropriate decisions for its use in diverse environments and circumstances. This can only be achieved if we are fully conversant with the ideas of the nursing process and its versatility in use. Being irresponsible when choosing or using a method of nursing can be just as damaging to patients as other forms of poor practice. For example, obtaining irrelevant assessment information by means of interrogation, or performing nursing actions which are not evaluated, could cause the patient as much harm and distress as administering an injection in the wrong site. On the other hand, a patient could feel more relaxed and confident if he is involved in the decision making and priority setting for his nursing care. This type of beneficial result is dependent on our skills in communicating and care planning.

Accountability and responsibility were discussed in Module I. You may wish to reread that section to help you recall the lines of accountability mentioned there. Although the nursing process is primarily for use by clinical practitioners it requires teaching, facilitating, supporting and monitoring by nurse managers and educators. The nursing process in use can, in return, provide them with feedback about clinical standards, workloads and resources and the learning progress of individual nurses. The management of change and the introduction of the nursing process will be discussed in Module 7.

> "You cannot teach a man anything; you can only help him to find it within himself" *Galileo Galilei.*

With these ideas in mind and using a sample nursing record, the purpose of this module is to present you with some challenges. It will offer a few ideas to set you on the road to your own practical use of the nursing process or will help you to review your progress in developing this approach.

Remember though, that this module – and indeed the whole course – is not intended as an end in itself and that you are likely to continue to adapt your views and discover alternative approaches as you gain more experience and confidence.

FLEXIBLE USE OF THE NURSING PROCESS

THE RELATIONSHIP BETWEEN THE STEPS OF THE NURSING PROCESS

The nursing process is sometimes described as a cycle but it is perhaps more accurate to liken it to a spiral. The practitioner winds continuously through the steps advancing through assessment, planning, implementation and, as evaluation takes place, it is followed, if required, by further assessment and amendments to plans and interventions. Each step can be returned to at any time, as the need arises. This has been illustrated in Figure 1.1 in Module I (p. 9).

Although the spiral commences with assessment and each step is dependent on the others, the time spent on each phase can be very variable. The collection and interpretation of information, planning, implementation and evaluation could be occurring simultaneously for different aspects of the same patient's care. For example, you may be changing a dressing on a patient's wound following his written care plan (*implementation*). At the same time, you are observing the patient and purposefully communicating with him verbally and non-verbally in order to gather new information about him (*assessment*). You may purposely be questioning him to ascertain or clarify information (*further assessment*). Perhaps you observe that the wound is not healing (*evaluation*), and as the dressing is completed you are already formulating in your mind an alternative plan of action (*planning*).

PACING THE STEPS OF THE NURSING PROCESS

You may be unable to spend much time on one phase of the nursing process before moving onto the next. For example, you would not attempt to complete an assessment interview with a patient who was tired or vomiting. You would however be able to use your senses of sight, smell, hearing and touch to gain some knowledge of the patient. If appropriate, you could gain further information from the patient's family, friends, or other professionals and helpers involved. If a patient were unconscious, had no family or friends and had received no previous health care, your plans for nursing intervention would have to draw substantially upon what you observed and your previous nursing knowledge and experience. These plans would be up-dated if, and when, new information came to light. Through observation and accurate recording, the patients' 'normal' patterns, likes and dislikes, and strengths and weaknesses can sometimes be established, even if they are unable to communicate. I nursed a patient who began eating, following many weeks of tube-feeding. He was unable to communicate because of brain damage, but over a few days his likes and dislikes were established by carefully recording the foods he accepted with relish, merely swallowed or spat out. Likes and dislikes were included in his care plan, thus avoiding the need for continuous trial and error. In this example, the patient's life depended on an improvement of his nutritional state which could best be achieved by a return to a naturally eaten diet. Although difficult to quantify, a great deal of nursing time and expense was probably saved by preventing his condition from deteriorating, as well as resulting in direct benefit to the patient.

A QUICKER PACE

With a patient having a cardiac arrest or being nursed in the immediate post-operative period, the steps of the nursing process spiral would be occurring very rapidly indeed. For high standards of nursing it is still necessary to make an assessment and plan, and to have specific objectives in mind. You would not have time in this situation, however, to record your thoughts before all the action has taken place. The usual practice in the example of cardiac arrest is to appoint someone to record events as they occur, but if only one or two people are present you may have to wait until the emergency is over and the events can be recorded in retrospect. A written record in these circumstances has two main purposes. Firstly, it gives nurses an opportunity to benefit from reflecting on the actions taken and considering the outcomes. Success or failure should deepen nurses' understanding and enhance their expertise when next faced with a similar situation. Secondly, permanent records are usually needed to document major events which happen to patients.

Often, where nurse-patient contact is brief, you will have to select priority areas for assessment and planning. For example, patients admitted for minor surgery as day cases may be asked if they have been in hospital before. They may need to be asked who is looking after their family and whether there is someone to take them home in the evening. It would be inappropriate in these circumstances to gather details of food preferences or hobbies, when they may already be fasting before a general anaesthetic and only be allowed a drink before going home. Their preference for what they drink on this occasion can be established at the time.

Even a day patient, however, may be looked after by two or more shifts of nurses, making nurse-to-nurse communication vital. The care plan itself should be simple, concise and pertinent if it is to be useful. Standard care plans, dealt with later in the module, may be of value in short-stay situations. If further information is required, because the patient has to stay longer in hospital, this can be ascertained later, building on the information already obtained.

A SLOWER PACE

There are numerous other occasions when a nurse may think it appropriate to spend time making and recording an in-depth assessment and making a comprehensive plan before most of the nursing action takes place. This will occur when it is anticipated that nurse-patient contact will be for a longer continuing period, such as with a district nurse whose patient is unable to walk and can perform few self-care activities, a patient being admitted to a psychiatric unit or a patient with kidney failure who could require a transplant and contact, for life, with a particular care team.

TIME WELL-SPENT

An in-depth *initial* assessment carried out by measuring, testing, listening, observing, and asking questions can often make better use of your time or in the long run save your time, by facilitating:

- the prevention of potential problems such as constipation, pressure sores or anxiety, thus saving a great deal of nursing time and patient misery
- the identification of appropriate goals by working with the patient
- the identification of priorities through greater understanding of the patient and his circumstances
- the selection of appropriate interventions for individual patients; written instructions, for example, are of no use to a patient who is later found to be illiterate
- the tackling of urgent problems at the earliest opportunity.

THE PATIENT AS A PARTNER

Problems which are urgent from the nurse's point of view may be seen in a totally different way by their patients. I recall a lengthy admission interview where I gathered a great deal of information about the patient's pain, nausea, diabetes, the death of her husband and her daughter, who had taken an overdose. When I asked, however, what she thought was her greatest difficulty, she replied without hesitation that she had forgotten to cancel the milk at home.

This experience was a good reminder, not only of the fact that patients' views may be different from those of the nurse, but also of the benefits of ensuring that the patient is a partner in care planning. This kind of partnership has been discussed in earlier modules.

Part of this nurse-patient partnership involves both encouraging the patient to ask questions and allowing flexibility within the assessment, as previously discussed in Module 2. An agenda for the interview that has been rigidly set by the nurse may be different from that anticipated by the patient. This could limit the scope of the assessment and could mean omitting matters of special concern to the patient. My interview, described above, did not include asking questions about uncancelled milk. Some open questions about possible social difficulties related to the hospital admission should have been posed earlier in the nurse-patient discussion; this could have helped to establish a course for continuing the assessment.

WRITTEN GUIDELINES FOR ASSESSMENT

To help less experienced nurses to be selective when undertaking assessment, more detailed guidelines written at ward or unit level can be useful. This can be particularly helpful where the same printed assessment document is used in a variety of specialties. It can guide staff in obtaining pertinent information for particular groups of patients, for example, short-stay gynaecological patients. Your Health Authority may have provided nursing assessment forms with printed headings or questions. These can be helpful as an aide-memoir or checklist for the various topics to be covered in your assessment. It is also quicker to retrieve information later if it is organised under discrete headings rather than being written as a narrative. You can use the same design of form for the assessment of a wide range of patients, but there is no one assessment style or content that is appropriate for all patients. You may therefore end up by adopting an almost blank sheet of paper on which to write your assessment but the assessment must still be appropriate, clear and concise.

APPROPRIATE ASSESSMENT

The focus of assessment should always be appropriate for individual patients. For example, it is important to identify the information needs of culturally and ethnically different patients in relation to health education. Patients from cultural or ethnic minorities may have life-styles, family patterns, dietary norms, priorities and expectations that differ from those of most patients. This can only be ascertained by appropriately focused and practised assessment.

> "Had I to carve an inscription on my tombstone I would ask for none other than 'The Individual'"
> *Soren Kierkegaard.*

Your decision about the content and style of assessment will be influenced in numerous ways. The nursing model which you use may affect the content, structure and approach. The patient's condition and anticipated length of contact have already been mentioned. The patient's responses and attitude to you and your questions should give you further clues as to the most suitable way to proceed.

Although your assessment form may have a list of headings under which information is to be recorded, this should not prevent priority information being gathered first. For example, during a busy admission morning on a surgical ward, a patient is welcomed into the ward at 11.55 am. You are about to serve the lunches. After showing him his bed and giving directions to the bathroom, it seems appropriate to ask first whether he is on a diet or dislikes any foods. At the first opportunity following the serving of the lunches at 12 midday, the information collected earlier can be recorded. You may also have gathered in the same five minutes' contact with the patient some details of his mobility, hearing, language, dress, family and worries and fears.

Effective use of the nursing process means making the most of every opportunity, rather than requiring excessive amounts of spare time or numbers of nurses on duty.

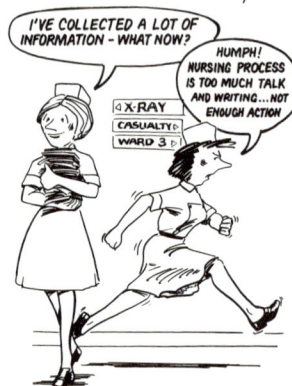

All information collected about a patient must be recorded for the purpose of planning care and not merely in order to fill an assessment form with writing. The nurse is in the privileged position of asking patients to share information which is personal, often intimate and confidential. If a patient responds to questions, then he will rightly expect action to be taken as a result of his replies. For example, if a patient is asked about his usual eating habits, likes and dislikes, then he will probably expect, if not informed to the contrary, that these details will be taken into account when food is served. If not, you may ask whether the question should have been asked in the first place. There is not one simple answer. You may, for instance, ask a patient about his fluid preference and learn that it is coffee. Ward stock levels, however, are not static and this particular item may soon be used up or become unavailable. I believe it may still be appropriate to make a note of the patient's preference because the aim is to meet patient's wishes when possible, and to give reasons to the patient when they cannot be met or find alternative routes to problem solving. For instance, you may have to discuss this issue with the supplies officer or catering manager; you could ask the patient to provide his own coffee or you could re-assess the situation with the patient. He may be satisfied with milk until the ward supplies arrive in a few days.

It is important that the patient understands *why* you are asking any personal questions. Introducing yourself as the patient's nurse, giving your name, grade and details of when you will be responsible for his care is one way to begin. It may be appropriate then to explain that you would like some information about his normal pattern of life so that, together, you can plan the most suitable nursing care and that this will be continued by other nurses involved with his care when you are off duty. The fact that the information will only be shared with other professionals and that the patient is free to refuse to answer questions, can be very reassuring to some patients.

The overall content and pacing of the process of nursing will always depend on the individual patient and circumstances, as well as the knowledge, judgment and creativity of the individual nurse involved in each instance.

THE NURSING PROCESS AND DOCUMENTATION

INTRODUCTION TO A SAMPLE NURSING RECORD

In this part of the module, you will find an example of a patient's assessment, care plan and progress record. There is nothing special about these particular records, either in their design or in the way in which they have been completed. They are similar to many other records currently being used in the United Kingdom and – even more importantly – are representative of the type of recording being produced by busy nurses. In other words, they are being used here not as an example of literary expertise but as an attempt by clinical nurses to communicate effectively about a patient. The purpose is to stimulate your thoughts about how you will use the nursing process.

Using a sample care plan for this purpose can have its dangers. You may be tempted to focus your attention on the patient's illness, which may not be the type usually treated in your work area. But try to overcome this by concentrating on the patient as a person and on the daily living activities that are applicable to all people, regardless of the type of their illness.

There is also a danger that you may concentrate on how these recordings differ from your own. It will help if you focus on the information collected, used and communicated.

You may be thinking that undue attention is drawn to the recording aspects of the nursing process. But by this stage of the course you will understand that the nursing process is much more than a new form of record keeping, although record keeping is, or should be, an integral part of nursing care reflecting nurse-patient activities. The purpose of having records is to make nursing explicit and to communicate it.

MEET MR KAPOOR

Mr Sunil Kapoor, aged 66, was admitted to a medical ward on 6 May because of a chest infection. The care plan presented is complete up to 20 May, at the stage of preparation for Mr Kapoor's discharge home on 22 May.

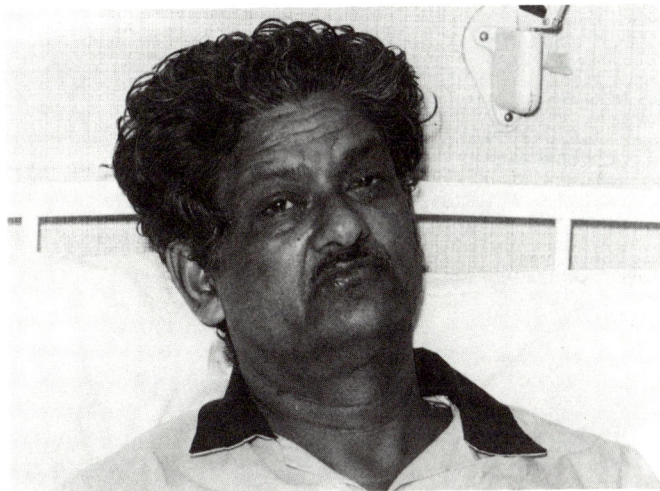

LOOKING CRITICALLY AT NURSING RECORDS

Activity 6.1   **Allow 45 minutes**

Making the most of records

Good nursing records should give enough information to plan and ensure continuity of nursing care. This activity should help you to make judgments about the quality of recordings and make the most of your own records.

Mr Kapoor's nursing records appear on pp. 134–141. For Activity 6.1, read through the complete set of records, covering the text beneath until you have completed the activity. Then continue working through the module text.

After reading Mr Kapoor's nursing records list your findings in relation to the following four questions:

1 In what ways do the records demonstrate the four steps of the nursing process and the links between them?

NAME Mr. Sunil Kapoor	**PROPERTY RETAINED IN HOSPITAL**	**DISCHARGE** ~~being planned for 22 May~~
ADDRESS 18, Jaffa Road, Catford, London SE28	Spectacles (Yes)/No	Date of Discharge ~~being planned for 22 May~~ ~~Transfer/Death~~
TEL. NO. 936-8420	Dentures Yes/(No)	Discharged/Transferred to
DATE OF BIRTH 23·2·1917	Hearing Aid Yes/(No)	Relatives informed (Yes)/No
RELIGION Hindu	Prosthesis (specify) Yes/(No)	Transport needed Yes/(No) — ordered
MARITAL STATUS Married	Valuables Yes/(No)	Escort needed Yes/(No) — arranged
HOSPITAL NO. 38521	Day Clothes Yes/(No)	

The form contains the following handwritten entries:

NAME Mr. Sunil Kapoor
ADDRESS 18, Jaffa Road, Catford, London SE28
TEL. NO. 936-8420
DATE OF BIRTH 23·2·1917
RELIGION Hindu
MARITAL STATUS Married
HOSPITAL NO. 38521

TYPE OF ADMISSION
Formal — Informal — (Urgent) — Routine
DATE OF ADMISSION 6 May

NEXT OF KIN NAME Mrs   **RELATIONSHIP** Wife
ADDRESS } as above
TEL. NO. }

CONTACT IN EMERGENCY NAME Wife or son
ADDRESS } as above

ARE NEXT OF KIN AWARE OF ADMISSION
(Yes)/No
Comments During the day Mon-Fri son can be contacted at 243-8971.

RELEVANT MEDICAL HISTORY
Was treated for tuberculosis in 1979.

PROVISIONAL DIAGNOSIS/REASON FOR ADMISSION
Chest infection

PROPERTY RETAINED IN HOSPITAL
Spectacles (Yes)/No
Dentures Yes/(No)
Hearing Aid Yes/(No)
Prosthesis (specify) Yes/(No)
Valuables Yes/(No)
Day Clothes Yes/(No)
Drugs Yes/(No)

COMMUNITY STAFF
G.P DR. M. DAVIS
ADDRESS 92, Broadbent Street, Catford, London SE28
TEL. NO. 936-8449
Other NAME
ADDRESS
TEL. NO.

HOSPITAL PERSONNEL e.g. Social Worker

Speaks Gujarati.
Understands little English - Interpreter Mr. Singh a patient on Florence Ward and son and daughter-in-law during visits.

DISCHARGE
Date of Discharge ~~being planned for 22 May~~ ~~Transfer/Death~~
Discharged/Transferred to
Relatives informed (Yes)/No
Transport needed Yes/(No) — ordered
Escort needed Yes/(No) — arranged

O.P.D. Appointment (Yes)/No
Date 29 May
O.P.D. Transport needed (Yes)/No — ordered ✓

Day Patient attendance Yes/(No)
Transport needed Yes/No — ordered

Doctor's Letter sent Yes/No
T.T.O's required (Yes)/No
Written   Dispensed

Home Help required Yes/(No)
Home Meals service required Yes/(No)
Community Nurse contacted Yes/(No) Not required
Nurses Letter sent Yes/No

DIAGNOSIS ON DISCHARGE

SURNAME KAPOOR   **FIRST NAMES** SUNIL   **AGE** 66   **CONSULTANT** DR. ROBERTS   **PERSONAL DOCTOR** DR. DEGAN   **HOSPITAL NO.** 38521

Fig. 6.1   Mr Kapoor's nursing records (continued on pp. 135–141).

2 Which aspects of the records indicate that the nurses are using an holistic view of the patient i.e. psychological, social, spiritual as well as physical aspects of him as a person? Are the records weak in any areas?

3 If you were a nurse working on the ward for the first time, could you give appropriate care from these nursing records? You have not previously met Mr Kapoor.

4 Do the records reflect an orderly progression of nursing care for this patient?

Author's comment

Your responses to the questions in Activity 6.1 may be variable, but probably the majority of you did see evidence in the records of assessment, problem identification, patient goal setting, planning of nursing action and some evaluation, under the relevant headings. You may have felt that the links between the steps could have been stronger. You may, for example, have thought that more assessment details should have been recorded about Mr Kapoor's home situation, in order to facilitate the plan for discharge. You may also have considered that evaluation was not adequately recorded. Was information available, for example, regarding the pain in his chest (problem 3). Problem 7 and the corresponding goal are 'woolly' and there is no clear link between "mobilisation" as the problem and "meeting usual hygiene and toilet needs" as the goal.

In response to Question 2, you probably identified some physical and social considerations and some evidence of family involvement, but you may not have identified any spiritual aspects. Your opinions may have differed as to whether all the necessary aspects had been covered with sufficient thoroughness to develop appropriate care for Mr Kapoor,

ASSESSMENT ON ADMISSION	BODILY FUNCTIONS	OCCUPATION Was an accountant. He has been retired since coming to Britain in 1981.

ASSESSMENT ON ADMISSION

OBSERVATIONS

T. 37 P. 128 R. 28 B/P 130/80

Height 5ft. 4ins   Weight 45.5 kgs

Urinalysis Ph 7.5 NAD

GENERAL APPEARANCE

Size — Normal — (Thin) — Emaciated — Obese

Mood — Anxious — Miserable — (Composed) — Euphoric

Remarks Short, thin looking man. Son says he has always been thin.

SKIN CONDITION

Broken areas   Yes/(No)
Bruises   Yes/(No)
Rashes   Yes/(No)
Oedema   Yes/(No)
Remarks

Condition of Mouth Moist and clean – Has own teeth.

MOBILITY — is help required with

Walking   Yes/(No)
Bathing   Yes/(No)
Dressing   Yes/(No)
Feeding   Yes/(No)

Other Activities

PAIN   Present (Yes)/No

Location Slight pain on inspiration – Rt. side chest.
Analgesic taken (if any) NO

ALLERGIES

None known

BODILY FUNCTIONS

Sight Good — (Poor) — Wears spectacles (Yes)/No

Any problems Eyes "water" if spectacles are worn for long periods.

Hearing (Good) — Poor — Wears aid Yes/(No)
Any problems NONE

Appetite (Good) — Poor
Special dietary requirements Does not eat meat. Eats fish and likes most other foods. Does not drink alcohol or smoke.

Elimination
Micturition — (Normal) — Frequency — Incontinence — Retention
Any problems

Defaecation — (Regular) — Diarrhoea — Constipation
                daily
Regular use of aperients — Yes/(No)
Any problems

Menstruation — Regular   Yes/No
Blood loss — Normal — Heavy — Light
Pain   Yes/No
Any problems

Sleep — Normal Pattern Usually wakes frequently and gets up at 6 a.m.
Sedation taken
What else helps Had sleeping pills from GP in the past but now prefers to do without. Gets up if he cannot sleep and makes a pot of tea.
For the past week has been breathless at night.

OCCUPATION Was an accountant. He has been retired since coming to Britain in 1981.

HOME SITUATION Lives with wife, son and daughter-in-law in son's 3 bedroomed terrace house.

DEPENDENTS Wife

OTHER RELEVANT SOCIAL ASPECTS

Born in Bombay, India. Came to live with son in UK (1981). He and his wife speak little English. Son and daughter-in-law speak good English.

History taken by (S/N SMITH) M. Smith
from Mr. Kapoor with help of his son and later through Mr. Singh, interpreter on Florence Ward.

Date 6.5.83

---

which should involve not only total care but the maximum self-care. Being human is being a whole person and being one's own agent or living one's own life. To what degree do you think that Mr Kapoor was assisted in caring for himself and did the records indicate that he was his own agent in respect of self-care?

Thirdly, could you carry out patient care from these records? You may have made criticisms of the records. You could have felt, for example, that the goals could have been more specific or the planned actions clearer. When I first read the plan, however, I thought it gave a good indication about the care required and the progress being made. Your response may have been that you could have done much better. As mentioned earlier, it was meant to represent a real, working record which would act as a focal point for your own thinking. Remember that there would have been various constraints on those nurses caring for Mr Kapoor in the form of time limits and the task of setting priorities for his

care alongside that of other patients. For example, the pressure of unexpected emergencies could have necessitated the involvement of the nurses caring for Mr Kapoor. Maybe each nurse's workload was increased because one nurse was absent or escorting a patient to X-ray or to another hospital.

DOCUMENTATION – WHAT AND HOW MUCH TO INCLUDE?

You may have felt that there was a great deal of information in these sample records, with some repetition. Record keeping itself should not become out of proportion to other nursing activities. The 'right' amount of writing, the detail given and the frequency of updating can only be judged in individual circumstances. Like any other nursing activity, a balance has to be achieved and priorities set. The trained

Name MR. KAPOOR

Problem No.	Date	Staff Assessment	Patient Assessment	Problem No.	Patient Goals	Signature
①	6 May	Breathlessness for past week probably due to chest infection. Respirations 28 on admission.	"I get more breathless at night. I slip down the bed and can't get my breath."	①	Mr. Kapoor to be less breathless. Respirations less than 28/min.	M. Smith
②	6 May	Language barrier. Speaks only Gujarati.		②	Mr. Kapoor to be able to communicate more easily.	M. Smith
③	6 May	Slight pain - right side of chest on inspiration and when trying to cough. Has difficulty in expectorating.	"My spit is green and I have difficulty in coughing it up."	③	Mr. Kapoor to be able to expectorate with less discomfort and effort.	M. Smith
④	6 May	Vegetarian but does eat fish. _Discont 8 May_	"I like most things to eat but have been off my food for the past few days."	④	Mr. Kapoor to eat a full vegetarian diet and at least maintain weight at 45.5 kgs. Review on Mondays and Thursdays.	M. Smith
⑤	6 May	Needs help with personal hygiene and toilet. (Bedrest ordered by doctor.)		⑤	Mr. Kapoor to have assistance with personal hygiene and toilet until he can give self-care.	M. Smith

nurse with overall responsibility for the patient may primarily be the best judge. I say 'primarily', as records have to mean the same thing to numerous other people who will also have a view on their usefulness. It's a good idea to question the night staff or the nurse who works the shortest number of hours about whether patient records are providing accurate, concise and good quality information which she can follow. You can further check, by asking how a particular item of information is interpreted, whether any omissions have been found or care perpetuated which is no longer required.

Nurse managers may also have to use records to answer queries about patient care. In this case, the records need to be sufficiently detailed to give the information required. The quality of record keeping should be continuously monitored by nurse managers as well as by clinical practitioners as a means of improving and maintaining a high standard of record keeping and clinical practice.

THE NURSING RECORD AS A PROFESSIONAL DOCUMENT

This is probably an appropriate moment to consider the main purposes of the nursing record (see King's Fund, 1983).

The nursing record is usually a professional document. For midwives it is a statutory requirement in their practice. What is recorded, by whom, and the frequency of recordings is a matter for professional judgment in the light of local circumstances. As with other areas of professional practice, the nurse will be expected to maintain records to professionally acceptable standards. In the same way, details of patient care recorded will be expected to meet up-to-date professionally accepted standards. Such standards have to be agreed and communicated to others and will probably involve those accepted nationally and locally. For instance, it is nationally

Nursing Care Sheet — Problems — On Going Assessments   Name MR. KAPOOR

Problem No.	Date	Staff Assessment	Patient Assessment	Problem No.	Patient Goals	Signature
⑥	6 May	Potential problem that Mr. Kapoor will not sleep at night due to breathlessness, cough or pain.	"I get more breathless at night because I slip down the bed. I have not slept well for many years".	⑥	Mr. Kapoor to sleep at night for at least as long as he does at home. To get a rest or sleep for 1 hour each afternoon.	M. Smith
⑦	8 May	Mobilisation to commence. (Ordered by doctor)		⑦	Mr Kapoor to meet usual hygiene and toilet needs independently.	T. Brown
⑧	20 May	Mr Kapoor for discharge on 22 May.	"I will be pleased to go home."	⑧	Mr and Mrs Kapoor to be aware of discharge date and preparations.	T. Brown

accepted that patients will have a nursing record but the frequency of recording is not prescribed. Ideally it should be left to registered nurses to make this decision for individual patients, but sometimes a policy about the frequency of recording is made within a particular Health Authority. For example, in a long-stay psychogeriatric ward the policy may be to record information about each patient on alternative days at least.

The main purposes of the nursing record are to:

- demonstrate that nursing care is planned and is not simply an haphazard series of events or tasks
- demonstrate that each patient appears to receive the appropriate nursing care at a professionally acceptable standard
- maintain continuity and provide a means of communication between nurses and other relevant disciplines
- record any changes in the condition or circumstances of the patient
- provide a continuous record when the patient is re-located or re-admitted
- provide a permanent record for future reference for research, teaching and/or investigation for legal purposes. It may be required for a local Health Authority investigation, an investigation by the Health Service Ombudsman or in a case brought to a Court of Law.

I have mentioned that records are necessary for communication and continuity where more than one nurse is involved with a patient's care, but they are also helpful for independent practitioners. Large case loads, long time intervals between patient contacts, as well as the normal frailty of human memory, are reasons why

Problem No.	Date	Nursing Care Plan	Signature	Date	Evaluation	Signature
					Name MR. KAPOOR	
① & ③	6 May	Sit upright in bed, support with pillows particularly at night. Instruct patient to take deep breaths and expectorate sputum at least hourly. Provide sputum pot – change 6 a.m. and 6 p.m. – Record amount and colour. To be seen later by physiotherapist. Record TPR 4 hourly and BP daily.	M. Smith			
②	6 May	Use sign language ie. point to objects and visual aids card kept on locker. Explain as much as possible when English speaking relatives visit. Try to understand and learn his language. Patient on Florence Ward will interpret also.	M. Smith			
④	6 May	Mr. Singh from Florence Ward will visit 10 a.m. daily and complete menu card for Mr. Kapoor. Weigh patient before breakfast on Mondays and Thursdays. Observe patient eating to make sure he is liking food. *Discontinued 8.5.83*	M. Smith	9.5.83 12.5.83	45 kgs. 45.5 kgs	
⑤	6 May	Mr. Kapoor may use the commode. Will need assistance with washing and bathing while in bed. Offer bedbath each morning.	M. Smith	8.5.83	Mr Kapoor can now walk to the toilet.	T. Brown

nurses such as district nurses and health visitors also need good record keeping. One example is monitoring the health status of elderly patients. Actually reviewing assessments, plans and care in a written form gives the lone nurse feedback and can trigger new ideas.

> E M Forster once said "How do I know what I mean till I see what I say?"

MONITORING DOCUMENTATION

Looking at records critically can be beneficial, not only for maintaining good standards of recording and reviewing standards of care, but also for monitoring the introduction of the nursing process.

These are the types of questions to ask about a patient's record where problem-oriented recording is being used:

1 Are the nursing process steps linked together?

2 Does the care plan result from information recorded in the assessment?

3 Is there a need for more or less or different information?

4 Are the problems identified as a direct result of a systematic nursing assessment of this patient, knowledge of usual problems for this condition or just guesswork?

5 Are the goals appropriate?

6 Would you know when the goals were to be achieved? Do you think that it is possible for the patient to reach these goals? Is there evidence of patient participation in goal and priority setting?

7 Are the nursing instructions sufficiently specific so that everyone nursing the patient has enough information to be able to carry out the correct care?

Problem No.	Date	Nursing Care Plan	Signature	Date	Name MR. KAPOOR	
					Evaluation	Signature
⑥	6 May	Nurse upright at night well supported with pillows. May sleep in other positions if patient prefers. Offer a cup of tea if patient does not sleep. Allow patient to sleep at other times of the day if possible.	M. Smith			
		Discontinued 10 May				
⑦	8 May	Mobilising commenced. Mr Kapoor can sit out of bed and walk to toilet. Observe for breathlessness. Allow Mr Kapoor to rest on his bed during afternoon.	T. Brown	10 May	Mr. Kapoor now less breathless and can attend to own hygiene and walk to toilet on his own.	M. Smith
	10 May	Mr. Kapoor to walk around ward as he wishes and take general bath.	M. Smith			
⑧	20 May	Prepare for Mr Kapoor's discharge on 22 May. Inform wife and son at visiting time. Discuss transport.	T. Brown			

8 Are the outcomes of care being recorded and do these permit comparisons with the pre-set goals?

9 Is there any evidence of goals not being achieved and further assessment and re-planning taking place?

10 Are there any alterations in the care plan following evaluation and further assessment?

Activity 6.2   Allow 25 minutes

Monitoring documentation

This activity is intended to build on Activity 6.1 by giving you more experience in looking critically at records.

Using the ten questions in the previous paragraph as a guide to your monitoring, look again at Mr Kapoor's records. Write down your comments in relation to each of the ten questions.

Author's comment

Asking these questions in relation to the sample record, or any other nursing records, can highlight strengths and weaknesses in techniques and streamline documentation.

My views of Mr Kapoor's records in relation to these questions, are:

1 The assessment, planning, implementation and evaluation steps are linked, but sometimes only weakly.

2 I would have liked more details of Mr Kapoor's normal pattern of life in areas such as diet and hygiene, in order to further personalise his care plan.

3 Although I would have liked more information, I am unaware of the constraints on time available to the nurse who carried out this assessment. Other priorities would have to have been balanced with assessing Mr Kapoor.

Date	Problem No.	Nursing Notes — see Ward Guidelines	Investigations	Signature
6 May	①	Breathless at times but not distressed.	CXR performed	M. Smith
		Respirations 26/28 min.	First sputum for AFB's	
	②	Mr. Singh has visited — Mr. Kapoor says he is feeling better and		
		has no pain.		
NIGHT	①+⑥	COUGHING WHEN HE SLIPPED DOWN THE BED. APPEARS TO HAVE SLEPT FOR	2ND SPUTUM FOR AFB'S	P. Fish.
		ABOUT 5 HOURS IN TOTAL.		
7 May	①	Respirations between 20-24min. Produced ½ pot yellow green sputum		T. Brown
		during past 12 hrs.		
	④	Taking most of his food yesterday but to-day has left most of his lunch.		
		Dietician requested to see Mr Kapoor.		
NIGHT	①+⑥	COUGH LESS PERSISTENT DURING THE NIGHT. SPUTUM NOW WHITE AND FROTHY.	3RD SPUTUM FOR AFB's	P. Fish.
8 May	① +	Not breathless to-day. Respirations 20-22min.		T. Brown
	⑤	Mobilisation started. Has walked to toilet on his own on a number of		
		occasions and attended to own hygiene.		
NIGHT	①+⑥	APPEARS TO SLEEP FOR LONGER PERIODS. LESS COUGHING.		P. Fish.
9 May	②	With the use of sign language and visual aids Mr. Kapoor	Results of sputum	M. Smith
		understands and can make most of his needs known.	specimens negative	
11 May		Observations are stable - No change in care plan.		M. Smith
13 May Night	①	Wakened by coughing at 2am. but went back to sleep after a cup		J. Wray
		of tea and change of position		
15 May		No change in care plan.		M. Smith

Surname	First Names	Age	Consultant	Personal Dr.	Hospital No.
KAPOOR	SUNIL	66	DR. ROBERTS	DR. DEGAN	38521

4 In most instances, the problems are identified from the nursing assessment. The recording of problem 7 is a doctor's order. You may be undecided about whether that was a suitable place to record the order, but it's an important part of the patient's total plan.

5 The goals are not always as clear or as concise as they could be. It would be difficult to know when patient goal 3 was achieved, for example. How will it be known that Mr Kapoor is expectorating with "less discomfort and effort"?

Goal 5 is written in terms of what the nurse will do and not as a patient outcome. "Mr Kapoor will bath himself each day" would have been clearer for all concerned.

6 Some of the goals in Mr Kapoor's plan have no target or review dates. Stated goals are set in realistic terms and should be achievable by Mr Kapoor, but with his language difficulties he may not have been involved in all stages of goal and priority setting.

7 If I were a nurse caring for Mr Kapoor, I think that the records would have provided a good guide for my actions and approach to him.

8 There are a few outcomes recorded. For example, on 10 May Mr Kapoor could now "walk to the toilet on his own". The goal for that outcome was stated as "Mr Kapoor to meet usual hygiene and toilet needs independently". In this case, it did allow a comparison.

9 There is no evidence in these sample records that goals have not been achieved and therefore further assessment or re-planning is not demonstrated.

10 There are few evaluation statements in these records although more may be added before Mr Kapoor is discharged. There are few alterations to the plan following evaluation.

Such questions may help nurses in your work area to monitor the quality and usefulness of the records in use.

Date		Signature
6 May	Mr. Singh, patient on Florence Ward will act as interpreter if English speaking relatives not visiting. Relatives are willing to be telephoned at any time if help is required.	M. Smith
8 May	Discussed with Mr. Kapoor, through interpreter, his diet. States he is liking the food presented but only enjoys it when less breathless. Agreed to send smaller portions and will provide Build-up to increase daily calorie intake.	J. R. Slim (Dietician)
12 May	Mr. Kapoor discussed at ward social meeting. Mr. Kapoor's family considered to be very supportive and will continue his care at home. No action at the moment.	M. Smith

SURNAME KAPOOR   FIRST NAMES SUNIL   AGE 66   CONSULTANT DR. ROBERTS PERSONAL DOCTOR DR. DEGAN HOSPITAL NO. 38521

STANDARD CARE PLANS

Advantages

One of the ways by which it may be possible to reduce the amount of writing when record keeping, is to use standard care plans, which were previously described in Module 3 (p. 78). The usual care can be pre-written and printed and unusual, personally-tailored care can then be written in for each patient. A comprehensive care plan is thus provided for patients; less time then has to be spent on writing anticipated problems and actions for certain parts of their care – such as pre- or post-operative care – or for certain conditions, a neonatal baby with respiratory distress syndrome, for instance.

The use of standard care plans is based on the recognition that, although people have many differences, they may also have many common characteristics, problems or needs and certain predictable responses, whether they are sick or well.

Figures 6.2 and 6.3 are two examples of standard care plans for general pre- and immediate post-operative care for patients having chest surgery. The plans have been devised by the ward staff and researchers involved in the World Health Organization (Europe) Medium Term Programme in Nursing and Midwifery. They are currently being tried out in practice and will be modified if the need arises. In use, a full and detailed care plan is maintained for each patient, with the exception of those aspects of care which are covered by the relevant standard care plan. Standard care plans for specific operations are also being used in some hospitals as part of the patient's total record. Individual modifications, patient problems, goals and interventions are added, and responses to care given are recorded in progress and evaluation notes.

STANDARD CARE PLAN:GENERAL ANAESTHETIC - PRE-OPERATIVE PREPARATION

NO.	PATIENT'S PROBLEM	DESIRED OUTCOME	RELATES TO P.NO.	PLAN OR NURSING INTERVENTION	SIGNATURE/ REVIEW DATE
1	Potential problems: Anxiety due to fear of anaesthetic/operation.	Patient will know operative procedure and its implications; will be able to express these when asked.	1	(i) Explain to the patient what to expect of pre-operative preparation, anaesthetic procedure, post-operative pain, dressing, drains etc. (ii) Ask patient to repeat the information.	
2	Wound infection from skin surface.	Patient will have clean and hairless operation site.	2	(i) Shave area around operation site. (ii) Patient to have bath prior to Theatre.	
3 (a) (b)	Post-operative chest complications due to: Inhalation of stomach contents during operation. Retention of chest secretions following anaesthetic.	Patient will have empty stomach prior to operation. Will have clear chest post-operatively - no excessive secretions and full ventilation. Will perform deep breathing exercises prior to operation.	3(a) (b)	No oral food or fluids to be given for 6 hours prior to Theatre. (i) Teach deep breathing exercises and explain their importance. (Liaise with physiotherapist where necessary.) (ii) Encourage patient to practise these exercises at least 2-hourly prior to Theatre. (iii) Observe amount and character of any sputum produced.	
4	Concern re damage/loss of property whilst patient absent from ward - in Theatre, Recovery Room or ICU.	Patient will know how/where property will be stored. No damage or loss to property will occur.	4	(i) Advise patient to send valuables home, if possible. (ii) Valuable items kept by patient to be stored in locked cupboard, before patient goes to Theatre. Give patient an itemised receipt. (iii) Remaining property to be placed in patient's locker.	
5	Hazards to well-being while under medication/ anaesthetised.	Patient will sustain no injury while anaesthetised.	5(a) (b)	Before giving premedication check: (i) False teeth, false limbs, false eyes, or any other prostheses are removed. (ii) Jewellery, hair grips etc. are removed. Wedding ring, if left on, must be covered with tape. (iii) Any make-up and nail varnish are removed. (iv) Patient has emptied bladder. After giving of premedication, explain to patient that he/she must not get out of bed and why.	

Fig. 6.2   A standard care plan for pre-operative care

Disadvantages

A word of caution is needed however. Standard care plans are useless if they are not used with the basic principles of the nursing process in mind. The individuality of the patient must be taken into account through assessment, a nurse-patient partnership should be established and, most important, the plans should actually be used to guide the nursing care.

Nurses new to the ideas or practice of the nursing process need to build up their knowledge and skills, and only then may they be ready to help to formulate and use standard care plans of their own.

It is not possible in this course to discuss in depth the formulation and use of standard care plans. If you wish to look at the subject further at some other time, some of the articles and books listed at the end of the module should help.

USING RECORDS ON SUBSEQUENT OCCASIONS

Where a patient has repeated admissions, the same nursing records can be used as a foundation for subsequent care. Depending on the length of the interval and changes in circumstances between admissions, a completely new assessment and plan may have to be

STANDARD CARE PLAN: GENERAL POST-OPERATIVE CARE					
NO	PATIENT'S PROBLEM	DESIRED OUTCOME	RELATES TO P.NO.	PLAN OR NURSING INTERVENTION	SIGNATURE/ REVIEW DATE
1(a)	Potential problems: Post-operative shock, as shown by rapid pulse, low BP and skin colour and condition.	To maintain: BP above 90/60mm. Hg. Pulse between 60-100 bpm. (limits are dependent on patient's baseline observations.) Skin to be dry warm and pink.	1(a)	(i) Record pulse, BP and respiration as soon as patient returns to ward - thereafter record observations $\frac{1}{2}$-hourly for the first hour, then hourly when observations stable. (ii) Report to Senior Nurse if beyond stated limits or any deviation from patient norm.	
(b)	Haemorrhage due to surgical trauma.	Blood drainage to be less than 500 mls. from drain/dressing site, in the immediate post-operative period.	(b)	Observe drain/dressing site at least hourly. Report heavy and/or rapid blood loss/drainage.	
2	Post-operative chest complications due to:				
(a)	Build-up of secretions post-anaesthetic.	Chest will be clear; no excessive secretions and full ventilation maintained.	2(a)	(i) When awake from anaesthetic, position patient upright - well-supported with pillows. (ii) Encourage patient to perform deep breathing exercises as taught pre-operatively, at least hourly when awake. Liaise with physiotherapist as necessary. (iii) Observe sputum/secretions produced for amount and character. Report abnormalities i.e. blood-stained, purulent sputum.	
(b)	Restricted chest movement due to pain from surgical wound.	Patient will not complain or show signs of pain.	(b)	(i) Assess patient's level of pain 3-4 hourly. (ii) Give post-operative analgesia as indicated - REGULARLY. (iii) To minimise discomfort, support wound during movement or coughing. If possible, teach patient how to do this.	
3	Temporary immobility due to surgery, leading to:				
(a)	Potential pressure sore development.	Pressure areas will remain intact, no signs of redness.	3(a)	(i) Give relief to pressure areas 3-4 hourly. (Or as individual plan). (ii) Report any signs of redness or breakdown of pressure areas. Change/review frequency of pressure area care.	
(b)	Inability to maintain own personal hygiene.	Personal hygiene will be maintained. Self-caring to be restored before discharge.	(b)	(i) Washing to be assisted by nurse, as indicated in individual care plan. (ii) Give regular mouth care as indicated in individual care plan. (iii) Assist hair care/facial shave (men) as patient norm. (iv) Restore dentures/spectacles etc. to patient as early as possible post-operatively.	
4	Concern re property which was stored for safety prior to operation.	Patient will resume responsibility for his/her property as soon as possible on return to the ward.	4	Return all property to patient as soon as he/she is fully conscious. Ensure that the patient checks valuable items.	

Fig. 6.3   A standard care plan for post-operative care

undertaken and written or the previous ones can be continued, with appropriate changes.

The same principles apply when patients move from one ward or hospital to another, or move between community and hospital care. In some instances, the assessment may be adequate for both situations but will be utilised in a different plan. For instance, information about the cat of a patient living alone may mean that it has to be cared for in a cattery while the patient is in hospital. On discharge home the patient will probably be able to care for the cat herself, but may need help with shopping for cat food. Special equipment in hospital to assist bathing may not be available at home, or the patient may be unable to manage his own medication. In either case, new goals and a new plan of action will be required.

IDENTIFYING THE THEMES OF A SYSTEMATIC APPROACH TO NURSING IN DOCUMENTATION

In the introductory group meeting, you were asked to identify the major themes associated with the nursing process, which then became the seven themes for this course. I will remind you of these in preparation for the next activity.

They were:

- problem solving
- people as patients
- the role of the nurse
- the nurse-patient relationship
- models for practice
- accountability
- nursing in an organisation.

Activity 6.3   Allow 15 minutes

Identifying nursing process themes in documentation

This activity should help you to identify these nursing process themes in practice, or at least see how the records reflect the practice.

Using Mr Kapoor's records as an example, make notes on when and where you can identify these seven themes being reflected in the records.

For example, in relation to problem solving there is evidence in the records of the use of all the four steps of the nursing process. In these particular records, there is no one column on the plan headed 'problems'. They have been identified instead under the heading 'staff assessment'. Some problems such as "Needs help with personal hygiene" can be followed through goal setting and the progress of Mr Kapoor to the step of evaluation and the discontinuation of the problem and nursing intervention as Mr Kapoor takes over his own self-care.

Author's comment

How many did you find? All the themes have been dealt with in other parts of the course, many on more than one occasion. To some degree they are all represented in Mr Kapoor's records. Here are notes on some of my findings and thoughts.

Problem solving: this has already been commented upon as part of Activity 6.3.

People as patients: numerous items of information are included which, in combination, are unique to Mr Kapoor, for example, his diet, language and usual sleep pattern. Social as well as physical aspects of Mr Kapoor, which contribute to him as a whole being, are also included.

The role of the nurse: these records identify the particular contribution of nursing to Mr Kapoor's total health care. Some of the items recorded relate to Mr Kapoor's daily living activities, as described by Virginia Henderson (1969) in Module 1 (p.12), as well as to the acts of helping and assistance which were also mentioned as important components of the role of the nurse. There is also evidence of other people's instructions being carried out (for example, bedrest ordered by the doctor), the nurse's collaborative role, and co-ordination of other professionals as well as of nursing activities (the organising of Mr Kapoor's diet).

The nurse-patient relationship: in these particular records, there are areas on the plan for recording both patient and nurse perceptions of Mr Kapoor's problems. Without working with Mr Kapoor, the nurses would otherwise only have been able to guess that Mr Kapoor had particular diet requirements or usually slipped down the bed at night, which made him more breathless.

Models for practice: did you identify that these records were based on any of the three models discussed in Module 1 – activities of living, stress-adaptation or self-care? You probably rightly felt that none matched identically. In this instance, it appears that aspects from more than one model have been used. The information obtained in the assessment covered many of the elements included in these three models. For example, information on elimination, sleep and mobility can be categorised as activities of living.

There is also some evidence of how Mr Kapoor has adapted to situations – for example, his poor sleeping; he now prefers cups of tea to sleeping pills. He has learned to cope with his problem and his nurses can make use of this for his care plan.

There is also evidence in the care plan of Mr Kapoor being unable to carry out aspects of his own self-care and of his progress back to independence in relation to personal hygiene and using the toilet.

A test of 'good' nursing might be construed in terms of the patient's ability to self-manage outside the hospital setting and the direct care of nursing staff. This particular record indicates some preparation for discharge but it could be continued by district nurses.

Accountability: *there is evidence of a specific nurse being responsible for completing Mr Kapoor's assessment and care plan and a full signature is included. Each nurse recording information about his care has also identified herself by a signature. In this way the nurses caring for Mr*

Kapoor could be traced at a later date and stand accountable for their actions. Through the records they have disclosed what they have done, why they did it and the results of the action.

Nursing in an organisation: *there is evidence in the records of the contribution to Mr Kapoor's total care by doctors and the dietician. The information sheet also mentions a 'ward social meeting' where there was a multi-disciplinary discussion about Mr Kapoor. There is mention of relatives visiting, which is an important organisational consideration if they are to be included in the nursing care in hospital and in preparation for discharge.*

USING THE NURSING PROCESS IN A MULTI-DISCIPLINARY SETTING

Although this systematic approach to care is called 'the nursing process', it also embraces the role of the nurse within a health team. Part of a nurse's work is to carry out prescriptions provided by medical staff. When the nurse writes a patient care plan this should be taken into account.

WORKING WITH OTHERS

There may be numerous people in the team involved with each patient, for example, nurses, doctors, a psychologist, a physiotherapist, a social worker and a dietician. Each has special knowledge and expertise which they will use to contribute to the patient's total care, as the dietician has in Mr Kapoor's plan of care. Some contributors will base their input on a problem-oriented framework. Social workers have been attempting to do this for some time and there is now growing interest and use of this approach in physiotherapy. There is also interest from medical staff. Some doctors already use the steps of assessment, planning, implementation and evaluation in their practice and may be making this more explicit by using problem-oriented medical records usually described as POMR (see Module 3, p. 76). Certainly many of the professionals will wish to make their own assessment of the patient before proceeding with their care and treatment. From the patient's point of view, it could be very frustrating and tiring if each team member independently collected the same information. Although each of the disciplines will require particular information on which to base their own actions, some of their assessment may overlap although ultimately it may be put to different use. For example, the doctor may want to know if a patient smokes as he is trying to diagnose the cause of his cough. The nurse may primarily want to know because it is a health risk, or may cause discomfort to other people or be a fire hazard, while the social

worker may be trying to estimate how much pension the patient has left for food each week, after he has bought his cigarettes. Some information can be shared amongst professionals, whilst other aspects will be obtained individually. Different staff may be concerned simultaneously about different steps of a problem-oriented approach. Various interactions will be occurring with the patient and between each other. The nurse is often required to be a co-ordinator for various other professionals' activities on behalf of the patient. It is therefore particularly important that the nurse is aware of the type of assessment being undertaken by others and in return, shares appropriate information with other team members.

LINKING OR SHARING PLANS

So that the patient receives co-ordinated and friction-free care, there must be collaboration between the various disciplines and their plans. Although each professional may keep his own in-depth records, there are now many instances where selected information is recorded by various professionals onto the nursing records, as in the case of Mr Kapoor. You will remember that the dietician had made comments on his record. The doctor may write a request to a physiotherapist for a patient to have breathing exercises following chest surgery. The doctor will make a note of this in his own records. The physiotherapist will then do her own assessment of the patient, formulate her plan and include this in her records. If the nursing staff have to continue the exercises with the patient during the night, this will be included in the patient's nursing care plan, where it may be recorded by the physiotherapist or the nurse. Likewise, as the plan is carried out, both nurse and physiotherapist may want to make comments about the patient's progress. Different professionals may use the same record, each being identified by a signature or, if many

Problem	Goal	Intervention	Evaluation
Potential problem of developing spasticity because of (R)CVA.	Patient spasticity will be minimal.	Inhibitory positioning while in bed and sitting.	Maintained full range of movements. Scapula remains mobile.
	Review daily.	Check with ward staff. Facilitate normal movement patterns.	Some control of scapular movements.
Hemianopia and left-sided neglect.	Patient will become aware of and use left side of body.	Teach nursing staff and visitors to approach from left side. Keep furniture on left side.	Patient taking weight on left side when sitting in chair. Posture more evenly balanced.
	Review daily.	Stimulate left hand, arm and hip. (Auto-assisted movements).	
Fully dependent in all bed activities.	Patient will be independent in bed and transfer activities.	Teach rolling, bed mobility with block. Transfer to and from bed.	Can roll with assistance and transfer with one helper if bed is low.

Fig. 6.4 Part of a physiotherapist's care plan

recordings are anticipated, a temporary division can be made in the progress notes so that the nurse's and physiotherapist's recordings can be seen simultaneously.

Figure 6.4 shows an extract from part of a physiotherapist's plan, which may be kept in her own records. The same areas of care recorded on a nursing record are shown in Figure 6.5.

In a few instances, a real attempt is being made to have more than one professional recording on a single patient record.

MULTI-DISCIPLINARY PLANNING

In some situations where there is already a cohesive multi-disciplinary approach to patient care, the formulation and agreement of the care plan may occur at a team meeting. This was mentioned in Module 3. At these meetings, each professional has a unique contribution to make based on their own assessment of, and involvement with, the patient. The nurse will probably also give feedback to the team about the patient's response to other professionals' treatment. For instance, the doctor prescribes drugs but it is likely to be the nurse who monitors a patient's pain or notices the patient's lethargy or nausea for a period following ingestion. The doctor is dependent on this type of feedback for his own evaluation purposes.

NURSING AUXILIARIES

Nursing auxiliaries form an important part of the nursing team. They meet a variety of needs and their role can be flexible, depending on individual capabilities and aptitude, the training provided, their experience and the nature of the work.

The nursing auxiliary needs to be taught about the purpose of the nursing process and the contribution which she can make. She needs to understand the responsibilities of the auxiliary and her accountability to the nurse acting as team leader, as well as the importance of patient information and its confidentiality.

Auxiliaries do not usually write in the nursing record, as it is a professional document. However, in long-stay areas mainly staffed by auxiliaries, or where there are only auxiliary staff on duty at night, nurse managers may have created a policy allowing auxiliaries to write in the nursing record. Their contribution to the record would usually consist of retrospective statements, such as a patient having opened his bowels, rather than the planning of care.

Problem	Goal	Intervention	Evaluation
Potential problem of developing spasticity because of (R) CVA.	Patient spasticity will be minimal. Review daily.	When in bed or sitting in chair, nurse with (L) arm on pillow and head forward. When in bed, place (L) leg on pillow.	Limbs are extendable and easily moved out of spastic pattern.
Hemianopia and potential left-sided neglect.	Patient to become aware of left-sided activities. Review daily.	Locker, TV and radio to be kept on left side. Touch, brush and lightly tap left hand when attending to patient. Teach relatives the importance of focusing on left side. Visitors to approach and sit on left side.	Patient turning head left towards patient in next bed without prompting.

Fig. 6.5   Part of a nursing care plan for the same patient

In each of the stages of the nursing process, the role of auxiliaries is that of assistants to trained nurses. As auxiliaries they do not have the education and knowledge base to make nursing decisions.

Auxiliaries can be involved in the steps of the nursing process as follows:

Assessment: it is nurses who know the importance of collecting relevant data and identifying patients' problems. Auxiliaries can play a part in gaining information for the initial or further assessment of the patient, and it is important that they understand the need to report relevant information which can then be corroborated, if required, by the nurse. Ultimate responsibility for the assessment must remain with the nurse.

Setting goals: goal setting is clearly the role of a nurse. It is useful for auxiliaries to understand some of the reasons for the care which they give and they should be kept informed of the care changes through verbal reporting and the written care plan.

Care planning: this again is part of the role of the nurse. However, an auxiliary has an important role in the provision of the care required and therefore needs to be familiar with care plans and be able to follow instructions under the supervision of a nurse. An unthinking auxiliary could otherwise undermine plans.

Implementation: auxiliaries can follow care plans and use patient's goals to guide their work and feed back information in relation to patients' progress.

Evaluation: the evaluation of nursing care given is the role of a nurse. Reporting on care given, the patient's response to care and observations on progress can all be contributed to by the auxiliary, for example, reporting that a patient feels sick after a meal, or that whilst bathing a patient a skin rash was noticed.

NURSE LEARNERS

Frequently, a concern of nurses is how learners will use the nursing process when they are unable to take full responsibility for total patient care. Nurse learners can be involved with the assessment, planning, implementation and evaluation of care for each patient to varying degrees, according to their knowledge and experience. As in any other aspect of nursing, they need to be taught, to observe other proficient nurses and to practise, with supervision, until they are capable and confident of acting independently.

The nursing process can have two main beneficial effects on nurse learners. Firstly, as a learning 'tool' it involves them in decision making, makes them aware of the rationale for nursing actions and can frequently challenge their knowledge, skills and attitudes.

Secondly, from the teachers' point of view – and I include ward sisters, charge nurses and staff nurses, as well as clinical teachers and tutors here – they become able to assess more accurately a learner's progress. Learners are more likely to be involved under supervision in decision making, setting priorities, writing records and giving verbal reports. It therefore becomes easier to identify areas where learners may be encountering difficulty or where they are making good progress and can be complimented on their work.

CONSTRAINTS ON NURSING CARE PLANNING

DIFFICULTIES ENCOUNTERED

Earlier in the module, the importance of flexibility when using the nursing process was discussed. Its use will be influenced by the grades, ability, permanence and numbers of nurses available, the rapidity of patient throughput and the repeated relocation of patients whilst in hospital. Progressive patient care through a pre-surgery ward, operating theatre, recovery room, intensive-care unit, and then a post-surgery ward and rehabilitation unit – or the movement of a maternity patient through attendances at ante-natal clinics, a pre-natal ward, labour ward and a post-natal ward – can actually inhibit personalised and continued care. So can movement in and out of hospital, to and from the care of nurses in the community. There is the chance, even a tendency in institutions, for nursing to become fragmented, given routinely when not required, or omitted because the need is unidentified or continuity is lacking.

On the one hand, these factors may appear to be constraints on the use of the nursing process but, on the other, the nursing process is greatly needed in these situations to give the maximum continuity and co-ordination. Using the nursing process is one way of meeting the challenge of the times and helping to avoid the danger of depersonalised care in large organisations.

When looking at Mr Kapoor's records, or indeed at any other patient's records in isolation, there may be no indication of all the constraints which have influenced care. In the type of record advocated in this course, however, nurses may be more likely to be honest about the care they were or were not able to carry out for a particular patient. Care not given is less likely to be hidden by blanket

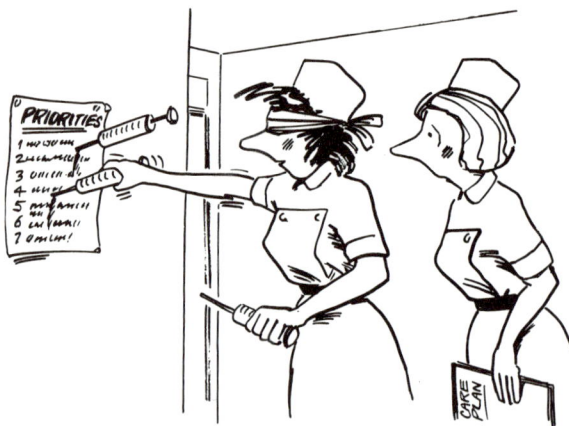

terms such as "all nursing care given". Comments of this nature are known to have been recorded, even though the patient may have been in the X-ray Department during the whole of the nurse's shift of duty. It would have been of help in this kind of situation if the nursing record had been with the patient, so that additions could have been made by the X-ray nurses if required.

OVERCOMING DIFFICULTIES – SETTING PRIORITIES

Setting priorities while identifying patient problems has already been discussed, but priorities also have to be set on numerous other occasions. They may have to be re-set within the individual patient's care plan if they are to remain realistic. Not only may the individual patient's condition or circumstances alter, but so may the overall workload for your group of patients or the whole ward change. You could be the sole nurse on night duty, for example. Priority setting in this way does not mean that lower priorities are ignored, but it works as a guide to putting them into realistic order for consideration, prevention, and solution. If nurses are more conscious of the decision making involved with these activities, it should become easier to pass this expertise on to future nurses. Nurses repeatedly have to set priorities, taking into account the greatest needs of the patient and the time and resources available. In this way, the time available to nurses can be put to the most effective use. Rather than perpetuating ritualistic activities which may or may not be affecting patient outcomes for the better, nurses now have the opportunity to be more selective and to achieve optimum standards of care within available resources, by planning care systematically. Lack of resources can then be identified more clearly and a clearer case made for improvements.

> "The worst boss anyone can have is a bad habit"
> Monta Crane.

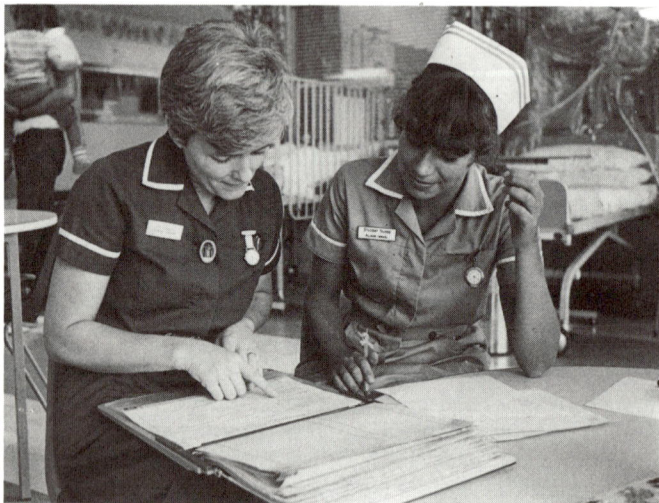

Sharing information helps to ensure continuity of care

THE NURSING PROCESS AS A PART OF NURSING'S DEVELOPMENT

It is about ten years since nurses in the United Kingdom first became interested and involved in the nursing process. There has been much discussion about its merits and demerits, whether it is really new or nurses have always used the approach intuitively, and whether they have time to use it anyway.

One of the complexities of the nursing process is that it has come to act as an umbrella title for numerous ideas and activities aimed at facilitating optimal personalised nursing for patients in a variety of circumstances. Ideas such as patient allocation, treating the patient as a whole, individual nursing orders for each patient, and flexibility in ward and hospital organisation continue to be new to some nurses, but the ideas have been considered 'good' for many years and nurses have been advised to adopt these practices.

"Man's fear of ideas is probably the greatest dyke holding back human knowledge and happiness" Morris L Ernst.

In 1958 the Standing Nursing Advisory Committee appointed a sub-committee to consider the in-patient's day. It suggested that ward work should be adjusted to enable a patient to be woken and have his day organised in a more normal pattern. It mentioned that one of the obstacles to such arrangements was the inclination of nurses to cling to traditional practices not always compatible with modern methods of treatment. It also mentioned that careful assessment of the total needs of patients was an essential preliminary to any reappraisal of arrangements. The report was published as *The Pattern of the In-Patient's Day* (Ministry of Health, 1961) and was followed by another report, *The Organisation of the In-Patient's Day* (Central Health Services Council, 1976). This emphasised the importance of taking into account the patient's point of view, effective communication with patients and relatives, and the need to preserve the individuality of each patient.

From the mid 1960s, nursing research in the United Kingdom has also been developing. The Royal College of Nursing was invited in 1966 by the then Ministry of Health to undertake studies to develop measures of the quality of nursing care. This work resulted in several studies, including ones on pre-operative fasting, the unpopular patient, admission to hospital, care of bowel function and nurses reporting (McFarlane, 1970). Many areas of nursing were highlighted where standards could be improved. An example is fasting patients pre-operatively. For many patients this fast was found to be unnecessarily long and not tailored to their individual requirements, yet how many patients are still prepared in this manner?

Advice was also forthcoming from the Standing Medical Advisory Committee (Ministry of Health, 1965). It was stated in what came to be known as *The Tunbridge Report* that "separate temperature and bathing books are traditional records outmoded by modern practice and should not be kept". This advice was reinforced further when Inspectors from the General Nursing Council visited nurse learner training areas to monitor, amongst other things, standards of nurse record keeping. The advice was not always taken and many nurses are still using outmoded record books.

The recent Office of the Health Service Commissioner's report (1983), and previous ones, states that many of the complaints received from patients and their relatives are due to a breakdown of communication between health care staff, and between them and patients and their relatives. One complaint described is of poor nursing care. "It was alleged, amongst other things, that her husband was left sitting out of bed for long periods; that nothing was placed on the chair to make him comfortable and that on one occasion he fell from it; that unsuitable food was given and bedsores and infection developed". After investigation the complaints were upheld and the Commissioner concluded that even with the staff available at the time, the care would have been much better if the patient's needs had been properly assessed and reviewed.

But what prevented widespread use of these ideas?

A continuing focus on physical tasks and routines based only on patients' mobility or medical diagnosis, the retention of outmoded recording practices and the deployment of nurses to 'jobs' rather than patients worked against the advocated individual and holistic approach. Other forces, such as increasing workloads, shorter-stay hospital admissions, the reduction in nursing hours and progressive patient care, had further negative effects.

"A habit cannot be tossed out of the window; it must be coaxed down the stairs a step at a time" Mark Twain.

The most important inhibiting factors, I believe, have been that the organisational approaches to nursing have not changed according to the new concepts. Task orientation is a method for delivering nursing care. Some nurses have tried to adopt a more personalised service, but sometimes without success. For example, if it is suggested that a ward no longer keeps a bathing book and that the routine of giving all patients confined to bed a daily bed bath is abolished, then nurses have to *think* and decide about the frequency, time of day and type of bath that each patient requires and ensure that the decisions are carried through. The nursing process is not a panacea for all nursing ills but it does provide a means of incorporating and facilitating the use of many of the ideas in a patient-centred approach. The decisions regarding bathing can, for example, be based on information about the patient's normal pattern of self-care, his views, needs and expectations in hospital, a written care plan for patient and nurses to share as a means of monitoring and adjusting the plan according to the patient's responses. Many nurses, through the attempted use of the nursing process, have already gained more self- and patient-awareness. There is more openness and sharing in discussions about clinical practice and a genuine attempt to maximise high quality nursing within a variety of constraints.

"The man who makes no mistakes does not usually make anything" *Edward J Phelps.*

What about future developments? The term 'nursing process' is common, but its practice is relatively new and at an early stage for many nurses. As experience is gained through continued practice and revision in one's work environment and with a personal responsibility for continued learning, its use will be refined and become a part of normal nursing practice. In this way it will contribute to the continuing understanding and development of nursing, as well as having direct beneficial effect on patients.

"Things do not change; we change" *Henry David Thoreau.*

An additional reason for good quality recording is the need for research to evaluate the effectiveness of different approaches to nursing, which could be based to some extent on information which nurses provide in their records.

For some nurses, this flexible approach, as opposed to set rules and routines, may require a reappraisal of their current views on nursing and a change in their practice. It can be a challenge, may be initially exhausting, but many nurses find that they gain job satisfaction whilst patients receive a more personalised service.

"Change is not made without inconvenience even from worse to better" *Richard Hooker.*

FURTHER READING

Bendle, M. (1983) 'Re-processing the process', *Journal of District Nursing,* June, pp. 11–16, 34. (Using standard care plans in district nursing)

Bridge, W. and Macleod Clark, J. (eds.) (1981) *Communication in Nursing Care,* London, HM & M Publishers.

Gibbs, J. (1983) 'A matter of convenience', *Nursing Mirror,* (156), 2, 12 Jan., pp. 61–3. (Using standard care plans in a neonatal unit)

Heath, J. and Law, G. M. (1982) *Nursing Process. What is it? A practical introduction,* Sheffield, NHS Learning Resources Unit.

Mayers, M. G. (1978) *A Systematic Approach to the Nursing Care Plan,* New York, Appleton-Century-Crofts. Ch. 7. (Standard care plans)

McFarlane of Llandaff and Castledine, G. (1982) *A Guide to the Practice of Nursing Using the Nursing Process,* London, C. V. Mosby Co., pp. 68, 85–87, 90–97.

McIntyre, N. and Petrie, J. C. (1979) *The Problem Orientated Medical Record,* Edinburgh, Churchill Livingstone.

MODULE 7
INTRODUCING CHANGE INTO NURSING PRACTICE

Prepared for the Course Team by Alan Pearson and Barbara Vaughan

CONTENTS

CONTENTS

OBJECTIVES

After studying this module, you should be able to:

1 Identify local problems in nursing practice which you feel might benefit by change.

2 Describe possible strategies for change which can be used by nurses.

3 Relate these strategies to your own work area as they apply to:
- the patients
- the individual nurses who make up the team
- the multi-disciplinary clinical team
- the organisation as a whole.

4 List the potential difficulties associated with introducing change and identify possible underlying causes.

5 Discuss ways in which these difficulties may be minimised or resolved.

6 Outline a plan for the introduction of a change in practice in your own clinical area.

7 Implement a planned change in your own clinical area.

8 Discuss ways in which you would evaluate the effectiveness of a change in practice.

IMPLEMENTING CHANGES IN NURSING PRACTICE

This final module is designed to help you to bring about any changes which you feel may be needed in your practice setting in order to make the ideas of the nursing process a reality. As you have worked through the course, you will probably have discovered that some of the ways in which you practise fit in well with the beliefs about the nursing process discussed in this course, whilst other ways in which you work clearly do not. Trying to introduce any new ways of approaching care means changing things which are accepted (at the moment) as the 'norm'. It may include changing attitudes as well as behaviour towards patients, colleagues and nursing work.

Changing the ways in which people think, feel about things and carry out their work is difficult, and introducing change in nursing is no different. All of us have difficulty with it. Of course, this module does not have all the answers. In discussing the problems associated with change, and in giving some concrete advice and examples, we hope that it will help you to be able to introduce, with the minimum of stress, some of the changes which you have identified as being useful in the place where you work.

A letter from a patient

We received this letter from a patient who knew that we were preparing this course.

Dear Course Team,

As a result of my recent experience as a patient in a surgical ward of a hospital ostensibly using the nursing process for the last year, I thought you may like to consider the following points. Maybe some or all of them have occurred to you, but I feel that they merit discussion.

Superficially, I was impressed and heartened by the more friendly and less rigid atmosphere in the ward than in ones I had previously encountered. But it soon became apparent that, despite the easing in atmosphere, there was still a sad lack of communication with patients – even with those like me who ask questions, but particularly with those who were confused by the uniforms and procedures and dared not ask.

One of the things that amused me was the irrelevance in practice of some of the questions in the assessment interview. As a small example, why ask patients what their preferred drink is when there can be no intention of meeting the preference? In my case, coffee (my preference) was only available twice a day. The example is negligible; but the principle needs further discussion. Why ask certain questions? To what use will the information given be put? Is the information required, and if so, why? Are there more ways in which we can make the system less rigid by being a little more imaginative?

What was the least well carried out, I thought, was the procedure of what I presume was meant to be re-assessment. This consisted of a group of learners and auxiliaries pushing a trolley with the record cards along the centre of the ward, calling to each patient "Any problems?", and then audibly discussing how to categorise this information in the right form for the records. I don't see this as an appropriate way to get good nurse-patient communication. Also it's only paying lip service to the philosophy behind the nursing process.

In the ward, the nursing process was being taught to learners. The staff nurses and sisters, however, had had it thrust on them, with the result that they were either antagonistic or threatened by it.

The nursing auxiliaries on the ward seemed to have been forgotten or ignored. Those who had worked there for many years seemed to be in an anomalous position: they had little official standing or responsibility yet, in practice, they were given responsibilities and duties beyond those officially recognised. If a ward is using the nursing process, what about the training of auxiliaries?

Now that I am recuperating from the knife, I wanted to put down a few thoughts arising from my first-hand experience. If you feel that there's any validity in my comments, maybe you will have time to think about these points.

Yours sincerely,

A non-nurse colleague interested in the nursing process.

It seems that, in this ward, whilst the documentation of the nursing process has been introduced, some of the underlying principles have not yet been developed. Several issues are raised which may be of some concern to you.

Activity 7.1   Allow 5 minutes
What issues are raised?

This activity gives you an opportunity to consider some of the issues raised by our colleague.

Having read the letter from a patient, quoted above, consider which of the issues raised indicate room for further development.

Authors' comment
The sort of issues which you have identified may include: meaningful assessment, where information is not only gathered but also used; a partnership relationship between nurses and patients; individualised patient care; and training needs for all members of the nursing team. Whilst many nurses are now using a more systematic form of documentation, they may only be at the beginning of their introduction to the nursing process. The letter may serve as a reminder to all of us that documentation is merely a tool to help us in our nursing practice. The important issues are the use which we make of information that has been gathered and the way in which we practise nursing.

WHAT CHANGES ARE NEEDED?

Module 1 introduced the seven basic themes of the course, and Modules 2–6 elaborated on the steps in the nursing process, their documentation and their integration. Depending on your own specific practice setting, any or all of the course themes may represent areas of needed change which you may wish to pursue. For example, you may already use documents which encourage you to assess, plan and implement, but you may feel that you are still limited in setting goals or in evaluation. In addition, it may be that the accountability of the nurse who gives direct care is not as explicit as it could be, or that you tend to direct the patient in his care, rather than to include him as a partner. You may, of course, be working in a way which reflects all that has been discussed throughout this course and your aim may be to explore further the subjects raised.

Many nurses who have been trying to implement a true nursing process approach to care for some years still find that, despite having moved ahead in many aspects of care, there is much to be changed and developed. A logical approach is to ask yourself, and your colleagues, whether or not the way in which you work fits in with each of the seven course themes, namely:

- problem solving
- people as patients
- the role of the nurse
- the nurse-patient relationship
- models for practice
- accountability
- nursing in an organisation.

Activity 7.2   Allow 10 minutes

Finding out what needs to be changed

This activity should help you to identify exactly what changes are needed in your work place, by working through our seven themes.

Thinking about your own day-to-day work, answer the following broad questions honestly:

1 Do you formally assess, plan, implement and evaluate the care which you give to each individual patient or client, and do your nursing records show that you do?

2 Is your approach to patients and your work pattern flexible enough to ensure that nursing care is geared to the patient/client as a person, or does he have to conform to a set routine?

3 In your work setting, is the role of the nurse clear and is it made explicit to other members of the health care team?

4 Is the patient/client always regarded as a partner in care, or do you encourage him to acknowledge that you know best when planning care?

5 Is your practice based on a model for nursing, which is agreed upon by the other members of the nursing team?

6 Is accountability for care clearly identified and understood by the nurses who give direct care or is one person, such as the sister, charge nurse or nursing officer always seen as the one who is accountable?

7 Is the nurse an equal member of the multi-disciplinary team and able to contribute effectively to patient care?

Authors' comment
Although these questions are very broad, they may give you an initial idea of where changes may need to be made. Answering such questions is the first step in the change venture – examining the practice in your area and identifying any changes needed.

A ward nurse from an acute general hospital studying this module may decide that:

- none of the four steps in the nursing process is explicitly carried out or documented in her work area

- although the patients in the ward are seen as 'whole' people by some of the staff, the way of organising care and the established routine do not reflect this

- the nursing care revolves around the medical diagnosis alone

- the nurses on the ward tell the patients what is planned for them, rather than taking them into partnership and planning care with them.

In consequence, the nurse may suspect that the ward team needs to:

- understand the problem-oriented approach to nursing

- introduce a patient-centred way of organising care: for example, primary nursing or patient allocation

- understand a number of nursing models, and select or develop one on which they can all agree

- explore their own attitudes towards patients, and move towards the adoption of a belief in nurse-patient partnership

- introduce a nursing process form of documentation.

Simple though these five areas for change may appear to be on paper, the actual approach to bringing about these changes needs to be careful and logical. Some people say that this first step in the change cycle – identifying the changes needed – is the easiest. It is certainly the most concrete, but it is often hard to be analytical enough to question seriously what we are doing. Being objective about both the way in which we currently view and carry out our work and the values and attitudes we possess is a task which none of us finds easy. To examine them objectively, and to find changes warranted, by implication means that something has been found to be less than good. Yet it is an exciting challenge which can be both rewarding and worthwhile.

In order to assist us to consider the steps in the change cycle logically and practically, let's meet an imaginary participant in this course. It would be really useful if she could be a super-nurse who worked in hospital/community/psychiatric/mental subnormality/paediatric/geriatric and all other areas of nursing rolled into one. But that would be just too imaginary.

Mary Thompson is a ward sister on an accident ward in a district general hospital. Although her situation may be somewhat different from yours, you all have much in common. For example, you are all nurses, you all have direct contact with patients and you are all studying this course. Two other major similarities may exist between you – an interest in providing the best patient care possible and a desire to introduce some changes in the practice setting.

Mary has discovered that she has been unable to answer any of the questions raised in Activity 7.2 with a resounding "Yes", so she wants somehow to bring about changes related to all of the seven course themes. How does she – or anyone who wishes to innovate change – set about it?

Although we have introduced Mary to you at this point in the module, we are initially more interested in the general principles of change. We will be referring to her occasionally to make these principles more concrete but will return to Mary's progress in more depth in the latter half of the module.

Activity 7.3   **We cannot specify a time for this activity since it may require varying degrees of thought and reflection.**

What do you want to do?

This activity asks you to consider your own area of practice in relation to the seven themes.

Identify one aspect of your practice which you would like to change and briefly outline the current state of affairs and how you would like it to be.

Authors' comment
You may well have identified any one of a number of issues ranging from something as complex as introducing primary nursing to something as simple as making sure that someone who prefers coffee can actually have it. As you work through the rest of this module, think about your response to this activity as we will be asking you to refer back to it when completing future exercises.

SOME THOUGHTS ABOUT CHANGE

Once you have decided on the value of something new or different, whatever it may be, the most suitable manner in which it can be brought into current practice has to be considered. It is at this stage that you can draw on the ideas and experience of others in order that the move can be wisely planned and purposefully structured. Without preparations of this kind, the results of an attempt to introduce change can be haphazard, ineffective or even dangerous.

The thought of trying something new is often viewed with caution or even fear. This caution, which is common to all of us, has been described as the "inherent conservatism of man" (Lupton, 1971). To lose something which is familiar to us can generate feelings which are similar to mourning. We grieve for old patterns of behaviour and find new ways difficult to accept and initially more demanding to apply. Yet as Sullivan (1977) says, "Nothing is exempt from change . . . change is innate and a normal and an expected process in individuals, institutions, organisations, and societies". Without change, no progress would be made and life would become stagnant. As the saying goes, change – along with death and taxes – is the only inevitable thing in life.

WHY CHANGE?

By 'change' we mean the process of bringing about an alteration or substituting one way of behaving for another. In some instances these changes can occur without being planned, but as a response to some external process. An example of a change of this kind is the ability of some bacteria to develop in such a way that they become resistant to certain antibiotics. This is not a planned event, but a response to things going on beyond the control of the bacteria. You may think that it would be a successful change for the bacteria – but certainly not for society.

Similarly, in nursing, some changes have occurred as a response to changes in areas other than nursing itself. For instance, with increased medical technology, nurses have had to learn new skills and to adopt new ways of practice. Social changes have resulted in a larger number of nurses continuing to work when married and thus wanting to work hours that are compatible with family life. Society itself has altered dramatically in the last century, with people becoming more knowledgeable and taking a greater interest in health.

These are all factors which have influenced nursing practice.

Besides these external factors, nurses themselves have become more knowledgeable about their own subject – nursing – and that new knowledge has led us all to look critically at our own practice and to see if there are ways in which we can develop and improve it.

WHO IS INVOLVED?

If you decide that you want to make some changes in your practice, it is not only the patients who will be affected but also the people with whom you work directly, the wider circle of people with whom you come into contact and the institution or organisation in which you work. Neither the individual people concerned, nor the organisation, can be considered in isolation. So, as a manager of care you cannot try to bring about a change in practice without considering the individuals that it will affect. Similarly, as an individual you cannot bring about change without considering the effect that it will have on the organisation.

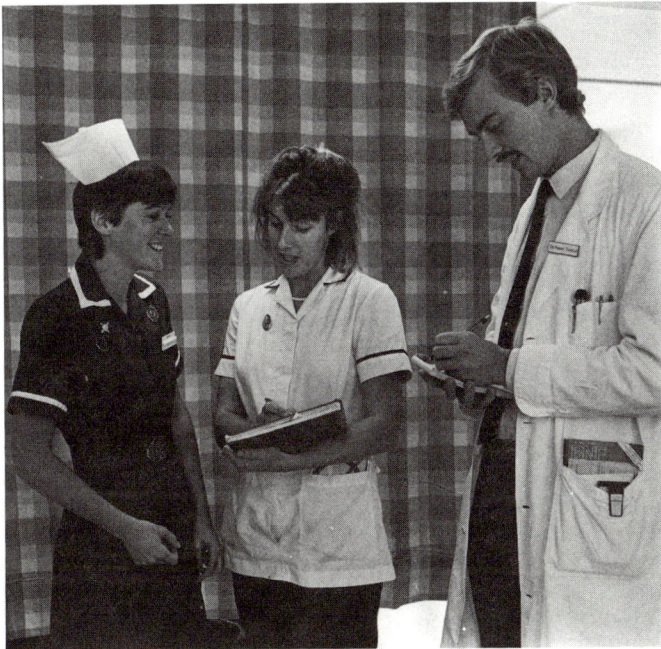

Change in nursing practice involves others

In considering changes at an individual level, Schein (1969) suggests that each person seeks a state of *balance* or *equilibrium* in himself. What he does has to match what he believes and values. If something occurs to disrupt this equilibrium, such as the acquisition of new knowledge, he will seek a way in which the balance can be restored, so that the way in which he behaves will again match what he believes in.

At the institutional level, Kurt Lewin (1951) says that organisations normally work in a fairly stable way. Each section has its own purposes, needs and difficulties but it is also pulled by the needs and constraints of other sections. For instance, a supplies service in a health organisation has to work out its own system of managing supplies, but also has to consider the demands made by the users of that service, including nurses. Similarly, doctors and nurses have to consider both their own function and that of each other. Lewin describes an organisation which is working in a stable way as being frozen. In many ways it resembles an ice cube which has shape and form, is tangible and can be grasped. Lewin suggests that if something happens in one section of an organisation, such as the appointment of a new leader or the recognition of a need for change, an imbalance occurs in the organisation as a whole and the situation becomes unfrozen. In the case of the ice cube it becomes fluid, intangible and can no longer be grasped. The second level in Lewin's description corresponds to the unfrozen ice cube: the whole institution will change or move until a state of equilibrium is regained. The final level is reached when the new state is stabilised and again becomes comfortable and refrozen in a new position.

Problem solving is a technique which was described in relation to the nursing process in Module 1. It was emphasised that the technique is not unique to nursing, but could be used in many other situations. One of these situations is the planning of change and each of the steps of problem solving can be matched, as shown in Figure 7.1, to those described by Lewin.

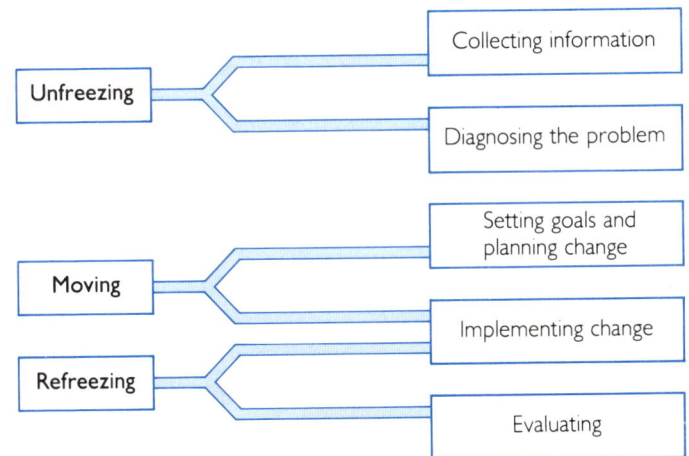

Fig. 7.1 Lewin's theory of change in relation to problem solving

Many people have used this problem-solving approach when describing how to plan and implement change. They have, however, frequently broken down each stage into a number of steps, in order to make it more explicit.

STEPS IN THE CHANGE PROCESS

The steps in the change process, related to the steps in problem solving which were described in Module 1, are shown in Figure 7.2.

In order to make each step clearer, we are taking one concrete example of a change with which you may be concerned. However, the principles illustrated in the example may be applied to any change situation in which you are interested. Suppose that one of the things you have decided that you would like to do is to introduce a new system of documentation in your clinical setting. The first question you may ask yourself is "Where did this idea come from?" Did it develop because you have acquired new knowledge or because you are aware that your current system does not work? There is a feeling of unrest in you as an individual. But you are not the only one affected. If you have altered your ideas, the way in which you interact with both your colleagues and the organisation itself will also alter. So change has begun, and the organisation has become unfrozen. But you are not prepared to leave the development to chance. You want to plan systematically the way in which this idea will be developed. So a series of activities must be considered.

ASSESSMENT

Initially, you must assess the situation and assessment itself can be divided into a number of smaller steps, which include:

Defining your broad purposes

At this stage, you have to clarify your own thoughts about the purpose of keeping records. Rather than making a woolly statement such as "Documents are for record keeping", you have to ask yourself several questions such as: "Why do I need to record?" "What do I want to record?" "How much do I need to record?" The answers to these questions will reflect your own personal beliefs about nursing, your beliefs about patients or clients, your relationship with them and, even more specifically, the model of practice from which you work. If you cannot answer some of these questions, it may mean going back to the drawing board. Did your initial feeling that you wanted to introduce a new system of documentation identify the real problem?

Gathering information

Once you have defined your overall purpose, then look at the situation as it exists at the moment. Gather all the documents available to you and consider ways in which they can be used. Do they match your requirements? Is there sufficient space? Do they reflect the model on which you base your practice or are they flexible enough to reflect several models? Is there a discrepancy?

It may be, at this stage, that no discrepancy is found and that no problem exists in the records themselves. It may be that the problem lies in their use. If the records themselves are clearly inappropriate you can proceed to the next step.

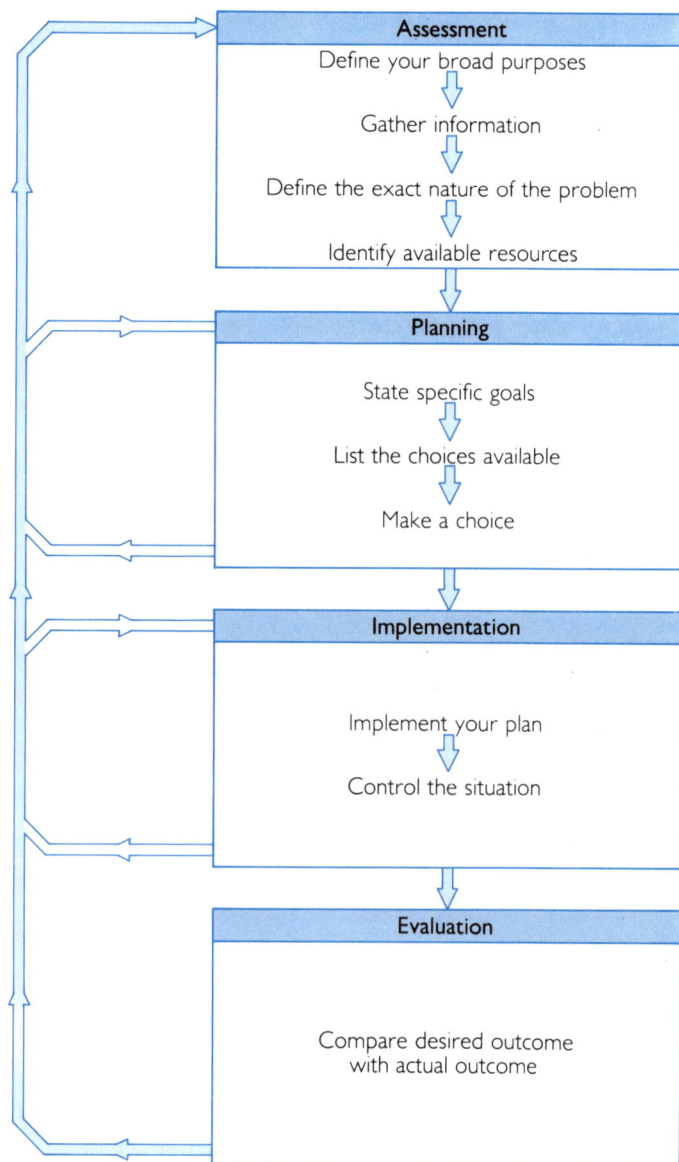

Fig. 7.2 Steps in the change process

Defining the exact nature of the problem

If you have decided that a discrepancy exists, its exact nature must be clarified. You may decide that the format of the documents is too rigid, that no consideration is given to particular areas of assessment highlighted in the model which you have chosen or that the system is too fragmented. You may even find that in your document there is no space for a nursing assessment or a care plan, and that it is merely used as a means of storing biographical data. Whatever the problem is, be specific in stating it, just as you would when identifying a patient's problem.

Identifying the resources available

Bearing in mind the needs of both the individual and the organisation, the next step is to consider what resources are needed and to find out whether or not they are available and how to get them. Your requirements for changing your system of documentation could include involving people with previous experience, printing new forms and developing new storage facilities and obtaining the necessary finance. Use of the new documents may also require the resource of educators and teaching and learning time, in order that they will be used as you would wish.

There may be a need for a flexible document which can be used by people working in different clinical settings, if there is a lot of movement amongst both patients and staff. Multiple interests have to be considered if you wish your plan to be effective.

These four steps will complete the phase of assessment.

PLANNING

The next stage to consider is the plan. There is rarely only one route by which your final goal can be reached and the way in which you plan your strategy will be dependent on both you as an individual and the situation in which you work. However, there are some basic steps to follow.

Stating specific goals

At this stage, you must state exactly what you want of the new documents. For instance, your specific goal may be that the documents will reflect one particular model of nursing. Alternatively, you may decide that your goal is that the documents will be sufficiently flexible to incorporate several different models. You may feel that the format for the assessment section should be linked specifically to one particular care plan format, or that it should allow for the use of a variety of different care plans. You may also decide at this stage on a specific time limit which you will set yourself for the completion of this work.

It is of little value simply to introduce new documents; they must also be understood and used correctly. Your specific goals may also relate to the behaviour of nurses and other staff who will use them, and may include the provision of some form of education.

Listing the choices available

Once the background work has been done, you are at the stage where all the options open to you can be listed. Look at what is available in other documents – do they meet your criteria? Or must you design a system of your own? Much valuable time may be saved if someone else has already prepared documents which suit your needs. However, it is inappropriate to accept other people's documents just for expediency; this will not save time in the long run.

What sort of storage systems are available? What are the training needs of the staff? How and when can they be met? Should the documents be tested in a pilot area? If so, which area should it be?

The alternatives are numerous and only you can know what opportunities are available to you personally. You will need to expend some time and imagination at this point in order to identify all the possibilities that are available, but it is time well spent since careful appraisal will, hopefully, lead you to the best available solution to your problem and ultimately may save you time.

Making a choice

Having listed all your options, there is a further series of questions to ask yourself. First of all, are all the options feasible and realistic? A ten page assessment form or a lengthy care plan would be of little use in a surgical day care unit where patients' length of stay is very short. Alternatively, when a nurse-patient relationship – such as that between a midwife and an expectant mother – will continue over a long period of time, there must be sufficient space to make accurate records.

Differing teaching strategies to introduce new documents may be required by different grades of staff, since they will all have different starting points. You may decide on one way of introducing the new system to the qualified staff, another for the auxiliaries and yet a third way for other health care workers, such as doctors or physiotherapists.

Several different approaches have been used when considering the training needs of staff and these will be discussed later in this module. The important thing is always to remember that, if you involve your colleagues at this planning stage, they are more likely to become committed and therefore successful in the future. Communication with, and involvement of, others is *crucial* and cannot be over-emphasised.

Having reached this stage, you will have completed your plan and will be ready to progress to the stage of implementation.

IMPLEMENTATION

Implementing your plan

Once your plan has been completed, it is time for action. Again, different approaches can be used. Small steps, one by one, may be best, in which case you may initially arrange some training for your colleagues to assist them to develop their assessment skills, and then change the assessment forms. Once everyone is happy with their use, progress towards using care plans may be made, each phase being supported by teaching. Alternatively you may choose to introduce the whole new system at one time, following a more intensive training programme. A third approach may be to introduce the documents and create a 'felt need' amongst the staff for more knowledge about their use, and then start the training once the staff themselves have recognised a need to acquire new skills. Ottoway (1982) is one person who recommends this strategy, but it must be pointed out that it is only successful if provision for learning is included at the planning stage.

Controlling the situation

There is no right or wrong way of introducing change – provided that the strategy, constraints and resources have all been considered.

What is important is that you *control* the situation. In order to control it, you need to establish:

1 A regular feedback system: for instance, ward meetings at fortnightly intervals, to air problems or difficulties at an early stage.

2 A follow-up system to make sure that directions have been understood: for instance, demonstrations of the use of assessment forms, or joint working sessions to draw up care plans.

3 A clear description of what you expect each person to do. This may be achieved not only by discussion but also by providing written instructions which have been prepared for each group of staff involved.

4 An 'early warning system' to indicate any difficulties at an early stage. Your feedback sessions should give you some indication of early signs of trouble, such as low staff morale or increased rates of sickness. But, bearing in mind that people are under extra stress, you need to be aware of the possibility of these situations occurring.

5 A specific review date to evaluate the system. This date could be decided between you and your colleagues and could take the form of a comparison between the information available from your old and your new record-keeping systems.

EVALUATION

As in any process, an evaluation system is essential if we are to know whether or not the change has been effected and is effective. Comparison of the old and new record-keeping systems is an approach that has already been mentioned. An alternative may be to consider the morale of your staff or possibly even to compare the reactions of patients who have had frequent hospital admissions, some experiencing the old system and some the new. Although this information would be subjective, it is always valuable to have the opinions of the people who are concerned.

THE PROCESS OF NURSING AND THE PROCESS OF CHANGE

As you can see, the steps in the change process which have been described are very similar to those used in a problem-oriented approach to nursing care. As we have already indicated, the problem-solving technique is not unique to nursing but may be used in many situations. Using this systematic approach of assessment, planning, implementation and evaluation increases your likelihood of successfully introducing the changes into your chosen area.

WHAT ROLE WILL YOU PLAY?

Once you have decided that you would like to become involved in the process of change, it is important that you identify what part you will be playing. This will obviously be partly dependent on your role within the health care setting – staff nurse, charge nurse, nurse manager or teacher. Whatever your role you will, in one way or another, become a 'change agent'.

Change agents can work in many different ways. Three basic groups have been described by Ottoway (1982): change generators, change implementers and change adopters.

CHANGE GENERATORS

These are the people who take an issue about which they feel very strongly and make their thoughts public in an attempt to influence other people. They achieve this mainly through open action of one kind or another, the suffragettes of the early twentieth century being a classic example. Alternatively, they may patronise the cause or act as a benefactor, either openly by attending public meetings or in a more discreet fashion, by donating money anonymously. In some instances, the change generators may be members of a minority group who feel that their needs are not being met. Some of the patient pressure groups may fall into this category. For example, some would say that members of the National Association for the Welfare of Children in Hospital (NAWCH) generated a change in paediatric care. Through their representations at public meetings and in the media, attention was drawn to the potential harm of separating children from their parents on admission to hospital. The eventual outcome has been a change in practice by the relaxation of visiting rules and the provision of accommodation for parents.

Change generators are, on the whole, people who have very strong feelings about the issues which they raise. They are independent and are prepared to withstand criticism by others. However, it may be difficult for them actually to bring about change, since they are often thought of with some misgivings by people who are resistant to change. Their role is to raise an issue and to create a feeling or recognition of a need for change.

Change generators have already played their role in relation to the nursing process. The subject is widely known about and discussed, often with a degree of hostility. It is not, however, always understood by those who criticise it nor practised by those who pay it lip service.

CHANGE IMPLEMENTERS

These are the people who are responsible for bringing about change in practice, once the need has been recognised. They fall into three main categories:

1 **External:** in this instance, an expert consultant is brought in to give advice on a particular situation and to assist in planning and implementing change. This is a fairly unusual situation in nursing at the clinical level. A consultant is sometimes used by nurse managers in such areas as staff planning. This is, however, a strategy which could be considered when plans are being made to implement the nursing process, as more people are becoming available who have both theoretical knowledge and practical experience of the situation.

2 **External/internal:** these are people who are employed by an organisation but do not necessarily have a designated role within the particular setting where change is desired. For instance, many health authorities now employ nurses designated as 'Nursing Process Co-ordinators' or 'Implementers', whose official role is to implement the nursing process by bringing about appropriate changes. This necessitates their working with staff from various units within the organisation. One of the difficulties which they face is that they have little or no official standing. Their contribution has to be negotiated on a contractual basis with the clinical staff and much depends on their ability to demonstrate competence.

3 **Internal:** the third category is those people who work within their own unit with their peers and colleagues. They are closely involved with the people with whom they work and with whom they have a more permanent relationship. This group will include any nurse working permanently within a clinical unit who, having recognised the need for change, works towards bringing about that change.

Change implementers are more readily accepted by those who are resistant to change than change generators are, since their function in keeping the organisation up-to-date can be recognised by those with whom they work.

CHANGE ADOPTERS

The majority of people are change adopters, that is people who hear about a change, try it in a limited way, accept it and incorporate it into their normal practice. Change adopters are willing to alter their practice because they have been convinced by the change implementers that it will be of benefit. Alternatively, they may feel committed to the group with whom they work and so conform to a new practice that the group agrees would be worthwhile. Finally, there may be those who find it least trouble just to follow everyone else rather than to maintain their old ways. These people are usually the slowest ones to change.

Each of these three categories – that is generators, implementers and adopters – is of equal importance, since they are all interdependent and none can succeed without the help and support of the others. If you decide your role is to be a change implementer, you will be dependent on the staff with whom you work for adopting your ideas. Similarly, if you are a change adopter the success of your new venture will be dependent on the plans devised by the change implementers.

Finally, a word about those who continue to reject new ideas. Occasionally you may come across people whose ideas and beliefs conflict so strongly with those which you are presenting that nothing will make them alter their ways. If all else has failed and they stand firm by their original beliefs and behaviours, we have no right to challenge them any further. It may be that the situation has to be resolved by finding another place in which they can work, where their beliefs are not in conflict with those currently being practised. This should not be considered as defeat, as it is important to recognise individual beliefs in nurses, as well as in patients, and to respect those beliefs. However, it must also be pointed out that, within the new United Kingdom Central Council *Code of Professional Conduct for Nurses, Midwives and Health Visitors (1983)*, there is a clause requiring every nurse to "be accountable for her practice and take every reasonable opportunity to sustain and improve her knowledge and professional competence". A nurse reluctant to consider new ways may find it difficult to fulfil this requirement.

Activity 7.4   **Allow 5 minutes**

Who has which role?

It may be useful to pause here and consider what role you will play, through the following activity.

1 Consider which type of change agent you will be when involved in the change within your own work area that you identified in Activity 7.3.

2 List the nursing colleagues with whom you have regular contact and identify which kind of role you think each one might play when introducing the change which you have identified.

Authors' comment

It is probable that you will be an implementer in your setting, but you may consider yourself to be a change adopter. Whatever role you have chosen it is important to remember that each is of equal importance.

THE DESIRE FOR CHANGE

Because change is ever-present in contemporary life, aspects of it are frequently welcomed. Certainly, labour-saving devices in nursing are usually welcomed by nurses; improved ward designs are changes most of us seek; and various re-organisations in nurse management are seen as opportunities for both improved nursing care and increased job satisfaction by many nurses. The rapid increase in knowledge and the resulting growth in technology have led to a situation where nurses are accustomed to the possibility of having to change various procedures and activities in the light of scientific advances.

Changes which require a shift in thinking, or an alteration in attitudes and values, are less easy to accept but, again, many nursing teams are either dissatisfied with current practice or simply wish to improve practice which is already of a high standard. There are numerous groups of nurses throughout the United Kingdom who wish to change, and who are highly motivated to do so.

Motivation is, of course, an essential ingredient if the effort to change is to be successful. What motivates people is a subject of much depth and breadth, and a host of theories have been expounded. For example, Maslow (1954), in his *hierarchy of human needs* illustrated in Module 1 (p. 10) sees Man as an individual who always has needs and, as one need is satisfied, another appears to take its place. For example, if the nurses in a team have their physiological and safety needs met, they may be seeking to meet social needs, and this in itself may motivate them towards the setting up of team meetings. McGregor (1960) also focuses on human needs, in the sense that organisations which consider the human needs of their members "get the best out of them". He believes that if people enjoy their work, if the working conditions are favourable and if opportunities exist for open discussion throughout the organisation, the individuals who work there are motivated both to practise well *and* to explore ways in which to improve practice. Numerous other theories exist, but general principles can be gleaned from all. In essence, a happy, communicating team of nurses, who are also able to communicate with their supervisors and those in other disciplines, are more likely to feel more personal worth, and are often more open to change. Furthermore, motivation is increased if the individual nurses in the team are all involved in the change process at all stages. Many of us work, or have worked, in such teams, and have experienced high motivation to implement a change. However, we probably all have experience of places where this ideal situation does not exist, or is less likely to develop quickly. Sometimes the unit may be under a lot of stress for various reasons, or one or two members of the team may be less motivated than the rest. It is therefore useful to consider resistance to change, bearing in mind that it is by no means inevitable that high levels of resistance will always be met.

RESISTANCE TO CHANGE

Some people, as we have said, may be eager for change and view it with excitement, whilst others may ignore new ideas and deny their existence; a third reaction, which is not uncommon, is to resist. Even when people want to change, the change must be planned and, whilst not all plans necessarily have to consider means of overcoming resistance, it is helpful to face up to the reality of this potential problem in order that it can be dealt with effectively should it arise.

It is often more comfortable to continue in a familiar way; the way in which we have always done things may appear to work all right, and changing things means that a bit of a risk must be taken. So resistance is a natural reaction to change, and is something to be expected. Duberley (1977) says that change "may even challenge the values and beliefs held; it threatens", and "whenever people are threatened, they mobilise various resources to resist the threat; they resist in order to protect themselves". It is probable that you will face resistance to a greater or lesser extent, depending on whom you work with and how radical the proposed changes are. Even the independent district nurse largely working alone in a single-handed practice may face some form of resistance from her colleagues.

We will be discussing how some of this resistance can be overcome, but an understanding of why we all resist change is often helpful in facing it when it occurs. If potential difficulties are considered from the outset by the promoter of change, plans to lessen or even prevent high levels of resistance can be made. Resistance can become less of a problem when the change promoter is aware of its causes and, even more importantly, when these insights about resistance can be shared with those who are being asked to change.

The 'unfreezing', which we mentioned earlier as an essential step in the change cycle, demands much from nurses and others working in a setting where their usual approach to nursing will be disturbed and re-established. Kelley and Conner (1979) describe how people react emotionally to change, and Figure 7.3 presents their picture of the emotional cycle of change.

This emotional cycle begins with optimism. The person who wants to introduce the change – and sometimes also those who are to be involved in the change – feels committed to it and confident that it will be implemented. But frequently, this first optimism moves on to a feeling of doubt, then hope and finally, if the change comes

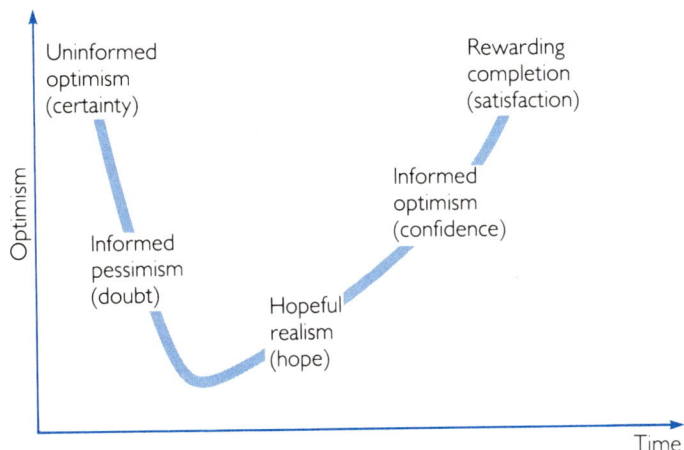

Fig. 7.3 The emotional cycle of change (modified from Kelley and Conner, 1979)

about, satisfaction at completing the cycle. Many of us who have been involved in change can testify to this cycle — and the eventual feeling of satisfaction is something which many people describe as one of the 'high points' of their life. However, enthusiastic attempts to introduce a nursing process approach to care can fail because of resistance to the change by nursing colleagues and other members of the multi-disciplinary team.

Resistance, on the whole, is based on an intense desire by people to maintain the status quo. They are either happy with the way things are or, if not exactly happy, not sufficiently unhappy to want to expend a good deal of energy on altering all that they are used to. They may also be unconvinced that the proposed change will be of any benefit and question whether there is any evidence of its advantage.

Why do we sometimes feel this way when faced with the suggestion of change? The practical and theoretical experience of others tells us much about why people resist.

FEAR

Lancaster and Lancaster (1981) suggest that resistance "seems to spring from fear". If the people who are expected to change resist, they may be afraid of the unknown, afraid that they will fail, or afraid that they will not know enough to be as useful a member of the team as they are now. *Very often, acceptance of change is expected without an adequate explanation of its nature and without education or training of those concerned.* Whilst talking and teaching about the change will generally help to lessen fear, many of the ideas associated with the nursing process and with individualised care need to be actually introduced before those involved can see that they are feasible and useful. For example, easing a ward routine to enable patients to wake at a time chosen by them may give rise to fears about whether or not the nurse will be able to fit in the work that has to be done.

Will it lead to chaos in a work environment which was previously well ordered and organised? Only by trying it out, and by seeing that it can work, will the nurses be able to resolve this worry. To make things more difficult, however, an attempt to change this routine in a team which strongly disagrees with it may lead to a self-fulfilling prophecy. They say it won't work — they believe it won't work — so they make sure that it doesn't when they try it out. A typical dilemma in changing things. Whilst most of us rarely consciously acknowledge that we really fear change since this could be seen as an admission of weakness, we can often sense it in others.

PERSONAL THREAT

Being told that changing the way in which we do things will result in higher standards of care may be seen by some to imply that the way in which they work now is not good enough. It can be interpreted as a challenge to years of trying hard to nurse well, and as an indication that the nurse managers or tutors are dissatisfied with the standards of care in that setting. Nurses with many years' experience sometimes say that they feel insulted about "introducing the nursing process" because they feel that its proponents are criticising their life's work. They frequently say that they "have always done it — it isn't new". This sort of change is threatening to the person who is being asked to change. Most of us have felt threatened by the prospect of having to function differently, for example, in moving jobs or moving to a new house. The kind of change involved in introducing the nursing process may relate to:

- alterations in work roles, for example, the role of the ward sister if primary nursing is to be introduced
- the content of the work, for instance, when staff nurses are expected to give total care, rather than to carry out complex tasks and to delegate other tasks to less experienced members of the team
- the knowledge needed to carry out the work, for example, knowing how to assess, plan, implement and evaluate, or understanding a nursing model.

If any of these areas is included the feeling of threat may arise. Because the nurse is expected to do things in a different — and to her, untried — way her previous integrity as an experienced and competent person, well used to the work, is shaken.

Mauksh and Miller (1980) say that maintaining the status quo is often important to nurses because it represents their position in the team, their span of control and their status. Changing this may, in the nurses' eyes, threaten their very being in the setting in which they work. This personal threat created by change, whilst understandable, is one of the prime causes of resistance.

LACK OF KNOWLEDGE

A knowledge deficit, already mentioned, can in itself lead to fear and a feeling of personal threat. Mauksh and Miller see "ignorance" as a frequent cause of resistance to change in nursing because "many nurses choose to live from day to day, not projecting future events or even preparing themselves for their inevitable occurrence". Although this may be somewhat of an overstatement in relation to the team with whom you work, it is not unusual to meet nurses who have a misguided impression of the nursing process and the changes which it suggests in today's nursing practice.

Duberley (1977) says that if nurses do not know and understand the nursing process, resistance can be expected "for people fear incomplete information, fear creates anxiety and this in turn gives rise to differing perceptions of the meaning of the nursing process and implementation". This resistance, caused by a lack of knowledge about what the nursing process is, can be exhibited by other members of the health team, and it is therefore essential to pass on this

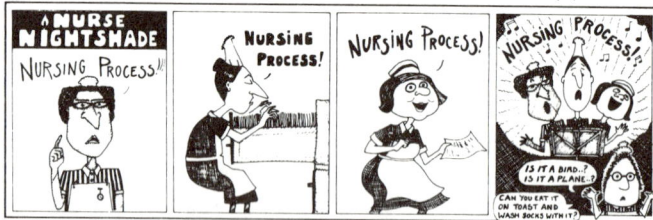

basic knowledge if these other groups are to accept and support it. For example, one group of doctors (British Medical Journal, 1982) are reported to have said that the nursing process serves to enhance the status of nurses, and that it takes nurses away from the patient, in order to write lengthy "histories" which have already been taken by junior doctors. These remarks represent a resistance to the nursing process, yet knowledge about the basic ideas on which it is based would refute these arguments. The nursing process focuses on patients, not nurses; nursing histories are written *with* the patient and focus *on* the patient as a basis for identifying his need for *nursing* care, whereas the medical history has a different emphasis.

An absence of the knowledge required to put the nursing process into practice will also lead to resistance. The basic philosophy of the nursing process summed up in our seven course themes and discussed throughout the course, incorporates a deepening of nursing knowledge and the acquisition of new skills. Nurses need to acquire new knowledge about such areas as nursing models, and about how they work, because accountability for our actions implies that we should possess the knowledge to justify them. We also need to become skilled in such things as interviewing, counselling and teaching. Not knowing about or understanding the changes must inevitably lead to a resistance towards accepting them. Only the most adventurous of us select the unknown dishes on a menu – many of us cannot resist the familiar and resort to the well-tried roast beef.

Similarly, even if we know what the change implies, we will resist it if we realise that we do not have enough knowledge and skills to carry it through. So even if we fancy an exotic dish, we will still plump for cooking roast beef if we think that we haven't the skills to flambé.

Lack of knowledge, then, may lead to:

- a concern about what the change implies for the individual and what its consequence may be
- an anxiety created by being asked to do something without having the knowledge to do it and without being offered help to acquire that knowledge.

CONFLICTING BELIEFS

The nature of a change may conflict directly with a person's strongly held beliefs. Duberley (1977) says that "resistant behaviour is present only when its sole function is an attempt to protect the resister against the consequences of change". If a nurse can give a well-reasoned and well-supported argument against a possible change, it may be that this is *not* evidence of resistant behaviour. As the change itself is usually based on certain beliefs, it cannot always be held that these beliefs are any more acceptable than those held by the people who are being asked to change. The changes which you may have identified as being necessary in your work place, as a result of this course, will probably be based on the beliefs about nursing proposed throughout it. The most basic of these is that Man should be viewed holistically and that nursing should centre its practice on this view. Some nurses may strongly believe that the traditional, biological, medical model is the most appropriate to nursing. Strongly held beliefs such as this may be changed through education and discussion but, in the end, if an individual chooses to reject the beliefs on which the nursing process is founded, and this choice is based on knowledge of the process, then rejection of the changes must be respected.

ENERGY

Moving away from the familiar, routine way of working in nursing requires an initial burst of real energy. Changing things means putting in more energy than one would if everything stayed the same, and this input of extra energy has to continue for some time until the change becomes established as the new norm. Owen (1983) refers to change as a "crisis" and outlines how it involves a high degree of stress. Stress in itself requires that a way of coping is developed and this, in turn, when tied to change, makes the work situation more exhausting than when there is the stability of a well-tried and established work pattern. Keeping up with this requires a commitment of extra energy. Because a series of small changes is the usual (and often best) way to introduce a big change – rather than the introduction of the whole change in one fell swoop – the energy input needs to last for some time. Change can thus be resisted because those who are asked to be involved in it are aware of the extra energy needed, and are unwilling to invest this to achieve the goal desired.

Sometimes change promoters are unrealistic in determining how much energy can be devoted to the change, and forget that the basic needs of the district nursing patch, ward or unit must first be met and that the nurses have to devote a certain amount of energy to these before they add on that needed to implement a change. They forget to ask how much effort can be devoted to certain parts of the work at any time, in order to balance work efforts which are routine with those which are innovative and creative. For example, in a busy rural area with one district nurse serving a largely elderly population, it may take some time before enough energy can be raised to design a new documentation system. The usual two nurses on duty on a thirty-bedded ward for the mentally handicapped may not easily be able to concentrate on actively involving relatives in care planning when all thirty patients have somehow to be given an acceptable level of care. Balancing the energy needed to maintain a service with the extra energy demanded by a change is of vital importance, if a high level of resistant behaviour is to be avoided.

Nurses asked to choose whether or not to implement major changes may indicate that they frankly "can't be bothered". They are saying that they are not prepared to invest the extra energy that the change demands. Others who are adamant that they "haven't time" may also be saying this, but their assertions may be valid. If there really isn't time, and the energy demands are too high, the change agent needs to explore how the balance can be achieved.

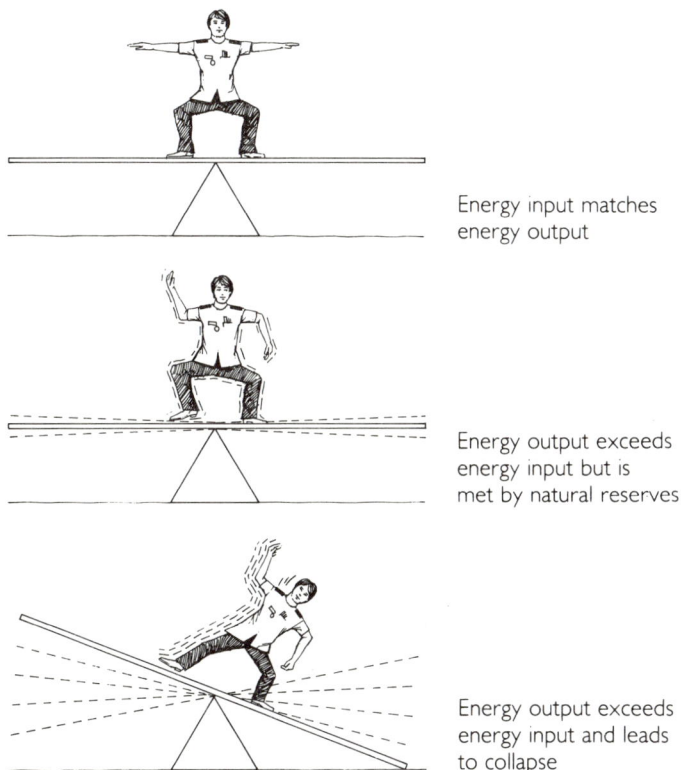

Is this what the nursing process is all about?

The changes associated with introducing the nursing process undoubtedly require a high level of energy and enthusiasm, both in actually implementing the changes and in acquiring the new knowledge and skills needed to do so. We may be prepared to spend time on introducing the nursing process 'forms', but not be willing to spend time on learning how to use them effectively. If the demand is too high, a nurse may give up because it is seen as impossible to put in so much effort continually, and the change cycle fails.

Many other factors may give rise to resistance, such as bad past experiences with change, personal factors, organisational factors and so on. The need to resolve resistance always has to be faced in a world currently acquiring a great deal of new knowledge and subsequently experiencing major change. Managing change includes an expectation of resistance and the plan must therefore incorporate strategies for coping with it.

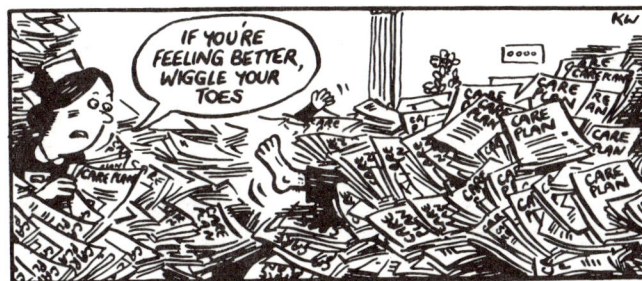

Energy input matches energy output

Energy output exceeds energy input but is met by natural reserves

Energy output exceeds energy input and leads to collapse

Fig. 7.4 Energy input must match energy output

Activity 7.5	Allow 10 minutes

Resistance to change in your practice setting

This activity is designed to give you an opportunity to consider whether you might meet some resistance to change in the area in which you work.

Thinking about the change area which you identified in Activity 7.3, consider whether the reaction of nurses and other team members (e.g. doctors, physiotherapists etc.) may be to:

● feel fear
● feel personally threatened
● feel a lack of knowledge
● have conflicting beliefs
● see it as a lot of extra work.

If so, for what reasons?

Authors' comment
Your answers to this activity are of course only supposition and may never become a reality. But it is as well to be prepared for them in order that you can minimise their effect, should they occur.

RECOGNISING RESISTANCE

Resistance can be manifested in a number of ways.

LIP SERVICE

This is a form of passive resistance probably well known to many nurses. When a change is suggested (or sometimes enforced), the people involved appear to go along with it, and may even discuss it as if they believe and accept it. Closer observation of their work, however, may make it clear that the change has either been misunderstood or is simply not being implemented. A ward team may nod in agreement when it is proposed that patients should be allowed to make decisions on how to organise their day, and may go on to claim strongly that this is what they will do. As a 'fly on the wall' you may still see them waking everyone at 5.30 am, giving them all a cup of tea, and showing signs of irritation when patients protest at being woken so early. 'Paying lip service' is a common way of passively resisting change which can sabotage the best worked-out change plan. However, one must always consider why the situation has occurred. It may be that the night nurses are expected to complete specific areas of work before the day staff arrive and that their behaviour is merely perpetuated through a desire to please.

LETHARGY

Those asked to participate in change may become overly tired and apathetic and disengage themselves from the change effort. Although they do not volubly object to the change, they do not become interested in it either. The change agent feels that it isn't worth going on because everyone is too apathetic, and changing their attitude is like 'flogging a dead horse'.

AGGRESSION

If people fear the change, feel threatened or are unwilling to give it the extra energy needed they may react by behaving aggressively towards both the idea and the promoter of change. This reaction may be manifested by obvious verbal aggression or a more subtle, less obvious, expression of anger. The change agent may find it too difficult to cope with apparent aggression towards himself and the effort may lessen. Those who wish to introduce change often need to understand that aggression may be a manifestation of resistance brought about by the insecurity of the aggressor, and is not always a personal attack on themselves.

DESTRUCTION

Change resisters can destroy attempted changes in many ways. They can consistently complain that the new method is not practical, perhaps expressing these feelings to key people in the organisation such as nurse managers, medical staff or even patients. They can use their skills in group situations to convince colleagues that these new ideas or practices are not useful or important. Using team nursing in a paediatric ward, for example, with the team leader having accountability for overall care strategies, may well be perfectly tenable. But if the ward sister is not committed to this change in work organisation and feels threatened by the change which it demands in her role, she may be able to resist. She may achieve this by making it known that this approach will not work and by ensuring that the team which she leads gives only a limited effort to making it work, thus undermining the effort.

LACK OF CONTINUITY

Resistance to a change is often manifested by the new practice being followed at certain times, and not at others. The written care plan may be effectively constructed and serve an extremely useful purpose, but it may be totally ignored by a relieving nurse on the district, or the staff nurse taking over on the evening shift. Primary nursing may operate when sister is on duty, but task allocation may prevail when she goes on holiday or has days off. This leads to confusion and dissatisfaction and the change fails to become an accepted norm in practice. One attempt to introduce total patient care in an intensive care unit failed because one charge nurse always dealt with patients' relatives when he was on duty, excluding the primary nurse from this activity. The primary nurses felt angry and were disappointed about the change which they had seen as being needed and beneficial, both to the patients and to their job satisfaction. Although the other sisters and charge nurses did not resist the change in this way, the idea was abandoned because of the lack of continuity.

Having to face resistance manifested in these ways is something which you may experience in your attempts to introduce change. In the later part of this module Mary Thompson, whom we introduced earlier as a typical nurse, faces such problems which may ring a bell with you. Knowing about and understanding these problems helps to overcome them but it doesn't, of course, give the needed enthusiasm to effect change.

Activity 7.6 **Allow 10 minutes**

You as a resister

The next activity gives you an opportunity to consider how you have reacted to change yourself in the past.

Consider one area of change which you have experienced in the recent past. It may be something that happened in your day-to-day work or which was even brought about through study of this course.

Consider whether you experienced any of the following feelings. If so, tick them and note how you responded to them:

- fear
- personal threat
- lack of knowledge
- a conflict in beliefs
- unable to gather up enough energy.

☐
☐
☐
☐
☐

Authors' comment

You would be an extremely unusual individual if you have never experienced any of these reactions when you have found yourself in a situation involving change. You may even be responding in one or more of these ways to some of what you have read in this course. If this is so, do not worry but stop and consider why you are feeling this way.

OBSTACLES TO CHANGE

We have stressed that change is not easy and that there are both difficulties and constraints which have to be faced and considered when introducing new ideas. Whilst some of these are related to resistance to change on the part of individuals, others are very practical and you may encounter real problems because of the kind of organisation in which you work. Some of these will be elaborated on when we return to Mary Thompson, but it is useful to introduce them briefly here.

SIZE OF THE TEAM

Nurses are the single largest group of people employed in health care, so we must bear in mind that any changes which occur in nursing involve a large number of people. The nature of our work often means that it is difficult to gather everyone together at one time for discussion, teaching or the sharing of ideas. This makes it awkward to arrive at cohesive ideas on the general pattern of practice in a ward or community setting. It is essential therefore to have a co-ordinator or leader who can communicate with all of those concerned.

Regardless of the large numbers of people involved, there are times when we look at staffing levels and wonder how we can ever find time to do anything but complete the most urgent work. Yet, if we want to be successful, it is crucial that enough time is made available to talk with the whole nursing team and somehow to meet the learning needs which become apparent. Both of us have tried and seen various methods being used to overcome this difficulty. On some occasions, we have managed to persuade nurse managers to supply an extra nurse either from another area or through the nurse bank or agency, or even to 'fill in' themselves. With this sort of help, the clinical area could be covered for a short period to allow for staff meetings. At times there have been anticipated 'lulls' in the work which have been used for discussion.

Other colleagues such as physiotherapists, occupational therapists or doctors have been prepared to stay in the ward to enable a nursing meeting to take place, provided that the nurses have been readily available if needed. A method which both of us have used on odd occasions has been to combine a staff meeting with a lunch break or supper in the evening. Whilst this is obviously not a technique of choice, if commitment to the new ideas is felt by all the staff the occasions can become both useful and enjoyable (sometimes more enjoyable than useful but excellent for team spirit).

HIERARCHICAL SYSTEMS

Traditionally, nursing has been structured in a rigidly hierarchical fashion with clearly defined rules and regulations applied to each level. Very often, senior nurses are themselves enthusiastic about innovations and new ideas. Indeed their support has often been the mainstay of clinical nurses who are attempting to introduce change. However, there are times when someone on a 'higher rung of the ladder' can appear to be blocking new ideas. There may be many reasons for this, such as financial constraints or limited resources. Other reasons may be those associated with resistance to change – fear of the unknown or personal threat. The underlying cause can often be overcome by a careful look at the communications network. The block can occur in either direction. When people above you in the hierarchy appear to block change and you have established that this is not occurring for any obvious sound reasons, it is useful to ask "Do I know all the causes which may lead to the blocking behaviour in this particular person? Have I spent time with the person to discuss these ideas and plans?" If a manager is responsible for standards of care within a unit, then it is clear that she will need to know about overall strategies rather than detailed plans, and making a point of continually informing her may lessen resistance and lead to positive support.

FINANCIAL CONSTRAINTS

In these days of economic constraint, we are continually forced to look at the costing of any new venture. Consequently, it may be necessary for you to 'do your homework thoroughly' and to estimate the cost of any innovation in your attempt to gain support and approval. For instance, it may be costly actually to introduce a new system of documentation. However, an initial trial of new document holders may lead you to find that they are more durable, provide easier access and are less time-consuming to handle than those currently in use. Such information would allow you to suggest that replacements would be required less often and would therefore cost less and that nursing time could be used more efficiently. So the high short-term costs would be balanced by long-term savings.

The major expenditure when introducing the nursing process is probably the time that is needed for staff development. If nurses spend time away from the clinical area, someone has to continue with the work. This is often a situation where management skills have to be brought into play. A careful review of the workload through the week may highlight spots when the pressure is less and the time can be used for teaching. From time to time colleagues may be prepared to work under slightly higher pressure, provided that they know that their turn will come and that they will be given the opportunity for 'time out' themselves.

WORKLOAD

We have already talked about the amount of energy required to introduce change. It is often difficult to see how you can possibly ask more of people when their workload is high and when they already appear to be using all their energy. Often there is little we can do to adjust the workload since it will always be there, so one way of coping with this problem is to look at the sources of energy. We don't mean that you offer doughnuts to everyone during their breaks, but rather that you look at the sources of support, help and guidance which can be offered in order to try to increase the motivation, job satisfaction and feelings of worth that the staff have. The effect of such improvements on working capacity has been well understood for many years. A famous series of experiments was carried out over a period of twelve years from 1927, which led to the description of a phenomenon known as the Hawthorne effect (Roethlisberger and Dickson, 1939). The experiments took place in a factory where a series of environmental factors such as lighting and temperature control were changed over a period of time. Each time a new factor was introduced the productivity was measured, and each time it had increased. Unable to explain what was happening, the experimenters withdrew all the new influences and yet again there was an increase in productivity. The conclusion to which they ultimately came was that the influential factor was that someone was paying attention to the workers and was interested in what they were doing. This simple strategy may be one that you can apply within the area in which you work. Greater attention to, concern for and interest in your staff may be that small additional factor which will enable them to cope with the extra demands imposed by the introduction of change. It is important, however, to remember that changes in practice can take a long time to be established and that

the extra supply of energy has to be continued for a long period of time.

The workload may also influence your decision about how much change can be managed at any one time. It may be the factor which will lead you to decide that a series of small steps taken over a period of time will be more appropriate than the introduction of a very big change all at once, on a pre-determined day. If you haven't considered the capacity of the individuals with whom you work and you then ask too much of them, they are likely to withdraw or become even more resistant. Levels of staff morale and sickness may be good guides to warn you if the pressure is becoming too high. Hopefully, open discussion and a good feedback system will have highlighted this problem before it becomes advanced.

It is equally important that you consider your own needs as well as those of others in this situation, particularly if the role which you have chosen to adopt is that of change implementer. You also need a constant extra supply of energy which you could find from your peer group, from colleagues in other areas and even from some outside sources. If you fail to do this and run out of energy yourself others are likely to follow suit, and however well you plan your change it is unlikely to succeed. Don't forget that all work and no play makes Jack a dull boy.

MULTI-DISCIPLINARY TEAM MEMBERS

One of the questions which we are commonly asked by people who are wanting to introduce the nursing process to their practice is "But what about the doctors?" Indeed, many comments have been made by doctors about the nursing process, both publicly and privately, which have not always been complimentary. Those doctors whom we have come across who are actually working with nurses who have introduced the nursing process find many points which are of help to them as well as the patients. The approach can lead to better communications and a shared approach of problem solving, resulting in a close working relationship and a single cohesive unit rather than segregated entities.

However doctors, like everyone else, may show some resistance to change and the major causes are often the same as those experienced by nurses. Through a lack of understanding, they may have a fear of the unknown and feel that the alteration in current practice is a threat. These worries are often founded in a concern that nurses will not only be taken away from direct patient care, but will be repeating a lot of work already undertaken by junior medical staff.

Recognising nursing as a separate but complementary service offered to patients, rather than as an adjunct to medical practice, may take some time to adjust to. What is needed is a clear understanding that the purpose of nursing assessment and planning is to focus on activities of living and an individual's ability to adapt to the effects of disease, rather than on the disease itself. This may help to right some of the confusion, since it can only lead to an improvement in standards of care. For example, whilst a doctor may be primarily concerned with helping a patient to control his high blood pressure, which has resulted in a stroke, the nurse may be primarily concerned with helping that patient to adjust to life with a paralysed limb.

Inevitably some conflict of opinion may arise from time to time between two groups working so closely together. It would be strange if it was otherwise and some degree of conflict is healthy, provided that it is dealt with openly and leads to discussion rather than to anger, resentment and withdrawal.

Another area of concern which was recently expressed by a medical colleague was the frequently heard description of nursing as *the* caring profession. He felt, quite rightly in our opinion, that everyone within the multi-disciplinary clinical team has the right to care. It is unlikely that any of us would consider that it is the nurse's sole prerogative to care. If this misunderstanding is widely held, then it must be clarified for all concerned.

The basic solution to this problem is to open up the communication channels and discuss your plans. It may be that you will have to modify your plans a little to meet others' needs. Similarly, it is likely that others will have to adjust to new ways as well. Through discussion you should be able to reach a position which will benefit everyone concerned, that is the patients as well as the doctors and the nurses. Our experience is that, if time proves you right and the services offered to the patients improve, resistance gradually decreases and a fruitful working relationship is established.

Activity 7.7   Allow 10 minutes

Obstacles to your change

In this activity, we would like you to consider some of the obstacles to your proposed change which you may have to face, in order that you can anticipate them and make plans to minimise their effect.

Returning again to the change which you identified in Activity 7.3, write down what obstacles you think may exist in relation to the following:

- size of the team
- hierarchical system
- financial constraints
- workload
- multi-disciplinary team members.

Authors' comment

Depending on your team and on the communication networks which you have established, you may predict various objections. Anticipation of such obstacles and consequent planning may help you in overcoming them before they even start. Initial careful assessment of all potential obstacles may help you to evolve plans which lead to support from unexpected places, rather than to resistance. For instance, early discussion with other members of the multi-disciplinary team and their involvement at the planning stage, may lead to their becoming supportive colleagues who can make positive contributions to assist you.

GETTING DOWN TO BASICS

So far, we have discussed some thoughts and ideas which are common to any change situation and have given a few concrete examples which relate to nursing and which may have sounded familiar to you. Now we would like to face some more of the realities, many of which we have experienced personally, which exist when nurses become involved in introducing a nursing process approach to care, with all its underlying implications. We hope that through our own experience we may be able to help you to find ways of overcoming any difficulties which may arise.

We have already introduced Mary Thompson earlier in the module. She is our imaginary nurse who, like you, is studying this course and who has decided that there is room for change in relation to all seven of the course themes. Following her as she goes through the change process will enable us to identify some of the practices which led her to consider the change, some of the difficulties which she experienced during that process and some of the ways in which she faced these difficulties. We hope that you will be able to relate some of her experiences to your own situation.

Having almost completed the course, Mary returned to her ward and took a critical look at how things were. She felt that many of the current practices in her team did not match up fully with the course themes.

PEOPLE AS PATIENTS

Mary noticed that, on her ward:

1 Conversation between nurses and patients was not encouraged, except when procedures were being carried out.

2 Visiting was strictly limited to direct family members, two to a bed, between 2.30 and 3.30 pm. and between 6.30 and 8.30 pm.

3 Great emphasis was laid on every patient having a bath every day, although she knew that this was not always their practice at home.

4 Patients going to theatre next day were always fasted from 12 midnight.

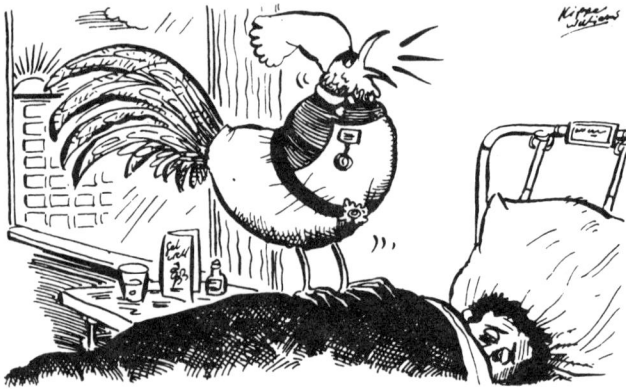

5 The night staff woke all patients at a set time, in order that they could complete certain tasks before their colleagues on day duty arrived.

6 Because the nurses were given jobs according to their experience, patients saw and were cared for by many different nurses and didn't relate to anyone in particular.

Mary realised that whilst the standard of physical care offered in the ward was high, all patients were treated in a similar way, regardless of their individual differences. Having recognised this as an area for change, she spent some time defining what she would like to achieve and writing down some specific goals. These goals were:

1 The pattern of each patient's day would be as similar as possible to the one followed at home. This would mean that there would have to be flexibility in the ward routine to allow patients to vary such activities as the time at which they would wake in the morning, and the time and frequency of bathing.

2 The patient's family and friends would be able to visit at times convenient to them and to the patient, rather than at those convenient to the ward. This would mean an alteration in the current visiting policy.

3 Individual plans would be made for each patient in order to meet their treatment and care regimes. This would mean that some of the established rigid routines would have to be modified to suit individual patients. For example, after consulting with the anaesthetist, it was decided that patients would be fasted for six hours before a planned operation rather than always from midnight.

4 Nurses would recognise that some of the needs of patients related to their social and emotional circumstances, which had been disrupted by their hospital admission, rather than just their physical disease. Mary realised that, in order to achieve this, focused social conversations between patients and nurses needed to be encouraged rather than criticised.

Mary had, in fact, undergone a considerable amount of change within herself, creating tension and an imbalance between her new beliefs and her current behaviour. In order to be able to resolve this situation, she needed to take some further action. Her first step was to discuss these ideas with the staff on her ward. With your knowledge of change you will probably realise that, initially, Mary's suggestions were not wholly accepted. The first reactions of her staff were to present Mary with a series of reasons why her ideas were unrealistic and impossible to bring into practice. The sort of comments which they made were ones which you may also hear if you find yourself in this situation:

"Nonsense, we'd never get the work done."

"But patients like a routine – it makes them feel secure."

"It's not safe – things will get missed."

"I can't cope with that – I don't want to get involved."

"What will the doctors think?"

"How can we let the visitors in when the work's not all done?"

"We have to do what the doctor says."

"Mrs Jones (the nursing officer) would go mad if they didn't all have a bath every day."

and finally

"What if there's an emergency?"

This list could be much longer, but maybe some of these remarks already sound familiar to you. They are comments that we have heard from many nurses with whom we have worked and are ones for which Mary, and you, may have to find an answer.

As far as getting the work done is concerned, gearing work to suit the individual patients, rather than to a routine, doesn't inevitably alter the amount of work involved – it merely redistributes it. In fact, life may be easier if we avoid the frantic rushes between 6 and 7 am, or having to get the baths done before lunch. What is more, if visiting is more flexible, friends and relatives may actually be able to give some of the care. This may help to meet their needs, as well as some of the patients' needs, since it would give them a purpose and feeling of usefulness. The benefits would then be felt by all concerned.

Next – the routine. In stating that patients like the routine, we are saying that they like *our* routine, whilst in fact we are disrupting theirs. Of course, this has been the pattern that they have been asked to follow for many years, and it has therefore become the expected norm. They are often unaware that variations are possible and when offered the opportunity for alternatives, their reactions may well be different. The only way in which you will discover whether or not this is true is by trying it, but in our experience patients welcome the opportunity to continue with their normal habits. The reaction of a gentleman, for whom one of us recently cared, when he realised that he could still have his usual gin and tonic in the evening, even when he was ill in hospital, was a delight to see.

Routine itself can put safety at risk, since practices can become so habitual that we fail to notice danger signals. Of course, throwing away a well-tried routine without replacing it with any organisation at all is dangerous. It is important that such routines are replaced by alternative safety mechanisms, such as individual responsibility for patients and unambiguous care plans for each patient. This may well involve a further change for Mary and will have to be considered as she plans the changes to meet her current goals. She will have to be careful not to throw the baby out with the bath water.

Our medical colleagues are as much concerned about the standard of patient care as we are, but, as people, they are also susceptible to concern when asked to adapt to new ideas. If Mary and the other clinical nurses who wish to implement change in nursing make a point of discussing their ideas with doctors so that fear, personal threat and misunderstanding are removed, the changes which they wish to implement are more likely to be seen to be beneficial to patients and complementary to medical care, rather than in opposition to it. The doctor's support would be a valued asset to Mary in her attempts to introduce her new ideas.

We have already said that nurses in supervisory roles such as Mrs Jones, the nursing officer, often feel threatened by changes in the clinical area. However, Mary may not yet have had a chance to check out how Mrs Jones does feel. Her resistance may be totally imaginary. If it is not, what can Mary do? Firstly, Mary's reasons for wishing to make these changes need to be presented to Mrs Jones in a well-reasoned and logical way. This may well be all that is required but, if Mrs Jones is not receptive to the arguments given, she may well be exhibiting a classical manifestation of resistance. If this is the case, alternative solutions must be sought.

Mary may decide that, as an autonomous practitioner accountable for her practice, she will continue with her plans without the support of the nursing officer. However, this is not the most desirable solution and she will probably choose to seek an alternative approach. One approach which she could try would be to seek the allegiance of a colleague whom Mrs Jones respects. This could be another member of the nursing team, another nursing officer or even a medical colleague. The important thing is to get this person on her side. However, if the resistance becomes destructive, Mary may choose to seek the support of a more senior nurse in order that she can continue with her new plan.

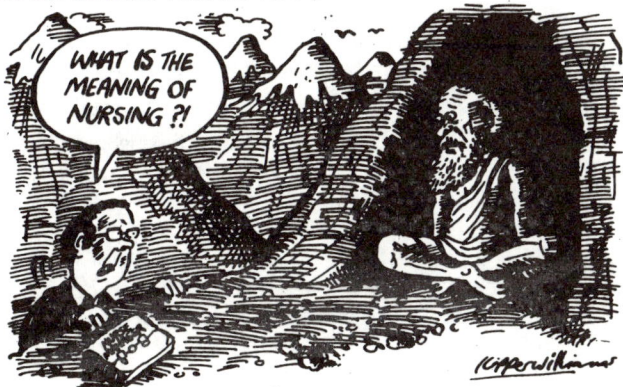

The next question that Mary had to face was "I can't cope with that – I don't want to get involved". This kind of attitude is a very real problem in nursing at the moment and it is difficult to cope with since, if her team is to change its practice, Mary is actually asking more from it. A comment of this kind is in fact quite healthy, since it shows that the nurse recognises the implications of the change that Mary has suggested and doesn't see it as something which is easy to achieve.

Full understanding of the implications of the desired change for both the patients and the nurses, in terms of job satisfaction, is vital. If the ward team fully appreciate the benefits for the patient and see the change as one which will give much greater satisfaction to them personally, this reluctance may well subside. Despite popular opinion, most people respond very positively to extra responsibility and involvement. They are able to see the outcome of their individual efforts and hence get better feedback, as well as a feeling of being able to control their own actions.

Finally, the familiar old chestnut "What if there is an emergency?" Nurses have always recognised that they must be prepared for unexpected crises. Relaxing a tight routine does not necessarily make coping with an emergency more difficult. Rigid routines can often be shaken when an emergency occurs and chaos can be the result. A flexible working pattern can usually absorb the unexpected occurrence more readily than one which is highly organised and ordered. Conforming to the individual patient's daily pattern does not inevitably lead to chaos. The care for each patient is still well-ordered and as reasonably predictable as a rigid ward routine; it just differs for each patient. Developing an understanding of this reality through discussion is essential, but it is often necessary to introduce the change before nurses can appreciate that the approach is perfectly reasonable in the busiest of wards, if managed properly.

Activity 7.8   Allow 15 minutes

Relating Mary's experience to yours

The experiences that Mary had may be very similar to ones which you will face. This activity gives you an opportunity to relate her situation to your own.

Do you expect similar reactions to the specific change you would recommend in your area?

Draw two columns in your notebook, heading one 'comments' and the other 'responses'. Write down in the first column the sort of comments you would expect to hear about your proposed change and, in the second column, your responses to those comments.

Authors' comment
Predicting and responding to these comments and thinking about the problems which they pose may help you to prepare for the realities of change in this area.

WHAT TO DO NEXT

Now that we have made some suggestions as to how Mary might respond to some of the questions posed to her, her next step is to consider all the resources she may need and what is available to her. Having recognised that this change demands an alteration in attitude, Mary may identify her major needs as teaching and learning resources. The resources could consist of teaching assistance and literature upon the subject concerned. She may have little difficulty in finding appropriate literature with the help of the librarian. She may also be fortunate enough to find a tutor, clinical teacher or a nursing colleague who holds similar convictions and who has already read widely around the subject. If this is not the case, Mary may well have to take on the responsibility of helping the team to learn for themselves.

Another resource on which she could draw would be the experience of nurses working in different units or districts who have already developed these ideas. She may be able to arrange visits to such units or for one of their staff to come and join a group discussion with her team.

Having determined what teaching resources are available, Mary will need to begin to consider how to release staff so that they can learn. Some of the strategies which she could use have already been suggested on p. 165, and she will have to explore the possibility of using any of them. She will also have to consider whether there are any financial implications. If this is so, she must find out where money is available for such things as photocopying, travelling expenses and lecture or course fees.

Once all these points have been considered, Mary must work out the feasibility of all her ideas and draw up a plan of action.

MARY'S PLAN

Mary's investigation into the possible resources have led her to decide that:

1 The teaching will be shared by Mary herself and a nurse tutor, who only has limited time available due to other commitments.

2 There is usually a lull in ward work on Monday afternoons and the nursing officer is prepared to help out on that day. Consequently she can draw up a planned teaching programme to take place each Monday during the shift overlap, arranging the duty rota so that as many staff as possible are available at that time, including part-time colleagues.

3 She will work a week of night duty herself in order to find time to talk to the night staff about her ideas.

4 Since she has not yet established formal written care plans, she will make fuller use of the nursing orders. Their new use will be included in the teaching programme.

5 After the teaching programme, she will change the pattern of work organisation to patient allocation.

6 Visiting hours may be extended as soon as she has talked to her team, nurse managers and colleagues. She will arrange a formal meeting with other members of the multi-disciplinary team to explain her plan and what she hopes to achieve. She will also make a special point of ensuring that all members of the multi-disciplinary team know with whom to link in discussing plans for individual patients and what to do if a patient's assigned nurse is not readily available.

This plan will take some time to put into action, and she and all her colleagues have agreed that they will aim for this new pattern of work to become normal practice after six months. The time at which they will change to patient allocation will be negotiated throughout the teaching programme and a date set when everyone agrees that they are ready.

Mary has also decided that, once changes have started to take place, she will hold fortnightly meetings to receive regular feedback. The times will vary so that staff on all shifts will have the opportunity of attending, but will be announced well in advance so that preparations may be made for the meetings. She also plans to use these sessions to give encouragement and support to her colleagues and to answer queries. Having recognised that the demands on all concerned will be high and will require extra energy, she hopes that this will be a way in which she can supply that motivation. She has recognised her tutor colleague as someone on whom she can personally rely and gain support herself.

During this planning stage, Mary has actively involved the rest of the ward team so that they feel part of the initiative. Because she has kept her manager fully informed, she also has Mrs Jones' support. She is now ready to begin the process of implementing the change which she has planned.

Planning, preparation and teaching are vital to the introduction of change. It is unfair to staff to expect them to carry out new ideas without them.

PROBLEMS FACED BY MARY

Because Mary had taken time and care in planning the change, she was eventually successful. However, this does not mean that she did not face many of the problems which we have already discussed. Some of the problems which she encountered were:

1 The cancellation of an occasional meeting due to a staffing crisis.

2 The continued resistance of one colleague throughout the programme. Through mutual agreement and the help of the nursing officer, this colleague eventually moved to another ward where her ideas did not conflict with current practice.

3 Some discomfort expressed by other members of the multi-disciplinary team when the changes were first introduced. The eventual outcome convinced them of the value of the ideas which Mary had introduced. The converted are most righteous and their support is now full.

4 Occasional 'hiccups' in the smooth running of the ward when the pattern of work was first changed, and an initial desire to revert to well-tried routines. This desire was overcome.

Now that Mary has successfully introduced this change and has achieved satisfaction from it, she is carefully planning her next step in moving towards the nursing process. Both she and the rest of the ward team have realised the benefits of their efforts and are eager to pursue their desire to introduce or develop the other six themes within their practice. The first step was probably the most difficult and yet the most rewarding, since it has led to a fundamental change in attitudes and a recognition of patients as people with individual needs.

INTRODUCING FURTHER CHANGE

The process which Mary has used to introduce change associated with seeing patients as people may also be applied in introducing all the other course themes into her practice. Many of the problems which she will face will be similar and many of the questions previously posed may be reiterated. Whilst some of the answers will likewise be similar, there are other considerations specific to each theme. We will deal with each one briefly.

PROBLEM SOLVING

A particular resource problem exists here because it involves the supply of a new set of documents and the storage facilities required. Some of these difficulties have already been highlighted in an earlier section, so we will not spend further time commenting here.

However, this is not the only consideration. The change also involves a considerable amount of expert teaching in problem solving and the use of the documents. The area which we have found most difficult is that of writing specific patient-centred goals and of promoting a recognition of their relationship to care and to evaluation. Some of the comments which we have heard include:

"But it isn't necessary."

"But it is too much writing."

"But we already do that – we just don't write it down."

The answers to these comments are given throughout the text of this course but, as a memory jolt, some responses may be:

- in the end, you will find that time is saved
- written communication overcomes the fallibility of the human memory
- accurate care plans avoid misunderstandings arising from varied perceptions or from people hearing inaccurately and ensure that everyone, including the patient, is working towards the same goals.

If the documentation system has been carefully planned and is designed to be flexible, Mary should be able to adapt it to the particular needs of her clinical setting.

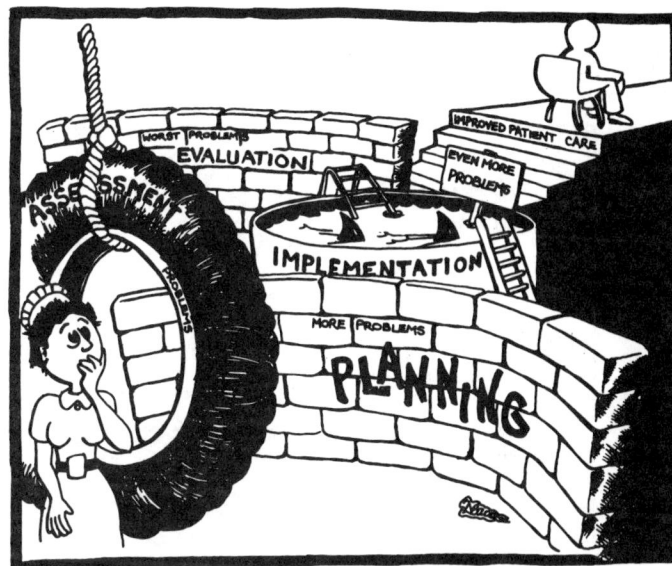

She will have to remember that, without the appropriate teaching about the plan, there is a risk that the new documentation system will become nothing more than an extra chore in the nurse's day and will be her master rather than her slave.

THE ROLE OF THE NURSE

A good deal of time and effort will need to be spent on discussions with both the nursing team and the multi-disciplinary clinical team. Mary may find that there are some conflicts of interest and there will need to be careful negotiation in order to overcome them. She must not forget that all members of the team have their own particular needs, and it may be necessary to be prepared to concede a little from her own ideas or ideals as well as to take from those with whom she works. Since the relationship which Mary is seeking is one of partnership between equals, there will probably need to be some movement on both sides.

Mary may also find here that her own learning needs relate to teaching and management, as well as to the development of her clinical skills. She may seek help and advice from both her tutorial and managerial colleagues for ways in which she can develop these skills. If this help is not forthcoming, however, her local librarian is yet again a useful resource person who could guide her to appropriate literature to help her to develop these skills herself.

THE NURSE-PATIENT RELATIONSHIP

This area of change revolves around attitudes and the acquisition of communication skills. In many ways it is the most threatening and it can be seen as the most demanding in the way of a teaching input. Learning to relate to patients in partnership, rather than as directors of care, also requires a new support system for nurses since they are being asked to expose some of their own personal self. In some units, special resources involving role play have been used to help nurses to develop these skills (Swaffield, 1982; Faulkner, 1980).

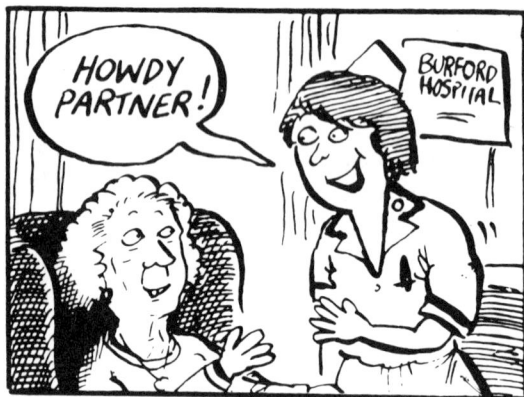

Other units have developed their own teaching or training programmes or have used locally based facilities. Role play is a learning technique which has played a large part in the development of these skills. If this technique is employed, however, it requires very skilful leadership as, without it, participants can be harmed. Personal feelings about oneself and one's view of other people are explored, and if this is poorly handled by the leader the experience can be traumatic. Yet again, Mary may seek the help and guidance of her tutorial colleagues in developing these skills.

Planning for this kind of change must include provision of adequate support to nurses who are prepared to become so closely involved with patients. This may take the form of peer group support, particularly of nurses who are experiencing similar desires for change. Mary may find that colleagues who have also studied this course are willing to share in her experiences and to form a continuing support group. Alternatively, support from the unit leader or the availability of an external counselling service may be considered. If a nursing process group is not already in existence in the district, it may be worthwhile considering setting one up.

MODELS FOR PRACTICE

The need for recognition of a model for practice within a team has already been mentioned in our discussion of documentation, of people as patients and, implicitly, in the section on nurse-patient relationships. Because of the relationship of the other course themes to the model on which you base your practice, it is probably the first change to be considered. As with all the others, adequate teaching, reading and the opportunity for group discussion are essential.

Nursing models are often thought to be particularly difficult to understand and their relevance is not always readily recognised. You may prefer to start by talking about your own ideas in relation to the three components of a model: that is, a belief about Man, the goals of nursing and the knowledge base from which you practise. Indeed, in working through Module 1 you may already have done this, but future modules could well have developed your ideas further. The literature available on nursing models is extensive, but as yet there is little written by British nurses. Some references for literature on nursing models were given in Module 1 and your local librarian should be able to offer suggestions for further reading, if you wish to look into the subject more thoroughly.

The only other point to make in relation to introducing this theme is that it is essential to have agreement amongst all your staff, so that the model which is selected is meaningful.

ACCOUNTABILITY

Mary may find that the changes concerning accountability relate very closely to the other themes which she has already considered, and that they will naturally come about with the introduction of change in other areas. However, two specific points must be borne in mind in introducing this aspect of the nursing process:

1 Every member of the nursing team must clearly understand the notion of accountability, and must be prepared to accept it.

2 It is sometimes necessary to engage in considerable negotiation within the organisation to establish clear lines of accountability.

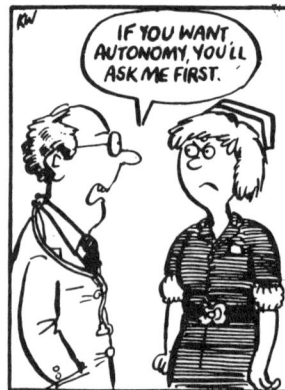

For example, if primary nursing is chosen as a method of delivering care it must be clearly understood within the nursing hierarchy, both at sister level and above, that the accountability for individual patient care lies with the individual primary nurse. The sister becomes accountable for the allocation of patients to the most appropriate primary nurse, for supporting her and for allowing her to practise safely by ensuring that she has access to both resources and expertise. These changes in role must also be understood by doctors and others.

In our experience, making accountability explicit is another means by which many nurses have found much greater job satisfaction. Not only are they able to be more creative in their work but they also gain satisfaction from the recognition which is given to them for what they have done.

NURSING IN AN ORGANISATION

Negotiation with and the involvement of the multi-disciplinary clinical team has already been mentioned a number of times and is essential. As far as the organisation is concerned, Mary must bear in mind that all the changes which she has planned may have an indirect effect on the whole organisation. For instance, the recognition of patients as people may mean that she will have to approach the catering department in order to see whether there is any possibility of flexibility in the meal services provided. Similarly the domestic services manager will need to be involved if the rigid routine of the day is going to be altered. The requirement for new documents may involve the supplies department and the local print shop, and the financial implications may be of concern to the administrators. This serves to emphasise Lewin's interpretation of change at an organisational level (p. 155) and the fact that adjustments may be necessary throughout the whole organisation. The skills which Mary may find helpful in managing this sort of change are mainly those of negotiation. These include being very clear about her own aims and how she hopes to achieve them, but also recognising the needs of other disciplines and taking their constraints into account when discussing plans with them.

DIFFERENT ROLES AND SETTINGS

Even if your clinical setting is different from Mary's, many of the strategies which we have suggested can be applied equally well. However, there are a few points which may help those of you who either have a different position or who work in a different setting.

If you are employed either as one of many sisters or as a staff nurse, you will inevitably face different problems should you wish to introduce change in your clinical setting. Without the support of your colleagues or the leader of your clinical team, it may be very difficult to change your own pattern of behaviour since it might lead to disruption of your own position and that of others in the group. This could lead to the formation of 'cliques' and the development of poor staff relationships, which are bound to have adverse effects on patient care. You will also have to consider how much authority you have to bring about change without the approval of your colleagues. In this situation, communications and negotiation may again be the key to success. If you meet resistance, the cause may be one of those mentioned previously, namely fear, personal threat, lack of knowledge, conflicting beliefs or lack of energy. In this case, it is again essential to be well prepared in presenting your ideas and to be in a position to point out the personal advantages to your colleagues or leader. Such advantages may relate to many of the arguments already suggested in relation to specific areas of change, but can also include the prestige resulting from the successful outcome of a plan. If lack of energy or lethargy is a difficulty with which you are presented, you may have to offer to undertake an active role as a change implementer, devising a suitable plan and taking a major part in the work involved in teaching and introducing the change.

Another point for discussion may be the national trend towards the introduction of the nursing process, supported by the United Kingdom Central Council for Nursing, Midwifery and Health Visiting, and reflected in the current examinations. In some health authorities, the practice of individualised patient care is already included in job descriptions and is, therefore, an accepted part of the agreement between the practitioner and the employer. However, many nurses would prefer to take some action themselves rather than to have ideas forced on them by others.

If your negotiations are successful, you could find that your colleagues are prepared to become change adopters, supporting your ideas and willing to participate in your plans but not to accept leadership of the project. If this is your situation, it is important that you consider the personal support which you can find for yourself since, if you are to be the change implementer, the demands on you will be very high.

If all your negotiations fail and you are unable to convince other people of the benefits of your plan, there are several approaches you can take. Initially you could reconsider your own plans and question whether they are too radical or major as a first step to change. A smaller, less threatening change may be more appropriate. Secondly, you could consider how you may adjust your behaviour within the structure of the team in which you work, without disrupting it entirely. For instance, you may lean more towards a partnership relationship with the patients with whom you are personally involved, without affecting other members of the team too much, whereas if you change the methods of work allocation when you are on duty whilst others adhere to old patterns, confusion could well arise. If none of these solutions are appropriate and you find that you can no longer work in the way that you wish, you may find yourself in the position of one of Mary's staff nurses who was unable to accept the changes introduced. In this case, it could be that your only solution is to look for another job in a situation where the beliefs are more in keeping with your own.

NURSES IN THE COMMUNITY

Nurses working in the community may have both advantages and disadvantages over Mary's position. The major advantage is that because of the nature of their work, much of it is carried out independently since it entails working alone. Because of this, there is less opportunity for others to challenge them on such issues as the relationship developed with patients or clients, or consideration of them from the holistic point of view, taking an interest in needs beyond their physical welfare.

District nurses, health visitors and community psychiatric nurses may all find a problem-oriented approach to care and a well-structured documentation system particularly helpful, since their lines of authority are less easily defined than those of nurses working in hospital settings. Their access to a patient or client at home must always be by invitation and their authority to act, and therefore their lines of accountability, need careful consideration. A systematic problem-oriented approach to care may help them to define such

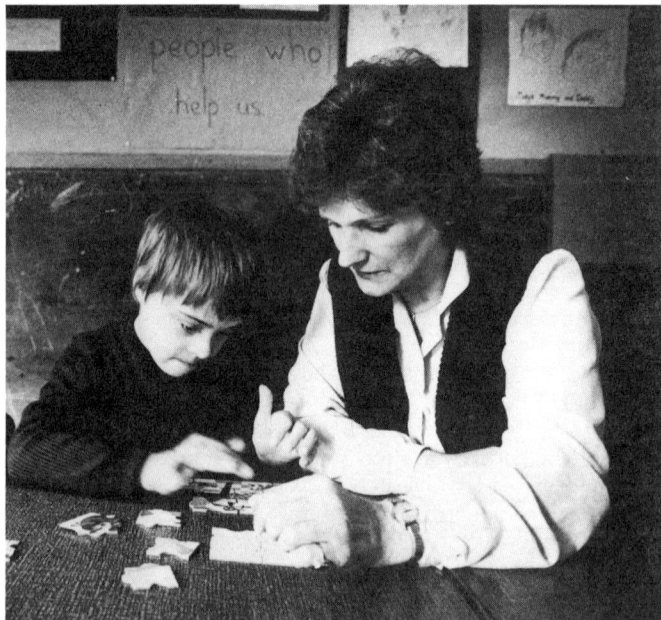

Health visitors maintain close involvement with handicapped children

lines. Since they work alone, they are in a position to devise and use documents which suit their own particular needs and to manage their work in a more autonomous way which allows them to adapt their practice more freely.

Such a position, although having advantages, can also have its difficulties, and the major one may be that of isolation. We have continually stressed the need for support from friends, colleagues or a peer group when trying to introduce change, and our personal experience has been that this is essential. If you work in a community setting where an obvious peer support group cannot so easily be identified, you may actively have to seek out others with similar ideas or to initiate a local support group yourself. The group with whom you have studied this course may wish to continue meeting regularly. Alternatively, other members of the practice in which you work, whether or not they are nurses, might be happy to listen and contribute to your plans and activities.

NURSES IN PSYCHIATRY

One of the comments which we have frequently heard from nurses working in psychiatric settings is that the nursing process may be alright for those nurses working in general fields, but that it is inappropriate for them. If you are working in psychiatry, this could be a remark that will become familiar to you too. The major cause of resistance here seems to be a lack of information, and hence understanding, about the interpretation and the flexibility of the nursing process, as it is presented in this course. There seems to have been an over-emphasis on the *process* and an under-emphasis on the *nursing* and the underlying issues that it represents.

The answer to this question, as with many others, seems to lie in open discussion about any changes which you think may be necessary. Our experience is that most nurses working in psychiatry have recognised the relationship between the nursing process and the underlying themes – particularly those of the nurse-patient relationship and accountability. They welcome it as a useful asset to their work.

NURSE MANAGERS AND TEACHERS

Many of the problems which both managers and teachers face are similar, in that they are not always in a position actually to practise and demonstrate the changes that they value. It is often difficult to recognise both the advantages and difficulties inherent in introducing new ideas, without actually experiencing them. However, the role that they have to play in a changing situation is vital to its long-term success. In the same way as the sister must reconsider her own role within the clinical setting should primary nursing be introduced, so nurse managers and nurse teachers must look at the contributions that they personally have to make to change within clinical areas.

From the managers' point of view, this may include a re-assessment of the lines of accountability within the nursing structure. They may also have to re-assess the support systems which they offer to the clinical nurses, in order to be able to help them to introduce the ideas that have been identified. Their role may involve supplying the right resources and negotiating for some of the services which support nurses throughout the organisation. In other words, they *enable* clinical nurses to develop and improve nursing care within their own units.

The teacher's role in many ways is similar. Having recognised that one of the biggest problems in a change situation is a lack of knowledge or understanding about some of the issues that have been raised, the teacher may be able to help and support clinical nurses in deepening people's knowledge. In a practical way, by offering to contribute to discussions and to give information about particular subjects, the teacher may act as a resource person, advising and supporting nurses at an individual level. She may also be in a position to supply other resources such as teaching materials, or have knowledge of where such things may be acquired.

Both these groups of people are at a disadvantage in that they are advocating some principles and ideas which they may not have had the opportunity to practise themselves. They may need to adjust their ideals in order that they can realistically be incorporated into day-to-day clinical work. However, in no way does this under-emphasise the value of the contribution that they have to make. Whatever change agent role you have decided to adopt, the whole process of change is only likely to succeed if each person's individual contribution is recognised.

LEGAL CONSIDERATIONS

Finally, a brief consideration of the legal aspects of introducing the nursing process into practice is important, when considering change. Some anxiety about the nurse's position in law has been expressed by legal advisers to health authorities, and this anxiety is sometimes expressed by nurses and other health workers. Nurses themselves are acutely aware of the legal value of nursing records, and of the need to be clear about their role in terms of whether or not they are doing what they should be doing in the eyes of the law. Scrivenger (1982) discusses the legal position of the nursing process at length, and clarifies a number of issues currently posing problems.

1 The way in which nurses practise is judged in law by asking 'nursing experts' if the approach taken was considered to be reasonable and acceptable. Thus, if the nursing process approach to care is used and those 'nursing experts' consulted deem such an approach to be reasonable, then, in law, it would be seen as such.

2 Gathering information from patients, relatives and others, for example, through interview, and recording it as a basis for assessment cannot be interpreted as a breach of confidentiality, although revealing such information indiscriminately would be. In fact, failing to record relevant information, or not even bothering to ask about it, could be seen as less than effective practice.

3 The use of nursing process documents is an attempt to improve nursing practice through a methodical and analytical approach and it requires careful recording and evaluating. This in itself may make it

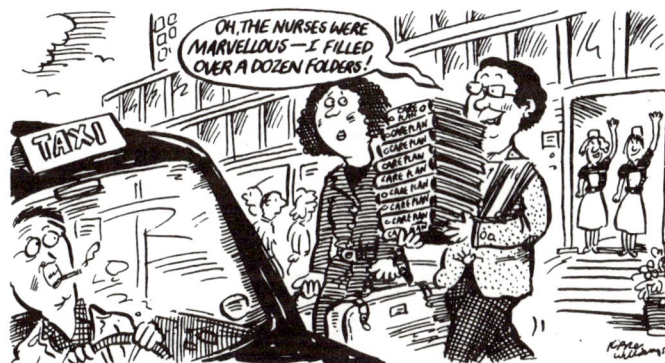

clear that the nurse involved has approached care in a proper, complete and reasonable way, much more than the conventional Kardex ever could.

Although the use of the nursing process cannot of itself ensure that care is approached systematically and documented accurately – in the final analysis, only the nurse can ensure this – it is a framework which promotes such an approach and which is both legally *acceptable* and often *desirable*. If legal objections to implementing the nursing process arise in your specific area of practice, legal advisers to trade unions or professional associations for nurses will be able to support its introduction from a legal point of view.

THE FINAL STEP

Now that you have nearly completed this course, we hope that you will have achieved two major things:

- firstly, a deeper understanding of the nursing process and some of the skills and attitudes on which it rests

- secondly, some thoughts about parts of your own clinical practice which are suitable for development and about the way in which you might introduce such developments.

As a final word, there are some brief comments we would like to make in order to summarise our thoughts about introducing such changes into your nursing practice.

1 Planned change, which follows the change process, is more likely to be successful than unplanned change.

2 *Communication* and *negotiation* are key words in relation to change.

3 Resistance to change is common and should be recognised, in order that it may be dealt with.

4 Never be in too much of a hurry – changes occur slowly rather than quickly.

5 Changes require energy, so consider both your own supply and that of others.

Activity 7.9

The end or the beginning?

This is the final course activity and it is impossible to set a time limit on it. It entails putting into action some of the things which you have read and thought about.

Neither we nor anyone else can tell you what to do, since it is up to you to decide whether there is any change which you would like to make. Nor can we tell you how to set about it. The initiative must lie with you.

Group Session 7 is the final group session which you will attend in connection with this course. It is slightly different from the others in that we hope that you will be able to consider not only the final module but the whole of the course, and to discuss some of your reactions to it. We hope that in this group session you will also be able to consider some of the ways in which you would like to progress in the future.

We would like to take this opportunity of saying that we hope that you have enjoyed working your way through the course and that it has been of benefit to you. We wish you every success in introducing the nursing process in its fullest sense in your own area of work.

REFERENCES

ALDERMAN, C. (1983) 'Individual care in action', *Nursing Times, 79:* (3), Jan. 19–25, pp. 15–17.

ALTSCHUL, A. T. (1972) *Patient–Nurse Interaction*, Edinburgh, Churchill Livingstone (University of Edinburgh Department of Nursing Studies Monograph – 3).

ASHWORTH, P. (1980) *Care to Communicate*, Edinburgh, Churchill Livingstone.

ASPINALL, M. J. (1975) 'Development of a patient-completed questionnaire and its comparison with the nursing interview', *Nursing Research, 24:* (5), pp. 377–81.

BATEHUP, L. (1983) How teaching can help the stroke patient's recovery, *in* Wilson-Barnett, J. (ed.) *Patient Teaching*, Edinburgh, Churchill Livingstone, pp. 119–36.

BATEY, M. V. AND LEWIS, F. M. (1982) 'Clarifying autonomy and accountability in nursing service: Part I', *Journal of Nursing Administration, 12:* (9), pp. 13–18.

BLAUNER, R. (1964) *Alienation and Freedom; the factory worker and his industry*, Chicago, University of Chicago Press.

BOND, S. (1978) *Processes of Communication about Cancer in a Radiotherapy Department*, unpublished PhD Thesis, University of Edinburgh.

BOND, S. AND HAGEL, A. B. (1982) *Selected Literature in the Management of In-dwelling Urinary Catheters*, Nursing Topics Project, Newcastle-upon-Tyne Polytechnic Library.

BOORE, J. R. P. (1978) *Prescription for Recovery*, London, Royal College of Nursing.

BRITISH MEDICAL JOURNAL (1982) 'Changing relations between doctors and nurses', *285:* (6348), pp. 1130–2 (Report of a meeting of the Central Committee for Hospital Medical Services, 30/9/82).

BYRNE, M. L. AND THOMPSON, L. F. (1978) *Key Concepts for the Study and Practice of Nursing*, St. Louis, C.V. Mosby (2nd. edn.).

CAVILL, C. A. AND JOHNSON, J. M. (1981) 'Steps towards the process', *Nursing Times, 77:* (49), Dec. 2–9, pp. 2091–2.

CENTRAL HEALTH SERVICES COUNCIL (MINISTRY OF HEALTH) (1963) *Communication between Doctors, Nurses and Patients; an aspect of human relations in the Hospital Service*, London, HMSO.

CENTRAL HEALTH SERVICES COUNCIL (1976) *The Organisation of the In-Patient's Day: report of a committee of the CHSC*, London, HMSO.

CLARK, J. (1982) 'Health visiting: a way to get organised', *Nursing Times, Community Outlook: 78:* (41), Oct. 13–19, pp. 287–97.

DOPSON, L. (1983) 'Every day is a bonus for us', *Nursing Times, 77:* (19), May 11–17, pp. 8–11.

DOWD, C. (1983) 'Learning through experience', *Nursing Times, 79:* (30), July 27–Aug. 2, pp. 50–3.

DUBERLEY, J. (1977) 'How will the change strike me and you . . . ?', *Nursing Times, 73:* (45), Nov. 10–16, pp. 1736–8.

ENGEL, G. V. (1970) 'Professional autonomy and bureaucratic organisation', *Administrative Science Quarterly, 15:* (1), pp. 12–21.

EWING, G. (1983a) *A Study of the Postoperative Nursing Care of Stoma Patients During Appliance Change*, unpublished PhD Thesis, University of Edinburgh.

EWING, G. (1983b) Personal communication from the author.

FAULKNER, A. (1980) 'Communication and the nurse', *Nursing Times, 76:* (36), Sept. 4–10, pp. 93–5 (Occasional Paper, Vol. 76, (No. 21).

FAULKNER, A. (1981) 'Aye, there's the rub', *Nursing Times, 77:* (8), Feb. 19–25, pp. 332–6.

FLEMING, I., BARROWCLOUGH, C. AND WHITMORE, B. (1983) 'The constructional approach', *Nursing Mirror, 156:* (23), June 8, pp. 21–3.

FLINT, C. (1981) 'Continuity of maternity care 1: our pregnant lady', *Nursing Mirror, 153:* (23), Dec. 2, pp. 22–3.

FLINT, C. (1981) 'Continuity of maternity care 2: Emma, Joan, Liz and A. N. Other', *Nursing Mirror, 153:* (24), Dec. 9, pp. 31–4.

FLINT, C. (1982) 'Get off the conveyor belt', *Nursing Mirror, 155:* (22), Dec. 1, pp. 37–8.

GALANO, J. (1977) 'Treatment effectiveness as a function of client involvement in goal setting and goal planning', *Goal Attainment Review, 3*, pp. 19–32.

GARRAWAY, W. M., AKHTAR, A. J., HOCKEY, L. AND PRESCOTT, R. J. (1980) 'Management of acute stroke in the elderly: follow-up of a controlled trial', *British Medical Journal, 281:* (6244), pp. 827–9.

GOLDIAMOND, I. (1976) Coping and adaptive behaviours of the disabled, *in* Albrecht, G. L. (ed.) *The Sociology of Physical Disability and Rehabilitation*, Pittsburgh, Feffer and Simons, pp. 97–138.

GRIFFITH, J. W. AND CHRISTENSEN, P. J. (1982) *Nursing Process: application of theories, frameworks and models*, St. Louis, C. V. Mosby.

HAMRIN, E. (1981) 'Activation of patients with stroke in clinical nursing care: effects on patients and staff', *Abstracts of Uppsala Dissertations*, University of Uppsala, Sweden.

HANLEY, I. G., MCGUIRE, R. J. AND BOYD, W. D. (1981) 'Reality orientation and dementia: a controlled trial of two approaches', *British Journal of Psychiatry, 138*, pp. 10–14.

HAYWARD, J. (1979) 'Can pain be measured?', *Nursing, No. 1*, April 1, pp. 32–4.

HEFFERIN, E. A. (1979) 'Health goal setting: patient–nurse collaboration at VA facilities', *Military Medicine*, Dec., pp. 814–22.

HENDERSON, V. (1966) *The Nature of Nursing*, London, Collier-Macmillan.

HENDERSON, V. (1969) *Basic Principles of Nursing Care*, Basel, S. Karger for the International Council of Nurses (rev. edn.).

HENDERSON, V. (1982) 'The nursing process – is the title right?', *Journal of Advanced Nursing, 7:* (2), pp. 103–9.

HOCKEY, L. (1968) *Care in the Balance; a study of collaboration between hospital and community services*, London, Queen's Institute of District Nursing.

HOLDEN, P. AND SINEBRUCHOW, A. (1978) 'Reality orientation therapy: a study investigating the value of this therapy in the rehabilitation of elderly people', *Age and Ageing, 7*, pp. 83–90.

HORSLEY, J. A. (1982) *Closed Urinary Drainage Systems*, CURN Project, New York, Grune & Stratton.

HUNT, J. M. AND MARKS-MARAN, D. J. (1980) *Nursing Care Plans: the nursing process at work*, London, HM & M Publishers.

INZER, F. AND ASPINALL, M. J. (1981) 'Evaluating patient outcomes', *Nursing Outlook, 29*: (3), March, pp. 178–181.

JOURARD, S. M. (1971) *The Transparent Self*, New York, Van Nostrand (rev. edn.).

KALISCH, B. J. (1973) 'What is empathy?', *American Journal of Nursing, 73*: (9), pp. 1548–52.

KELLEY, D. AND CONNER, D. R. (1979) The Emotional Cycle of Change, *in* Jones, J. E. and Pfeiffer, J. W. (eds.) *The 1979 Annual Handbook for Group Facilitators*, La Jolla, California, University Associates, pp. 117–122.

KING'S FUND (1983) *A Handbook for Nurse to Nurse Reporting*, London, King's Fund, (Project Paper No. 21).

KRON, T. (1981) *The Management of Patient Care: putting leadership skills to work*, Philadelphia, W. B. Saunders (5th. edn.).

LANCASTER, J. AND LANCASTER, W. (1981) *Concepts for Advanced Nursing Practice: the nurse as a change agent*, St. Louis, C. V. Mosby.

LELEAN, S. R. (1973) *Ready for Report Nurse?; a study of nursing communication in hospital wards*, London, Royal College of Nursing (Study of Nursing Care Research Project Series 2, No. 2).

LESNIK, M. J. AND ANDERSON, B. E. (1955) *Nursing Practice and the Law*, Philadelphia, J. B. Lippincott.

LEWIN, K. (1951) *Field Theory in Social Science*, London, Tavistock.

LEWIS, F. M. AND BATEY, M. V. (1982) 'Clarifying autonomy and accountability in nursing service: Part II', *Journal of Nursing Administration, 12*: (10), pp. 10–15.

LITTLE, D. E. AND CARNEVALI, D. L. (1976) *Nursing Care Planning*, Philadelphia, J. B. Lippincott/Harper & Row Medical Division (2nd. edn.).

LUKER, K. A. (1979) Evaluating nursing care, *in* Kratz, C. (ed.) *The Nursing Process*, London, Baillière Tindall, pp. 124–146.

LUKER, K. A. (1982) *Evaluating Health Visiting Practice*, London, Royal College of Nursing.

LUPTON, T. (1971) *Management and the Social Sciences*, Harmondsworth, Penguin (2nd. edn.).

MAGER, R. F. (1972) *Goal Analysis*, Belmont, California, Pitman Learning.

MANCHESTER STROKE STUDY (1978) *Medical, Social and Psychological Aspects of Stroke*, Department of Geriatric Medicine, University of Manchester.

MANTHEY, M., CISKE, K., ROBERTSON, P. AND HARRIS, I. (1970) 'Primary nursing – a return to the concept of "my nurse" and "my patient"', *Nursing Forum, 9*: (1), pp. 65–83.

MARKS-MARAN, D. (1983) 'Can nurses diagnose?', *Nursing Times, 79*: (4), Jan. 26–Feb. 1, pp. 68–9.

MASLOW, A. H. (1954) *Motivation and Personality*, New York, Harper.

MAUKSH, I. G. AND MILLER, M. H. (1980) *Implementing Change in Nursing*, St. Louis, C. V. Mosby.

MAYERS, M. G. (1978) *A Systematic Approach to the Nursing Care Plan*, New York, Appleton-Century-Crofts (2nd. edn.).

MCFARLANE, J. (1970) *The Proper Study of the Nurse*, London, Royal College of Nursing (Research Project Series 1 Introduction).

MCFARLANE, J. (1980) 'Essays on nursing', London, King's Fund Centre, (Project Papers based on the Working Papers of the Royal Commission on the National Health Service, No. RC2).

MCFARLANE OF LLANDAFF AND CASTLEDINE, G. (1982) *A Guide to the Practice of Nursing Using the Nursing Process*, London, C. V. Mosby.

MCGREGOR, D. (1960) *The Human Side of Enterprise*, New York, McGraw-Hill.

MENZIES, I. E. P. (1960) 'A case study in the functioning of social systems as a defense against anxiety; a report on a study of the nursing service of a general hospital', *Human Relations, 13*: (2), pp. 95–121.

MINISTRY OF HEALTH, CENTRAL HEALTH SERVICES COUNCIL (1961) *The Pattern of the In-Patient's Day*, London, HMSO.

MINISTRY OF HEALTH, CENTRAL HEALTH SERVICES COUNCIL, Standing Medical Advisory Committee (1965) *The Standardisation of Hospital Medical Records Report of the Sub-Committee*, London, HMSO, (Tunbridge Report, 1965), paras. 18–28, 85.

NIGHTINGALE, F. N. (1859) *Notes on Nursing; what it is and what it is not*, London, Harrison (reissued Blackie, 1974).

NORTON, D. (1975) 'Research and the problem of pressure sores', *Nursing Mirror, 140*: (7), Feb. 13, pp. 65–7.

NORTON, D. (1981) 'The nursing process in action – 1. The quiet revolution: introduction of the nursing process in a region', *Nursing Times, 77*: (25), June 17–23, pp. 1067–9.

NORTON, D., MCLAREN, R. AND EXTON-SMITH, A. N. (1962) *An Investigation of Geriatric Nursing Problems in Hospital*, National Corporation for the Care of Old People (reissued Churchill Livingstone, 1975).

OFFICE OF THE HEALTH SERVICE COMMISSIONER (1983) *Report of the Health Service Commissioner: selected investigations completed October 1982– March 1983* (1st. Report for Session 1983/84), London, HMSO.

OREM, D. E. (1980) *Nursing: concepts of practice*, New York, McGraw-Hill (2nd. edn.).

OTTOWAY, R. N. (1982) Defining the change agent, *in* Evans, B., Powell, J. A. and Talbot, R. (eds.) *Changing Design*, London, Wiley.

OWEN, G. M. (1983) 'The stress of change', *Nursing Times, 79*: (8), Feb. 23–March 1, pp. 44–6, (Occasional Paper, Vol. 79, No. 4).

PARKES, C. M. (1979) Evaluation of a bereavement service, *in* de Vries, A. and Carmi, A. (eds.) *The Dying Human*, Ramat Gan, Israel, Turtledove Publishers.

PEARSON, A. (1983) *The Clinical Nursing Unit*, London, Heinemann Medical.

PHANEUF, M. C. (1972) *The Nursing Audit: profile for excellence*, New York, Appleton-Century-Crofts.

PUNTON, S. (1983) 'The struggle for independence', *Nursing Times, 79*: (9), March 2–9, pp. 29–32.

REVILL, S. AND BLUNDEN, R. (1980) *Goal Planning with Mentally Handicapped People in the Community: report on an evaluation of the use of goal planning techniques by health visitors*, Report No. 9, Mental Handicap in Wales – Applied Research Unit.

ROETHLISBERGER, F. J. AND DICKSON, W. J. (1939) *Management and the Worker; an account of a research program conducted by the Western Electric Company, Hawthorne Works, Chicago*, Cambridge, Mass., Harvard University Press.

ROGERS, C. R. (1967) *On Becoming a Person: a therapist's view of psychotherapy*, London, Constable.

ROPER, N. (1976) *Clinical Experience in Nurse Education*, Edinburgh, Churchill Livingstone.

ROPER, N., LOGAN, W. AND TIERNEY, A. (1980) *The Elements of Nursing*, Edinburgh, Churchill Livingstone.

ROPER, N., LOGAN, W. AND TIERNEY, A. (1981) *Learning to Use the Process of Nursing*, Edinburgh, Churchill Livingstone.

ROPER, N., LOGAN, W. AND TIERNEY, A. (eds.) (1983) *Using a Model for Nursing*, Edinburgh, Churchill Livingstone.

ROYAL COLLEGE OF NURSING AND BRITISH GERIATRIC SOCIETY (1975) *Improving Geriatric Care in Hospital: report of a working party of the British Geriatric Society and Royal College of Nursing of The United Kingdom*, London, Royal College of Nursing.

ROYAL COMMISSION ON THE NATIONAL HEALTH SERVICE (1978) *Patient Attitudes to the Hospital Service*, London, HMSO (Research Papers, No. 5).

SAXTON, D. F. AND HYLAND, P. A. (1979) *Planning and Implementing Nursing Intervention: stress and adaptation applied to patient care*, St. Louis, C. V. Mosby (2nd. rev. edn.).

SCHEIN, E. H. (1969) The Mechanisms of Change, *in* Bennis, W. G. et al (eds.) *The Planning of Change*, New York, Holt, Rinehart and Winston (2nd. edn.).

SCRIVENGER, M. J. (1982) *The Legal Implications of the Nursing Process*, (Unpublished Royal College of Nursing Discussion Paper).

SKEET, M. H. (1970) *Home from Hospital: the results of a survey conducted among recently discharged hospital patients*, London, The Dan Mason Nursing Research Committee.

SULLIVAN, M. E. (1977) 'Processes of change in an expanded role in nursing in a mental health setting', *Journal of Psychiatric Nursing and Mental Health Services*, 15: (2), pp. 18–24.

SUNDEEN, S. J., STUART, G. W., RANKIN, E. D. AND COHEN, S. A. (1981) *Nurse–client Interaction – implementing the nursing process*, St. Louis, C. V. Mosby (2nd. rev. edn.).

SWAFFIELD, L. (1982) 'Spanner in the works', *Nursing Times*, 78: (25), June 23–29, pp. 1049–54.

SWAFFIELD, L. (1983) 'Change for the better', *Nursing Times*, 79: (16), April 20–26, pp. 59–61.

TEASDALE, G. AND JENNETT, B. (1974) 'Assessment of coma and impaired consciousness', *The Lancet*, 7872, July 13, (Vol. 2), pp. 81–4.

TEASDALE, G. (1975) 'Acute impairment of brain function – 1. Assessing "conscious level"', *Nursing Times*, 71: (24), June 12–18, pp. 914–7.

TEASDALE, G., GALBRAITH, S. AND CLARKE, K. (1975) 'Acute impairment of brain function – 2. Observation record chart', *Nursing Times*, 71: (25), June 20–26, pp. 972–3.

UNITED KINGDOM CENTRAL COUNCIL FOR NURSING, MIDWIFERY AND HEALTH VISITING (1983) *Code of Professional Conduct for Nurses, Midwives and Health Visitors*, London, UKCC.

WAINWRIGHT, P. AND BURNIP, S. (1983a) 'Qualpacs at Burford', *Nursing Times*, 79: (5), Feb. 2–8, pp. 36–8.

WAINWRIGHT, P. AND BURNIP, S. (1983b) 'Qualpacs – the second visit', *Nursing Times*, 79: (33), Aug. 17–23, pp. 26–27.

WANDELT, M. A. AND AGER, J. W. (1974) *Quality Patient Care Scale*, New York, Appleton-Century-Crofts.

WEED, L. L. (1969) *Medical Records, Medical Education and Patient Care; the problem-oriented record as a basic tool*, Cleveland, Ohio, Press of Case Western Reserve University.

WILLER, B. AND MILLER, G. H. (1976) 'Client involvement in goal setting and its relationship to therapeutic outcome', *Journal of Clinical Psychology*, 32: (3) pp. 687–690.

ZIGMOND, A. S. AND SNAITH, R. P. (1983) 'The Hospital Anxiety and Depression Scale', *Acta Psychiatrica Scandinavica*, 67: (6), pp. 361–70.

ACKNOWLEDGEMENTS

Grateful acknowledgement is made to the following sources for material used in this *Workbook:*

Text

Figure 1.3: data based on a Hierarchy of Needs in 'A Theory of Human Motivation' in *Motivation and Personality,* 2nd. edn. by Abraham H. Maslow. Copyright © 1970 by Abraham Maslow. By permission of Harper & Row Publishers Inc.; *Figures 1.6(a) and (b), 2.3 and 2.4* from N. Roper, W. W. Logan and A. J. Tierney, *Using a Model for Nursing,* 1983, Churchill Livingstone, reprinted by permission; *Figure 1.12* adapted with permission from Dolores F. Saxton and Patricia Hyland, *Planning and Implementing Nursing Intervention,* 2nd. edn., 1979, The C. V. Mosby Co., St. Louis, Missouri, USA; *Figures 2.2, 2.9, 3.6, 4.8(a) and (b)* reproduced with permission from McFarlane of Llandaff, Baroness and George Castledine, *A Guide to the Practice of Nursing Using the Nursing Process,* 1982, The C. V. Mosby Co., St. Louis, Missouri, USA; *Figure 2.5* from *Nursing Times,* 1979, Macmillan Journals Ltd.; *Figure 2.6* from G. Teasdale, S. Galbraith and K. Clarke, 'Acute impairment of brain function – 2. Observation record chart' in *Nursing Times,* 71: (25), 1975, Macmillan Journals Ltd.; *Figure 2.7* from J. Hayward, 'Can pain be measured?' in *Nursing,* 1st. series, Vol. 1, 1979, Medical Education (International) Ltd.; *Figure 2.8* from A. Zigmond and R. P. Snaith, 'The Hospital Anxiety and Depression Scale' in *Acta Psychiatrica Scandinavica,* Vol. 67, 1983, 361–370; *Figure 3.3* from S. Revill and R. Blunden, *Goal Planning with Mentally Handicapped People in the Community,* Research Report No. 9, 1980, Mental Handicap in Wales, Applied Research Unit; *Figure 4.2* from T. Kron, *The Management of Patient Care: putting leadership skills to work,* 5th. edn., 1981, W. B. Saunders Publishing Inc.; *Figure 4.5* from L. Batehup, 'How teaching can help the stroke patient's recovery', in J. Wilson-Barnett (ed.) *Patient Teaching,* 1983, Churchill Livingstone; *Figure 7.3* from D. Kelley and D. R. Conner, 'The Emotional Cycle of Change' in John E. Jones and J. William Pfeiffer (eds.) *The 1979 Annual Handbook for Group Facilitators,* 1979, San Diego, CA, USA, University Associates Inc. Adapted with permission.

Cartoons

pp. 86 and 162: Cath Jackson/Nursing Times; *pp. 132 and 148:* Steve Gleadall/DHSS; *p. 171:* J. P. Deacon/Nursing Times. Our special thanks go to Kipper Williams and the Editor of the Nursing Times for permission to reproduce the cartoons on *pp. 36, 66, 70, 71, 75, 88, 95, 99, 107, 119, 163, 168, 169, 172, 175.*

Photographs

Cover photographs Top right: PACE; middle left and right: Andy Burridge/Nursing Mirror; bottom left: Tony Sleep/UKCC; bottom right: Roger Tooth/Nursing Mirror; *p. 61:* Senga Bond; *p. 133:* Ray Leng; *p. 174:* Tony Sleep/UKCC.